Evaluation, Stabilization, and Transport of the Critically Ill Child

Evaluation, Stabilization, and Transport of the Critically Ill Child

BYRON Y. AOKI, M.D.
Director, Critical Care
Kapiolani Medical Center
Associate Professor
John A. Burns School of Medicine
University of Hawaii
Honolulu, Hawaii

KARIN McCLOSKEY, M.D.
Assistant Professor
Department of Pediatrics
University of Alabama
Medical Director, Critical Care Transport
The Children's Hospital of Alabama
Birmingham, Alabama

Mosby
Year Book

St. Louis Baltimore Boston Chicago London Philadelphia Sydney Toronto

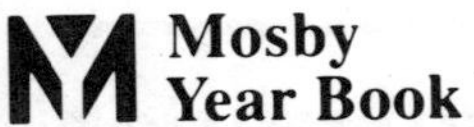

Dedicated to Publishing Excellence

Sponsoring Editor: Stephanie Manning
Assistant Editor: Jane Petrash
Assistant Managing Editor, Text and Reference: George Mary Gardner
Production Manager: Nancy C. Baker
Proofroom Manager: Barbara Kelly

A Year Book Medical Publishers imprint of Mosby-Year Book, Inc.
Mosby-Year Book, Inc., 11830 Westline Industrial Drive, St. Louis, MO 63146

1 2 3 4 5 6 7 8 9 0 CL/ML 96 95 94 93 92

Library of Congress Cataloging-in-Publication Data
Aoki, Byron Y.
Evaluation, stabilization, and transport of the critically ill child / Byron Y. Aoki, Karin McCloskey.
p. cm.
Includes bibliographical references and index.
ISBN 0-8151-0114-7
1. Pediatric emergencies. 2. Critically ill children—transportation. I. McCloskey, Karin. II. Title.
[DNLM: 1. Critical Care—in infancy & childhood. 2. Critical Care—methods. 3. Emergencies—in infancy & childhood. 4. Transport of Patients—in infancy & childhood. 5. Transport of Patients—methods. WS 366 A638e]
RJ370.A55 1992 91-44505
618.92′0025—dc20 CIP
DNLM/DLC
for Library of Congress

ACKNOWLEDGMENTS

In acknowledgment of

all who served as teachers, knowingly and otherwise; the recent journey that accompanied the writing of this book—the Loma Prietas, the probing, the proffered kindness, the new insights.

Thank you.

Byron Y. Aoki

CONTRIBUTORS

Angela Anderson, M.D.
Instructor in Pediatrics
Brown University School of Medicine
Attending Physician
Pediatric Emergency Medicine
Rhode Island Hospital
Providence, Rhode Island

Byron Y. Aoki, M.D.
Director, Critical Care
Kapiolani Medical Center
Associate Professor
John A. Burns School of Medicine
University of Hawaii
Honolulu, Hawaii

Parvin H. Azimi, M.D.
Director, Infectious Diseases
Children's Hospital Oakland
Oakland, California
Clinical Professor of Pediatrics
University of California at San Francisco
San Francisco, California

Steven Baldwin, M.D.
Instructor in Pediatrics
University of Alabama School of Medicine
Fellow in Emergency Medicine and Critical Care Transport
The Children's Hospital of Alabama
Birmingham, Alabama

Jonathan Cronin, M.D.
Instructor in Pediatrics
Associate Neonatologist
Joint Program in Neonatology
Harvard Medical School
Assistant in Medicine
Children's Hospital of Boston
Boston, Massachusetts

Luigi D'Orsogna, M.D.
Consultant Cardiologist
Princess Margaret Hospital for Children
Perth, Western Australia

Laura Lee Dyer, R.N.
Assistant Director
Critical Care Transport
University of Alabama Hospital
Birmingham, Alabama

Lisa Etzwiler, M.D.
Clinical Fellow in Pediatric Emergency Medicine
Harvard Medical School
Assistant in Medicine
Children's Hospital of Boston
Boston, Massachusetts

Jim Fackler, M.D.
Instructor in Anesthesiology (Pediatrics)
Harvard Medical School
Medical Director
Multidisciplinary Intensive Care Unit
Children's Hospital of Boston
Boston, Massachusetts

Gary Fleisher, M.D.
Associate Professor of Pediatrics
Harvard Medical School
Chief, Division of Emergency Medicine
Children's Hospital of Boston
Boston, Massachusetts

Hope Friedman, R.N., M.S.
Pediatric Intensive Care Outreach Coordinator
Children's Hospital Oakland
Oakland, California

Michele Holloway, M.D.
Assistant Professor of Pediatrics
University of Alabama School of Medicine
Attending Physician
Emergency Department
The Children's Hospital of Alabama
Birmingham, Alabama

Gary Lee, M.D.
Director, Pediatric Intensive Care Unit
Sacred Heart Hospital
Spokane, Washington

Dennis Lund, M.D.
Instructor in Surgery
Harvard Medical School
Director, Trauma Program
Assistant in Surgery
Children's Hospital of Boston
Boston, Massachusetts

Faye Lundergan, Pharm.D.
Pediatric Clinical Pharmacist
Children's Hospital Oakland
Oakland, California

Karin McCloskey, M.D.
Assistant Professor
Department of Pediatrics
University of Alabama
Medical Director, Critical Care Transport
The Children's Hospital of Alabama
Birmingham, Alabama

Maggy Myers, M.D.
Staff Pediatrician
Brigham and Women's Hospital
Children's Hospital of Boston
Boston, Massachusetts

Richard Orr, M.D.
Assistant Professor of Anesthesiology/Critical Care Medicine and Pediatrics
University of Pittsburgh School of Medicine
Associate Director
Pediatric Intensive Care
Medical Director
Pediatric Transport
Children's Hospital of Pittsburgh
Pittsburgh, Pennsylvania

Robert Pascucci, M.D.
Instructor in Anesthesiology (Pediatrics)
Harvard Medical School
Associate Director
Multidisciplinary Intensive Care Unit
Children's Hospital of Boston
Boston, Massachusetts

Richard Saladino, M.D.
Clinical Instructor
Harvard Medical School
Assistant in Medicine
Children's Hospital of Boston
Boston, Massachusetts

PREFACE

Pediatric intensive care is a relatively new subspecialty, but has developed rapidly and become the standard of care for the critically ill or critically injured child. It is now the expectation that critically ill children* will be cared for in pediatric intensive care units (PICU) that can provide the expertise and coordinated, comprehensive care that these patients need for best outcome.

The number of critically ill children is small. The Pediatric Intensive Care Network of Northern and Central California study found that only 230 of 100,000 children receive intensive care annually.[1] For comparison, approximately 4,800 of 100,000 children are hospitalized annually in the United States,[2] and California's CCS estimated that 8 neonatal ICU beds were needed for every pediatric ICU bed in 1984.

This small critical mass is sufficient to support only a limited number of PICUs. There are approximately 300 to 350 PICUs in the United States (vs. 6,500 hospitals), most of which are located in tertiary pediatric centers where the extensive and comprehensive services that PICUs require can be found. The small numbers of critically ill children and PICUs therefore raise two significant problems: patient access to PICUs and acquiring and maintaining pediatric critical care skills.

PICU Access. Large numbers of critically ill children present emergently to facilities without PICUs or develop critical illness while in such facilities. In these situations, emergency stabilization must be initiated at the first facility; then the child must be *transported* to a PICU for definitive care. Critical care therefore is commonly divided into three phases:

1. *Presentation and stabilization:* Critical illness is recognized and stabilization is initiated. The child frequently presents to a non-PICU setting, for example, an emergency department or a general inpatient (pediatric) ward.

*The term *critically ill children* in this book refers to both critically ill and critically injured children.

2. *Transport/transfer to a PICU:* Interfacility transport—a mobile PICU setting—is the second phase when the child must be transported to another facility for care in a PICU. Intrafacility transfer is phase 2 when the PICU is located within the same facility.
3. *Care in the PICU:* Definitive pediatric intensive care is delivered.

Acquiring and Maintaining Pediatric Critical Care Skills. As care of the critically ill child advances and increasingly falls under the domain of pediatric intensivists and PICUs, it is increasingly difficult for nonpediatric intensivist personnel to acquire and maintain the necessary skills to provide pediatric critical care. Paradoxically, all medical facilities and first responding physicians and other medical personnel are expected to provide appropriate initial care for the critically ill child up to the time the child either reaches a PICU or is picked up by a transport team. Paradoxically, too, the situation is frequently among the most uncontrolled: the sudden and unexpected appearance of such a child, with multiple problems that need to be identified, in a setting that lacks many of the diagnostic and therapeutic supplies available in a pediatric tertiary center.

This book is directed to those who provide the first two phases of critical care—presentation/stabilization and transport/transfer—before the child reaches the PICU. Specifically, it is directed to emergency departments, inpatient wards where children are hospitalized, and transport teams. It is especially written for the first responders, who must initiate care, many of whom have limited experience in pediatric critical care: physicians (such as nonintensivist pediatricians, family practice physicians, emergency department physicians, surgeons, any physician who cares for children), nurses, and respiratory therapists. It is also written for the transport personnel who must provide intensive care in a setting without access to the full resources of a PICU. The book aims to be a readily usable resource that helps the user initiate the key medical interventions that maintain and protect the child until he or she reaches a PICU.

The book is written with the assumptions that (1) the reader has medical experience; (2) there are numerous resources one can consult for more detailed information regarding diagnoses, pathophysiology, therapy, and PICU care after the crisis has passed; (3) a regional poison control center will be consulted for specific advice in ingestion of poison cases. The book presents an approach for use in the frequently chaotic critical situation where the principles of emergency medicine must prevail and where a few fundamental concerns always remain central in thinking and action.

For these purposes, the book is organized in the following manner. The book begins with the basic principles that govern emergency medicine. Chapter 1 includes a discussion of oxygen delivery, because this is the key aim of emergency therapy. Subsequent chapters are presented by organ system or by problems when the former grouping is not applicable. Presentations are organized in the following scheme: (1) reviews of relevant, clinical pathophysiology provide the rationale for recommended interventions (these are meant to be read at nonemergent times); (2) quick reference therapy outlines, tables, and formulas for use in the emergency situation are presented in individual chapters; (3) the critically needed references, such as weight-specific resuscitation sheets, are placed in the Appendixes for rapid access.

It has been our aim to write a book that will provide the reader with the information essential for stabilizing the critically ill child, a book that provides not only "recipes" for critical problems but also a working understanding of fundamental pathophysiology that can help one better assess and treat such children in the future. We realize that we can only provide guidelines that will be fairly easy to utilize when the clinical problems/responses can be recognized; they will be difficult to apply when the problems are not well-defined because they are either subtle or extreme or because multisystem problems confuse the picture. We are unable to convey the numerous other nuances utilized in assessment and therapy that come only with experience. For this reason, we strongly emphasize the importance of conferring with the regional PICU or Pediatric Emergency Department (whichever handles consultations and transports) when encountering these patients, to obtain recommendations specific for the individual patient, an action that will allow the best possible outcome for the patient.

Last, most of the contributors to this manual are both experts in their own subspecialties (e.g., cardiology, neonatology) and active transport team members. Therefore they are able to offer the unique perspective of in-depth knowledge of a given topic coupled with a practical understanding of the limitations of treating patients during stabilization and transport without access to the sophisticated technology of a PICU.

Byron Y. Aoki, M.D.
Karin McCloskey, M.D.

REFERENCES

1. Pettgrew A, Singer J, Falade E, et al: *The Pediatric Intensive Care Network of Northern and Central California: A Regional Approach*. Pediatric Intensive Care Network, 150 Felker St., Suite H, Santa Cruz, CA 95060. DHHS Grant MCJ-063336, Aug 1986.
2. US Department of Health and Human Services. *Health United States 1987*. Public Health Service, Centers for Disease Control, National Center for Health Statistics, Hyattsville, Md. DHHS Publ (PHS)88-1232, March 1988.

CONTENTS

PRINCIPLES OF STABILIZATION 1

I. Approach to Critically Ill Child

The situation surrounding the initial encounter with the critically ill child frequently is chaotic and accompanied by discomfort. One obvious cause of discomfort is the limited experience most people have with critically ill children. The prospect of having to arrive at the appropriate diagnosis and treatment plan can be overwhelming. The discomfort is further compounded by the wide ranges of age and size of the patients, the diseases and responses unique to children, the frequent absence of a direct history, and the need to tailor therapy to patient age and size. An approach to effectively manage these children in the face of realistic limitations is the subject of this chapter.

The primary diagnoses of 200 critically ill children admitted initially to local emergency departments or hospital wards are presented in Table 1–1. By primary diagnosis, the two most commonly encountered critical pediatric problems are respiratory and neurologic (55%). In contrast to adult medicine, primary cardiovascular problems account for a relatively small proportion of cases. Many diagnoses are limited exclusively to pediatrics. Not indicated in the data is the multisystem nature of many critical illnesses. The data from this transport series point out the wide range of pediatric problems one must be prepared to deal with.

By age, the patients tend to be very young:

<1 year: 40%
1–5 years: 30%
6–10 years: 10%
11–15 years: 5%
>15 years: 5%

One can therefore anticipate treating a predominance of

TABLE 1–1.
Primary Diagnoses in 200 Critically Ill Children Seen in Emergency Departments or Hospital Wards*

CNS disease	60	**Trauma/accident**	44
Meningitis	16	Drowning	13
Seizures	16	Ingestion	12
Head trauma	13	Automobile accident	10
Shunt failure	6	Child abuse	5
Reye's syndrome	6	Gunshot wound	2
Spinal cord injury	1	Burns	1
Myelomeningocele	1	Snake bite	1
CNS bleed	1	**Surgical**	7
Respiratory	50	Acute condition of the abdomen	7
Arrest	16	**Infection**	5
Croup	9	*Meningococcus*	2
Pneumonia	7	*Pseudomonas*	1
Asthma	6	Diphtheria	1
Apnea	4	Virus	1
Bronchiolitis	3	**Miscellaneous**	17
Pertussis	3	Sudden infant death syndrome	4
Epiglottitis	2	Diabetic ketoacidosis	2
Cardiovascular	16	Hemorrhage	2
Shock		Anaphylaxis	1
Hypovolemic	6	Inborn error of metabolism	1
Septic	5	Other	7
Congenital heart	4		
Arrhythmia	1		

*From Children's Hospital Oakland, 200 consecutive transports to the pediatric intensive care unit from surrounding hospital emergency departments/wards.

young children with respiratory and neurologic problems; one must, however, be prepared to treat the complete spectrum of problems, in patients of all ages.

If the critically ill child is to be cared for effectively, urgency of intervention dictates that a different approach be used than in the nonemergency situation. *A pathophysiologic and organ systems approach is used to rapidly identify the major problems and their likely sources of origin; this information is then used to direct therapy.* Diagnosis and therapy are largely directed at the organ system level:

1. Findings are described pathophysiologically.
2. Therapy tends to be broad rather than specific in aim, and its goals are twofold:
   a. Reverse the life-threatening condition.
   b. Treat the likely causes of the problem.

   Example: A 2-year-old child has cyanosis, marked retractions, and inspiratory stridor. Diagnostically, cyanosis indicates hypoxemia and inspiratory stridor localizes the problem at the level of the upper airway (croup syndrome); he is likely to have either viral croup or epiglottitis. Therapeutically, the child first needs oxygen. He needs to be kept in an upright position and may benefit from a trial of racemic epinephrine aerosol if he has croup. If he does not improve or if he worsens, he needs to be taken to the operating room for direct airway visualization and intubation if he has epiglottitis, probable intubation if he has worsening croup.

In the emergency situation, management of life-threatening problems is given first priority: urgent therapy must be provided expediently. Other less emergent problems, more specific diagnostic evaluation, and therapeutic intervention can wait to be addressed in the more stable setting of the pediatric intensive care unit (PICU).

A. Goals in care of critically ill child

1. Initial stabilization in the medical facility to which the child is admitted.
2. Safe and expedient transfer to a PICU after the child is stabilized (or is as stable as possible). The child is transferred or transported to a PICU accompanied by a medical team that can continue to provide necessary care in transit. The child should be stabilized before departure to minimize the need for complex intervention en route and to decrease the transit time for the patient.
3. Definitive care with the fine tuning of diagnosis and therapy in the PICU.

II. Operating Principles In Stabilization of Critically Ill

Because this book focuses on the initial stabilization and transport phases of critical care, the principles that operate in the emergency situation follow. They provide the framework on which to approach the assessment and treatment of the critically ill child.

A. Focus assessment and therapy on life- and organ-threatening problems

Problems of nonvital importance, such as fine tuning of therapy and diagnosis, are left to be addressed at a later time (i.e., in the controlled setting of a PICU).

Life- and organ-threatening problems must be treated urgently. In this situation, therapy may very well have to be provided in the absence of a specific or definite diagnosis. Usual diagnostic tests may also have to be deferred if the time used to perform them will delay critically needed therapy or if the test may further compromise the patient.

Examples:

Case 1: Spending 30 minutes to obtain a blood culture before starting antibiotic therapy in a child with fever, purpura, and shock delays the administration of critically needed therapy. In this situation, antibiotics should be given as soon as possible, before a blood culture is drawn if the specimen proves difficult to obtain. Identification of the causative organism can possibly be made later by bacterial antigen tests; if these studies fail to identify the causative organism, the child will empirically receive the full course of antibiotics to which he or she is responding.

Case 2: Performing a lumbar puncture (LP) in a febrile child with meningismus who is now postictal and hypoventilating is not recommended because this puts the child at great risk of having a respiratory arrest when curled up for the LP. If the child is believed to have meningitis, appropriate antibiotics in meningitic doses should be given empirically. At a later time, when the child is stable, an LP can be performed to confirm the presence of meningitis because the cerebrospinal fluid (CSF) cellular response persists for more than 1 week. Decisions about further antibiotic therapy can be made accordingly.

The primary life-threatening problem in all emergencies is oxygen deficiency; therefore, the first goal of emergency therapy is to rapidly restore and maintain oxygen delivery to the cells. Attention must first focus on the respiratory and cardiovascular systems in all emergencies.

Adequate oxygen delivery to the cells requires the simultaneous functioning of three systems:

1. Respiratory system (partial pressure of oxygen [Po_2])
2. Cardiovascular system (cardiac output)

3. Hematologic system (hemoglobin [Hgb])

Medical attention is therefore first directed to these systems, especially the respiratory and cardiovascular systems. When all three systems are functioning adequately, one can usually be assured of adequate oxygen delivery to all tissues.

When the brain is injured, oxygen delivery to the brain may become dependent on meeting one additional condition: maintenance of adequate cerebral perfusion pressure. Brain injury and cerebral perfusion pressure are discussed in Chapter 5.

Oxygen supply must be greater than or equal to oxygen needs to avoid tissue oxygen deficits and further tissue damage. When the body's ability to supply oxygen is limited or oxygen needs are increased, measures that reduce oxygen needs should be used to maintain oxygen balance in favor of supply over demand.

Situations in which oxygen delivery is limited include shock and respiratory failure. States in which there are high oxygen needs include high fever, multiple trauma, and sepsis. In these situations, the use of measures that reduce oxygen needs decrease the risk of oxygen deficit states and the risk of further damage. Measures that reduce oxygen needs include temperature control and measures that decrease body work, such as mechanical ventilation and neuromuscular paralysis.

B. Provide specific disease-directed therapy

The underlying problem needs to be treated (e.g., provide antibiotics for the child in septic shock whose cardiovascular system is already being treated).

By using this framework, one can begin to approach the critically ill child in a systematic manner and provide the crucial therapy needed for stabilization.

In addition to these stabilization principles, the following guidelines are suggested if the patient is to be transported.

III. Operating Principles in Transport of the Critically Ill

The patient should be transported to the receiving hospital in as stable a condition as possible. For most patients stability and level of care during transport will be the major goal, superseding speed of departure from the referring hospital.

Pediatric intensive care is begun when the transport team assumes care of the patient. Except for the infrequent case when the physical facilities of the tertiary care center are needed immediately (i.e., for evacuation of an epidural hematoma or surgical intervention in multiple trauma), there should be no rush to leave the referring hospital until the transport team has fully stabilized the patient.

The transport team will need a report of the course of the patient's illness and interventions provided. The team will need to obtain vital signs and secure all lines and tubes because of the movement associated with transport. They will attach transport monitors and may obtain additional data, including laboratory data and x-ray studies, as part of the stabilization process. Consultation with the receiving hospital may be needed.

As opposed to the "swoop and scoop" philosophy of scene trauma flights, the mobile intensive care provided during interfacility transport generally requires 45 to 60 minutes of in-hospital stabilization time. Very critically ill patients may need more time. All activities should be performed in an efficient and coordinated manner, but neither the team nor the staff of the referring hospital should feel pressured by the clock.

During transport the level of patient care should maintain or exceed that provided by the referring hospital during initial stabilization.

A transport mode should be chosen that can either maintain the referring hospital's level of care or elevate the level of care by provision of a sophisticated intensive care team. For this reason local ambulance transport, especially without a physician, is not usually appropriate for a critically ill child.

IV. Oxygen Delivery and Administration

Oxygen delivery, which is the prime concern in critical care medicine, is achieved only through the simultaneous functioning of three systems:

1. Respiratory system (Po_2)
2. Cardiovascular system (cardiac output)
3. Hematologic system (Hgb value)

The Po_2 and Hgb values determine the amount of oxygen (i.e., *oxygen content*) of the blood. The cardiac output determines the amount of blood (i.e., oxygen) that is *delivered* to the cells. Oxygen delivery is therefore the product of oxygen content and cardiac output. The following equation illustrates the **conceptual relationships** among these factors in determining oxygen delivery; it will be the fundamental equation to which problems regarding oxygen delivery will be referred:

$$\text{Oxygen delivery} = \text{Oxygen content} \times \text{Cardiac output} \quad (1)$$

$$\text{Oxygen delivery} = P_{O_2} \times \text{Hgb} \times \text{Cardiac output}$$

When any one of these systems falters, oxygen delivery is diminished. Correcting the problem that has decreased oxygen delivery, such as raising the P_{O_2} value in the hypoxemic patient, is the ideal means of restoring oxygen delivery. There are times, however, when adequate correction cannot be achieved for the moment, so oxygen delivery remains impaired; compensatory mechanisms must be sought to remedy the situation. An understanding of the interrelationships among the three systems that determine oxygen delivery allows one to use compensatory measures that improve and restore adequate oxygen delivery in the face of a system failure.

These concepts form the foundation for the principles of resuscitation.

A. Physiology: Oxygen content of blood

Oxygen exists in two forms in blood:

1. *Dissolved* in plasma: a small amount
2. *Hgb-bound oxygen:* the majority of oxygen in blood

The amount of oxygen that is present in each form is related to the P_{O_2} value but in differing ways. The absolute amount of oxygen in each form can be calculated (expressed as milliliters of O_2 per 100 mL of blood).

1. *Dissolved oxygen:* linear relationship with P_{O_2}.

$$\text{Dissolved oxygen} = P_{O_2}\ (\text{mm Hg}) \times 0.003\ \text{mL}$$

2. *Hgb-bound oxygen:* related to P_{O_2} value by O_2 saturation. The Hgb-O_2 dissociation curve is represented in Figure 1–1.

$$\text{Hgb-bound oxygen} = \text{Hgb} \times 1.34 \times O_2\ \text{saturation}$$

3. Determination of oxygen saturation: 1 g of Hgb is capable of carrying 1.34 mL of oxygen. For each P_{O_2} value, the amount of oxygen 1 g of Hgb carries (× milliliters) has

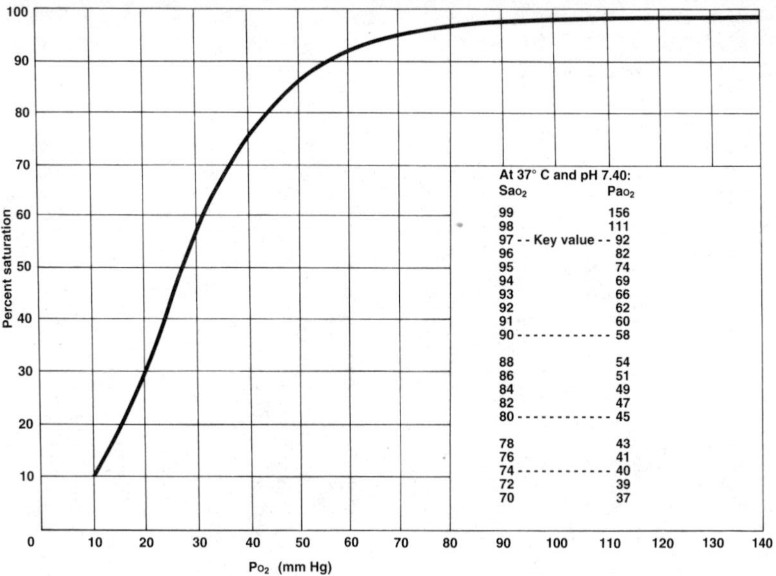

FIG 1–1.
Oxygen dissociation curve for human blood.

been measured and compared with the amount 1 g of Hgb is capable of carrying (1.34 mL). The resulting value ($\times$ $\div$ 1.34) is the oxygen saturation.

Example: When Po_2 is 40 mm Hg, 1 g of Hgb carries 0.99 mL of oxygen. Oxygen saturation is therefore 0.99 mL/1.34 mL = 0.74 = 74%. The significance of this value is that at a Po_2 value of 40 mm Hg, each gram of Hgb carries 74% of the oxygen it is capable of carrying and approximately 74% of what it carries normally when the Po_2 is 100 mm Hg (oxygen saturation 98%).

4. Calculation of Hgb-bound oxygen from O_2 saturation: For a given Po_2 value, the corresponding oxygen saturation is obtained and used to calculate Hgb-bound oxygen (see Fig 1–1).

   Example: For a Po_2 value of 40 mm Hg, the oxygen saturation is 74%. The amount of oxygen carried by 1 g of Hgb = (1 g of Hgb) $\times$ (1.34 mL/g) $\times$ (0.74) = 0.99 mL O_2.
5. Oxygen content of blood:

$$\text{Blood } O_2 \text{ content} = \text{Dissolved } O_2 + \text{Hgb-bound } O_2$$

B. Normal oxygen content

1. *Normal child:* Hgb = 12.0 g, Po_2 = 100 mm Hg, oxygen saturation = 0.98.
2. Calculation for oxygen content of blood:

$$\begin{array}{lr}
\text{Dissolved } O_2 = (100 \text{ mm Hg}) \times (0.003 \text{ mL/mm Hg}) = & 0.30 \text{ mL} \\
+ \text{ Hgb-}O_2 = (12 \text{ g Hgb}) \times (1.34 \text{ mL/g}) \times (0.98) & = 15.75 \text{ mL} \\
\hline
\text{Oxygen content of blood} & = 16.05 \text{ mL}
\end{array}$$

The majority of oxygen in the blood is bound to Hgb (15.75 mL/16.05 mL = 98%); the amount contributed by dissolved oxygen is negligible. The oxygen content of the child's blood is closely approximated by reporting 12 g of saturated Hgb. *The oxygen content in the blood of well children is usually an amount equal to 10 to 12 g of saturated Hgb* (usual Hgb 10–12 g, Po_2 100 mm Hg, O_2 saturation 0.98).

Pulse oximeters report oxygen saturation values (i.e., the relative amount of oxygen each gram of Hgb is carrying). When the oxygen saturation value is multiplied by the child's Hgb value, one has a good approximation of the number of grams of saturated Hgb the child has and, therefore, the oxygen content of the blood. This is the great value of pulse oximeters.

C. **Pathophysiologic states of decreased oxygen delivery** (Relationships between Po_2, cardiac output, and Hgb)

1. **Hypoxemia:** low Po_2 secondary to pulmonary disease or cyanotic heart disease.
   Example: Child has Hgb 12 g, Po_2 40 mm Hg, O_2 saturation 0.75.
   a. Calculation for oxygen content of blood:

Dissolved O_2 = (40 mm Hg) × (0.003 mL/mm Hg)	=	0.12 mL O_2
+ Hgb-O_2 = (12 gHgb) × (1.34 mL/g) × (0.75)	=	12.06 mL O_2
Oxygen content of blood	=	12.18 mL O_2

   Compared with the previous normal child, this child's oxygen content is only 12.18 mL/16.05, or 76% the amount of the normal child. Referring to equation 1, if the Po_2 cannot be returned to normal levels, oxygen delivery can be maintained only by increasing cardiac output or by increasing Hgb levels. These compensatory efforts are reviewed.

   b. Acute situation: increased cardiac output. The cardiovascular system increases its output to compensate for the diminished oxygen content. Cardiac output will have to increase by at least 1.3 times to deliver the same amount of oxygen to the tissues. Because cardiac work is increased, the child has limited reserve for further stress and may develop cardiac fatigue, then decompensation if this state persists, with further drops in Po_2 levels or increase in energy needs. If cardiac function becomes impaired, measures to support the cardiovascular system, as inotropes, are crucial to maintain cardiac output.

   c. Chronic state or acute intervention: Increased Hgb value. If hypoxemia persists over time, the Hgb value increases to raise oxygen content; cardiac output can decrease correspondingly. A transfusion of red blood cells (RBCs) acutely is another way to increase oxygen content acutely when the Po_2 value cannot be raised further; this will also decrease cardiac work. If the Hgb value is raised to 15 g and the Po_2 value remains 40 mm Hg:

$$
\begin{aligned}
\text{Dissolved } O_2 &= (40 \text{ mm Hg}) \times (0.003 \text{ mL/mm Hg}) = 0.12 \text{ mL } O_2 \\
+ \text{ Hgb-}O_2 &= (15 \text{ gHgb}) \times (1.34 \text{ mL/g}) \times (0.75) = 15.07 \text{ mL } O_2 \\
\hline
\text{Oxygen content of blood} &= 15.19 \text{ mL } O_2
\end{aligned}
$$

The oxygen content is now comparable in amount with that in the normal child even though the Po_2 value is much lower.

2. **Severe anemia**
   Example: Child has Hgb 4 g, Po_2 100 mm Hg, O_2 saturation 0.98.

$$
\begin{aligned}
\text{Dissolved } O_2 &= (100 \text{ mm Hg}) \times (0.003 \text{ mL/mm Hg}) = 0.30 \text{ mL } O_2 \\
+ \text{ Hgb-}O_2 &= (4 \text{ gHgb}) \times (1.34 \text{ mL/g}) \times (0.98) = 5.25 \text{ mL } O_2 \\
\hline
\text{Oxygen content of blood} &= 5.55 \text{ mL } O_2
\end{aligned}
$$

The child's blood has 5.55 mL/16.05 mL = 35% the amount of oxygen that the normal child has. The oxygen content can be raised by transfusing Hgb, but until a transfusion of RBCs can be provided, raising either the Po_2 value or cardiac output (refer to equation at beginning of chapter) will improve oxygen delivery to the cells.

a. *Increased cardiac output:* Increased cardiac output is the immediate response to the decreased oxygen content. Cardiac output must increase by about 300% to provide the oxygen the tissues need. The increased work, if excessive, results in cardiac fatigue, congestive heart failure (CHF), then shock. When CHF and shock are present, until the Hgb can be raised, diuretics and inotropes are needed to support the heart and cardiac output.
b. *Acute intervention: Increased Po_2 value and dissolved O_2 level:* If the lungs have adequate to good function, increasing the Po_2 value in this situation can raise the dissolved oxygen in the blood and oxygen content substantially. When one provides a patient with fractional

concentration of oxygen in inspired gas (FiO_2) 100%, it is possible to reach PO_2 values to the 600 mm Hg level. Assume that the PO_2 value is increased to 600 mm Hg, O_2 sat = 100%.

$$
\begin{array}{lr}
\text{Dissolved } O_2 = (600 \text{ mm Hg}) \times (0.003 \text{ mL/mm Hg}) & = 1.80 \text{ mL } O_2 \\
+ \text{ Hgb-}O_2 = (4 \text{ gHgb}) \times (1.34 \text{ mL/g}) \times (1.0) & = 5.36 \text{ mL } O_2 \\
\hline
\text{Oxygen content of blood} & = 7.16 \text{ mL } O_2
\end{array}
$$

The significant increase in PO_2 value has increased the level of dissolved O_2 by 1.5 mL, the equivalent of having increased the Hgb value by slightly more than 1 g.

The oxygen content of the blood has increased by 30% before a transfusion has been given. The cardiac output needs are decreased, and there is more time available to provide definitive therapy.

c. *Intervention: Increase Hgb value (transfusion):* This increase is the ultimate correction, but when CHF is present or incipient, a transfusion cannot be performed rapidly without risk of cardiac decompensation from volume overload. When a transfusion is performed in this situation, it must be performed very cautiously, either very slowly or via partial exchange.

3. **Diminished cardiac output (shock)**
   Normal oxygen content of the blood (normal PO_2 and Hgb values) with low cardiac output will result in inadequate oxygen delivery to the tissues. Interventions to correct this situation or to compensate for it when cardiac output cannot be fully restored follow; they include interventions that involve all determinants of oxygen delivery (refer to equation 1).
   a. *Inotropes:* Inotropes in the form of vasoactive infusions or metabolic agents are provided acutely to restore cardiac output.
   b. *Increased hemoglobin values:* Increasing the Hgb value acutely will increase the oxygen content of the blood and decrease the cardiac output needs and cardiac work. This is a very important intervention when cardiac function is limited (see p. 10.)
   c. *Increased PO_2 values:* When possible (e.g., in noncy-

anotic heart disease), increasing the Po_2 value to very high levels to increase dissolved Po_2 values will increase the oxygen content and again diminish cardiac output needs and work (see effect of Po_2 on oxygen content, p. 11).

d. *Reduction of oxygen needs:* Take steps to reduce oxygen needs that will reduce cardiac output requirements. This is especially important when cardiac output remains limited in spite of aggressive therapy. Measures include fever reduction, mechanical ventilatory support, and sedation.

D. Summary of acute compensatory interventions for states of decreased oxygen delivery

1. Interrelationships between determinants of oxygen delivery:

$$\text{Oxygen delivery} = Po_2 \times \text{Hgb} \times \text{Cardiac output}$$

(A conceptual equation)

2. Hypoxemia: when Po_2 values cannot be returned to normal:
   a. Increase Hgb levels.
   b. Support increased cardiac output.
3. Anemia
   a. Increase Fio_2 (Po_2) levels.
   b. Support increased cardiac output.
   c. Increase Hgb levels cautiously.
4. Decreased cardiac output
   a. Provide inotropic or volume support to improve cardiac output.
   b. Increase Hgb levels.
   c. Increase Po_2 levels.

   NOTE: *Always remember to use measures that will decrease oxygen needs when oxygen delivery is limited.*

E. Oxygen administration in nonintubated patients

There are many methods one can use to administer oxygen to patients with nonintubated airways. The method used is not crucial in patients with only modest Fio_2 requirements because all methods provide some elevation of Fio_2. The method of administration becomes critical, however, in the hypoxemic patient who has high Fio_2 requirements because the simple provision of 100% oxygen from the source (tank or outlet) does not provide assurance that the patient is breathing high-concentration oxygen. Effective methods of providing FiO_2 concentrations for the child who needs them follow. Patient size and tolerance must be considered in selection of the method that will produce maximum FiO_2 values.

1. **Suggested methods to provide maximum FiO_2 values for children of different sizes:**
   a. Small, quiet neonates and young infants: hood oxygen.
   b. Infants, small toddlers: nasal cannulas (NCs).
   c. Toddlers, preschoolers: NCs; if NCs alone are not sufficient, supplement with plain mask (if tolerated) or oxygen blown over the face.
   d. School-aged children, adolescents who are cooperative: nonrebreathing masks.

   These guidelines will need to be modified for the individual situation, as for the infant who is mouth breathing. Use of the pulse oximeter will help assess adequacy of oxygen therapy.
2. **NC oxygen: Relationship between NC flow and patient size in the determination of FiO_2 values**

   The use of NC oxygen can provide high FiO_2 values in small children. A simplified review of the basic factors involved in determination of FiO_2 values is presented to illustrate why and in whom NCs may be beneficial. (NOTE: The calculations presented in the cases are ideal values and are subject to many factors that lower the final FiO_2 value; they do, however, illustrate the impact of patient size on the effectiveness of NC oxygen.)
   a. Definitions
      (1) Lung volume:
         (a) Inspiratory reserve volume (IRV)
         (b) Tidal volume (TV) = 6–7 mL/kg
         (c) Expiratory reserve volume (ERV)
         (d) Residual volume (RV)
      (2) Vital capacity = IRV + TV + ERV = 50–70 mL/kg
   b. Assumptions
      (1) NC flow rate: amount of O_2 passing by/into the nostrils:
         (a) 1 L/min = 1,000 mL/min = 16.5 mL/sec

(b) 6 L/min = 6,000 mL/min = 99 mL/sec
(c) ¼ L/min = 250 mL/min = 4 mL/sec

(2) TV:
(a) 2 kg infant: TV = 12–14 mL.
(b) 70 kg male: TV = 420–490 mL; 450 mL used for cases.

(3) Fio_2:
(a) Fio_2 of supplemental oxygen = 1.0.
(b) Fio_2 of room air = 0.21.

Examples:

Case 1: NC flow = 1 L/min (16.5 mL/sec)
Inspiratory time = 1 second

2 kg infant: TV = 12 mL. The NC flow rate exceeds the infant's TV, so the Fio_2 value can theoretically be 100%. Because of turbulence and other factors, however, some room air is entrained, and the final Fio_2 level is lower. But the infant is clearly provided with a high Fio_2 value because a large portion of its TV is composed of 100% oxygen.

70 kg male: TV = 450 mL. Fio_2 value is:

$$\begin{array}{rl} 16 \text{ mL} \times Fio_2\ 1.0 & = 16 \text{ mL oxygen} \\ + 434 \text{ mL} \times Fio_2\ 0.21 & = 91 \text{ mL oxygen} \\ \hline 450 \text{ mL TV} & = 107 \text{ mL oxygen} \end{array}$$

Fio_2 = 107 mL O_2/450 mL = 0.24.
For a given flow rate, the Fio_2 value in the small child will be much higher than the Fio_2 value for the larger child. Also note other factors that will decrease the Fio_2 value: (1) a shorter inspiratory time and (2) an increased TV.

Case 2: NC flow = 6 L/min (99 mL/sec)
Inspiratory time = 1 second

2 kg infant: TV = 12 mL. The inspired Fio_2 value is again close to 1.0 because the NC flow greatly exceeds the infant's TV.

70 kg male: TV = 450 mL. Fio_2 value is:

99 mL × Fio_2 1.0	=	99 mL oxygen
+ 351 mL × Fio_2 0.21	=	74 mL oxygen
450 mL TV	=	173 mL oxygen

Fio_2 = 173 mL/450 mL = 0.38
Nasal cannulas generally do not provide high Fio_2 concentrations for larger children and adults.

Case 3: NC flow = ¼ L/min (4 mL/sec) Inspiratory time = 0.5 seconds. With an inspiratory time of 0.5 seconds, 2 mL of Fio_2 1.0 will be flowing by the infant's nostrils.

2 kg Infant: TV = 12 mL. Fio_2 value is:

2 mL × Fio_2 1.0	=	2.0 mL oxygen
+ 10 mL × Fio_2 0.21	=	2.1 mL oxygen
12 mL TV	=	4.1 mL oxygen

Fio_2 = 4.1 mL/12 mL = 0.34

This example illustrates why very low flow NC oxygen can be a very important source of supplemental oxygen to small infants and why these small amounts cannot be removed abruptly without producing hypoxemia in the small infant who still needs some supplemental oxygen.

In all instances an arterial blood gas (Po_2) and/or pulse oximeter must be used to monitor the effectiveness of any regimen of oxygen administration.

RESPIRATORY SYSTEM — 2

I. Primary Respiratory System Functions

The arterial blood gas is the measure of the adequacy of the respiratory system. The three parameters are partial pressure of oxygen (Po_2), partial pressure of carbon dioxide (Pco_2), and pH. Of these, Po_2 and pH are of paramount importance.

The respiratory system has two primary physiologic functions:

1. Oxygenation
2. Maintenance of normal pH

A. Oxygenation

The most important function of the respiratory system is to *get oxygen into the blood*. Normal Po_2 value is 90 to 100 torr. However, increasing numbers of children are seen whose usual Po_2 values are substantially lower: children with uncorrected cyanotic heart lesions whose Po_2 values run in the 40 mm Hg range and children with advanced chronic lung disease whose usual Po_2 values run between these numbers, frequently in the 60 to 70 mm Hg range.

B. Maintenance of pH

The second important function of the respiratory system is to *maintain blood pH in the 7.35 to 7.45 range;* this is a fairly universal value that the body aims to maintain. The respiratory system maintains pH by regulating the Pco_2 level. Normal Pco_2 value is 35 to 40 mm Hg. When, however, the acid-base status is disturbed, the respiratory system attempts to alter the Pco_2 value secondarily to maintain normal pH. With successful efforts, the Pco_2 value is low in the presence of metabolic acidosis and high in the presence of metabolic alkalosis. There are also increasing numbers of children whose usual Pco_2 values are significantly elevated above normal on a primary basis as a result of advanced chronic lung disease such as bronchopulmonary dysplasia and cystic fibrosis. These children can have Pco_2 values as high as 70 to 80 mm Hg, can tolerate them and not need mechanical ventilation because the kidneys have had time to retain enough bicarbonate to get the pH into the 7.35 to 7.45 range. The Pco_2 value is therefore variable and must be interpreted in the context of the pH.

Therefore, the two primary goals of treating respiratory problems are restoring and maintaining:

1. *Usual or higher Po_2 values for the child*
2. *Normal pH by using the intervention(s) required to accomplish them.*

Maintaining an adequate Po_2 value takes highest priority and remains a constant concern in the care of the critically ill child. A key rule to remember about oxygen therapy in the critical situation follows: **Provide supplemental oxygen for the critically ill child. Use fractional concentration of oxygen in inspired gas (Fio_2) 100% throughout the stabilization and transport phases to assure good oxygen levels. Do not attempt to wean the Fio_2 until the child is in a controlled setting.**

In the emergency situation, the risk of oxygen toxicity posed by the use of high Fio_2 levels and the potentially adverse effects of high Po_2 levels are not significant, whereas the risk of damage from hypoxia is great. Attempts to wean the Fio_2 in the unstable and uncontrolled setting are associated with a high risk of inadvertent hypoxia. For this reason, Fio_2 weaning is left to be done in the controlled setting of the pediatric intensive care unit (PICU). The uncommon situation where supplying high concentration oxygen is potentially detrimental exists where the child with very advanced pulmonary disease breathes on hypoxic drive.

II. Approach to Respiratory Problems

To achieve desired pH, Pco_2, and Po_2 values, air must move through the respiratory tree to reach the alveoli where gas exchange takes place. Problems at any level that interfere with the ability of fresh gas to reach the alveoli or for gas exchange to occur across the alveoli can produce hypoxemia, hypercarbia, and respiratory failure.

The altered breath sounds that arise from problems at different levels of the respiratory tract are fairly distinct. They should be used to identify the level of respiratory involvement. This identification is useful because it enables one to direct more specific evaluation and therapy to problems likely to be encountered at that level. Table 2–1 provides an overview of respiratory problems, clinical findings characteristic of pathologic conditions at each level, and approach to therapy.

Problems arising anywhere in the respiratory tract will, when severe enough, interfere with final gas exchange and result in hypoxemia and/or hypercarbia and acidosis. Significant interference with gas exchange produces a generic picture of *respiratory distress* superimposed on the primary respiratory problem. Prompt recognition of this state and intervention at this time are important.

A. Findings in child in respiratory distress

1. Cyanosis (hypoxemia), pallor (acidosis)
2. Tachypnea
3. Dyspnea (use of accessory muscles: retractions, grunting)
4. Tachycardia
5. Upright position: effort sought to maintain position of comfort and least respiratory work
6. Anxiety, agitation; concentration on respiratory efforts
7. Signs of severe respiratory distress and impending arrest
   a. Decreasing level of consciousness or responsiveness
   b. Falling respiratory rate and effort
   c. Falling heart rate

III. Initial Nonspecific Therapy for Child in Significant Respiratory Distress

A. Provide oxygen.

1. Use Fio_2 100%; administer oxygen using optimum method for patient size and situation (see p 14).
2. Monitor patient with pulse oximeter and cardiac monitor.

B. Maintain patent airway and adequate air movement.

1. Support upper airway as needed; use jaw lift as needed.
2. Suction nasopharynx/oropharynx as needed.
3. Provide airway adjuncts as needed: oral airway, oropharyngeal or nasopharyngeal airway.

TABLE 2–1.

Respiratory Tract Problems

Structure	Problem	Physical Findings	Therapy (general approach and for respiratory failure)
Nasopharynx			
Nose *Nasopharynx* *Oropharynx*	Choanal atresia, stenosis; thick secretions; enlarged adenoids, tonsils, tongue; tumor	Snoring, mouth breathing	Surgical intervention; *provide airway*
Upper Airway			
Epiglottis *Larynx*	Epiglottitis, croup, laryngomalacia, laryngitis, vocal cord problems, foreign body	Stridor (inspiratory), barking cough, obstruction	Vasoconstrictor aerosol; removal of foreign body; *provide airway*
Lower Airways			
Trachea	Tracheitis, tracheomalacia, compression, foreign body	Rhonchi	Nonspecific; *airway and mechanical ventilation*
Bronchi *Bronchioles*	Bronchitis, bronchomalacia, foreign body, bronchiolitis, asthma	Wheezes/rhonchi (pronounced on expiration), prolonged expiration	Bronchodilators; *airway and mechanical ventilation*

Alveolus			
Alveoli *Interstitium*	Pneumonitis, pulmonary edema, atelectasis, hemorrhage, fibrosis	Crackles, decreased or absent breath sounds	Medications; *airway and mechanical ventilation*
Non–Respiratory Tree			
Pleura	Pneumothorax, chylothorax, hemothorax; pleural effusion, empyema	Decreased breath sounds, mediastinal shift	Surgical drainage
Chest wall, central nervous system	CNS depression, Guillain-Barré, myasthenia gravis, botulism, spinal cord injury, muscular dystrophy, flail chest, rib fractures	Decreased respiratory movements, efforts	*Airway and mechanical ventilation*

C. Maintain patient in upright position.

1. Do not force the severely distressed patient to lie down, especially the patient with stridor who may have epiglottitis.

D. Minimize patient disturbances, discomforts.

E. Reduce fever to decrease metabolic needs.

1. Use antipyretics; remove excess coverings.
2. Avoid the use of external cooling devices in the unparalyzed patient: shivering results, which increases the metabolic rate by 200% to 300%.

F. Provide intravenous (IV) fluid therapy

1. Restore and maintain good circulation. Provide volume expanders in the patient with volume depletion.
2. When circulation is good or restored, it is advisable to limit fluid intake to an amount ranging from restricted to just slightly over the usual maintenance rate for the following reasons:
   a. Syndrome of inappropriate secretion of antidiuretic hormone (SIADH): common problem in moderate to severe respiratory distress.
   b. High negative intrathoracic pressures (retractions) may pull fluid out of the capillaries into the pulmonary interstitium and produce pulmonary edema, aggravating the primary respiratory problem.
   c. Consider furosemide (0.5–1.0 mg/kg IV) in the *hydrated* patient. It will be beneficial for the patient with pulmonary edema, pulmonary vascular congestion on chest radiograph and it may be beneficial for the patient who has extra interstitial water without overt pulmonary edema on chest radiograph.

G. Identify the level of respiratory involvement.

1. Provide specific therapy available for the disease. Using these measures may provide stability and the time needed to administer more specific therapy that can prevent progression to respiratory failure (e.g., asthma, croup). In other instances, where respiratory failure exists, these measures provide critically needed support until an airway and assisted ventilation can be provided.

IV. Evaluation of Child in Respiratory Distress

A. Arterial blood gas

1. A capillary blood gas is a good alternative if the extremity is warm and the blood specimen flows freely. It can provide valid pH and P_{CO_2} values.

B. **Complete blood cell (CBC) count: The hemoglobin (Hgb) value is especially important.**

C. **Electrolytes**

D. **Glucose: Hypoglycemia is a common finding in very young and very ill children.**

E. **Chest x-ray studies**

1. For diagnostic purposes
2. Investigation for complicating problems
   a. Pulmonary edema.
   b. Extrapulmonary air: pneumothorax, pneumomediastinum.
   c. Atelectasis.

F. **Other laboratory work as indicated (e.g., cultures)**

G. **Noninvasive monitoring**

1. Pulse oximeter
2. Transcutaneous monitor for CO_2, if available

V. Criteria for Intubation

A. **Respiratory failure: defined by one or more of the following factors**

1. Hypoxemia while receiving high levels of Fio_2.
   a. $Po_2 < 60$ mm Hg in a previously normal child.
   b. Po_2 value not clearly established for child with chronic hypoxemia; suggest consulting receiving hospital.
2. Acidosis: pH < 7.25.
   a. For pH values between 7.25 and 7.30, clinical judgment is required; suggest consulting receiving hospital.
   b. NOTE: No specific mention is made about the Pco_2 value at which intubation is required because there are increasing numbers of children with chronic CO_2 retention who function well and do not need mechanical ventilation as long as the pH value is 7.35 or more.
3. Increasing fatigue, absence of improvement with therapy.
4. Transport considerations: The child who fails to meet the criteria of respiratory failure but has significant potential for deterioration during transport should have his or her airway intubated in the sending medical facility before departure rather than risk failure and the need for intubation in transit.

B. Neuromuscular weakness: respiratory failure may not be present

1. Clinical criteria
   a. Bulbar dysfunction: poor or absent cough, gag, swallow
   b. Chest wall weakness: neurologic or muscular origin
2. Physiologic criteria
   a. Vital capacity < 12 mL/kg
   b. Maximum inspiratory force < -20 mm Hg.

VI. Endotracheal Tubes (Table 2–2)

A. Cuffed vs. uncuffed ETTs

Uncuffed ETTs should be used in children less than 7 to 8 years of age because the subglottic space, which is the narrowest part of the airway in children of this age, provides a good seal around the ETT. Use of a cuffed ETT in children in this age group may put enough pressure on the tracheal mucosa to interrupt its blood flow and produce necrosis, eventual scarring, and subglottic stenosis.

B. ETT size in upper airway obstruction (croup, epiglottitis)

Because the upper airway is significantly narrowed, these patients require a smaller-sized ETT than usual to avoid pressure necrosis and subsequent airway problems. Suggestions for ETT choice are:

1. Use an ETT smaller than usual for age by 1 mm or more.
2. Use uncuffed ETT.
3. Use *nasal-length ETT*. Do not use an oral length or ETT that has been precut to prevent right mainstem intubation. Because a smaller than usual ETT is used for this patient, oral length and precut ETTs are frequently too short to allow these critical airways to be positioned securely: The tip of the ETT is frequently far above the carina and at great risk for accidental dislodging.

C. ETT insertion distance (lip-to-tip guideline)

Incorrect ETT tip placement is common in children; right main stem bronchus intubation is especially common in young children. To minimize this complication, use the following guideline. When the appropriate-sized ETT is used

TABLE 2–2.

Guidelines for Pediatric Endotracheal Tube Size

Patient Age	Internal Diameter (mm)	Distance to Lips (cm)	Suction Catheter
Newborn	3.0 uncuffed	9	6 F
1–6 mo	3.5 uncuffed	10	8 F
6–18 mo	4.0 uncuffed	11	8 F
1.5–2 yr	4.5 uncuffed	12	8 F
3–4 yr	5.0 uncuffed	14	10 F
5–6 yr	5.5 uncuffed	16	10 F
7–8 yr	6.0 uncuffed	18	10 F
9 yr	6.0 cuffed	18	10 F
10–11 yr	6.5 cuffed	20	10 F
12+ yr	7.0 cuffed	22	10 F

Mnemonic for endotracheal tube (ETT) size in children ≥2 yr of age:

$$\text{ETT (mm ID)} = \frac{16 + \text{Age (yr)}}{4}$$

Laryngoscope blades for intubation:
- Straight blade, for use in children ≤4–6 yr of age:
  - Miller 0, 1, 2
  - Wis-Hipple 1.5
- Curved blade, for use in children ≥4–6 yr of age:
  - Macintosh 2, 3

for age and with the ETT tip in good position, *the distance at the lip (in centimeters) is usually about 3 times the ETT size (which is given in millimeters).* Auscultation of the breath sounds and a chest radiograph are used to confirm correct position.

Example: A 4-year-old requires a 5.0 mm ETT. When it is positioned correctly, the ETT mark at the lips is usually about 15 cm.

VII. Pediatric Emergency Intubation and Ventilation Guidelines

A. Oxygen: Use Fio_2 100% throughout resuscitation, stabilization.

B. Bag-valve-mask ventilation.

1. Uses and indications
   a. Before intubation is attempted to improve oxygenation, ventilation.
   b. In between unsuccessful intubation attempts.
   c. While awaiting experienced intubator to arrive; it can maintain the patient for long periods of time if necessary.
2. Technique
   a. Open airway: jaw thrust, sniffing position; suction secretions.
   b. Maintain the airway: may need oropharyngeal or nasopharyngeal airway.
   c. Assist ventilation: Provide tight seal with mask, ventilate with adequate volume to cause chest to rise, maintain cricoid pressure; see p. 27 for respiratory rate.

C. Intubation

1. Use *oral* route for intubation.
   a. Nasal intubation is more difficult to perform in small children than in adults because of the anterior and cephalad location of the larynx.
   b. Do not attempt blind nasal intubation in small children; these attempts are almost always unsuccessful.
2. Suction equipment: essential to visualize the airway.
3. Stylet: Use of a stylet may increase the chance of successful intubation in small children (but may also increase the risk of damage to a small trachea).
4. Consider use of a neuromuscular relaxant to facilitate in-

tubation (to be used only by a person skilled in intubation). (See Appendix A.)

D. Ventilation: Ventilate manually

1. Tidal volume (TV) and pressures
   a. *Chest movement* is the criterion by which to judge adequacy of tidal volume. Use whatever pressure is required to produce good chest movement.
   b. Positive end-expiratory pressure (PEEP): Physiologic PEEP equals 3 to 4 mm Hg pressure.
2. Ventilation rate: suggested initial rates
   a. Minimum initial ventilation rates
      Neonate, young infant: 30–40 breaths/min
      Toddler, preschooler: 20–30 breaths/min
      School age (Preadolescent): 16–20 breaths/min
      Adolescent: 12–16 breaths/min
      (1) *For the child without cardiorespiratory failure: Use the previously listed rates.* ***Examples:***
         (a) The child with neuromuscular weakness (e.g., infantile botulism).
         (b) The child who needs to be sedated and ventilated for a computed tomography (CT) scan.
      (2) *For the child with cardiorespiratory failure, other problems:* Use rate 1.5 to 2 times those listed earlier.
         (a) Respiratory failure
         (b) Circulatory failure
         (c) Acidosis of other origins
         (d) High metabolic needs (e.g., high fever)
         (e) Increased intracranial pressure

E. Guidelines for ventilation adjustments

1. Obtain arterial blood gas (ABG) values. The two goals of ventilation are:
   a. Po_2: ≥80 mm Hg. (Do not be concerned about very high Po_2 values.)
   b. pH: ≥7.35.
      (1) pH up to the 7.5s is generally safe.
      (2) A Pco_2 value as low as 20 mm Hg is safe. Use hypocarbia (respiratory alkalosis) to compensate for metabolic acidosis during this phase.
2. Clinical assessment of ventilation needs in the responsive (i.e., moving) patient
   a. Central pinkness and minimal to absent patient respi-

ratory efforts suggest that the two drives to breathe (hypoxemia and acidosis) have been met.

(1) Po_2 value is adequate to high.

(2) pH value is adequate to high.

b. Persistent patient respiratory efforts above the mechanically provided breaths suggest:

(1) Respiratory drive(s) has (have) not been met:

(a) Poor central color: suggests Po_2 value is low.

(b) Good central color: suggests pH value is low, that the respiratory rate (RR) and/or TV need(s) to be increased.

(2) The patient is uncomfortable: need to provide sedation.

F. Mechanical ventilator choice when patient is stable

One may choose to use a mechanical ventilator or continue with manual ventilation at this stage.

1. *Pressure ventilator:* for use in infants up to 5–10 kg

a. Select the pressure that produces adequate chest movement. The pressure required to move the chest may be very high when compared with neonates.

(1) After adequate chest movement is attained, adjust rate to change Pco_2 and pH.

2. *Volume ventilator:* for use in children >5 kg

a. Use *delivered* (vs. "set") TV 10–15 mL/kg.

(1) Confirm good chest movement with the selected TV.

(2) After adequate TV is selected, adjust rate to change Pco_2 and pH.

G. Controlled ventilation

(i.e., mechanically providing all or most of the patient's breaths) is highly recommended even for the patient who has respiratory efforts. Rationale: The patient's own efforts may be ineffective; the increased oxygen needs resulting from respiratory work may increase the risk of developing oxygen deficits.

1. If the patient continues to struggle or fight the ventilator, use:

a. Sedation (see below)

(1) Morphine sulfate, 0.1 mg/kg IV q1–2h, and/or

(2) Diazepam, lorazepam, or midazolam, 0.1 mg/kg IV

b. Neuromuscular relaxant
   (1) Pancuronium bromide (Pavulon) or vecuronium bromide (Norcuron), 0.1 mg/kg IV prn movement, *plus* sedation
   NOTE: See management summary of emergency intubation and ventilation in Appendix A.

VIII. Postresuscitation: Maintenance of the Airway and Ventilation

A. Secure the endotracheal tube

1. Use bite block or oral airway if patient is biting the ETT.
2. Tape ETT securely; use benzoin for improved adhesiveness and skin protection.
3. Restrain the patient's limbs and head.
   a. Elbow restraints: provide greater security; especially useful when ETT maintenance is critical.

B. Insert nasogastric (NG) tube

Empty stomach, leave open to gravity.

C. Sedate the agitated, uncomfortable patient.

1. Morphine sulfate (MS): 0.1 mg/kg IV q1–2h.
   a. Good first choice: analgesic (ETT hurts) and sedative.
2. Benzodiazepines: Add if morphine is not sufficient.
   a. Diazepam: 0.1 mg/kg IV q1–2h as needed.
   b. Lorazepam: 0.05–0.1 mg/kg IV q6–8h as needed.
   c. Midazolam: 0.1 mg/kg IV q1h as needed.

D. Neuromuscular relaxants

Use when sedation is not sufficient to control patient activity that poses risk to the patient and/or interferes with mechanical attempts to oxygenate and ventilate the patient. *Sedation (listed earlier) must be provided when a neuromuscular relaxant is used.*

1. Pancuronium bromide
   a. Dose: 0.1–0.2 mg/kg IV; repeat whenever patient begins to move.
   b. Duration of action: 30–120 minutes.
   c. Side effects
      (1) Tachycardia
      (2) Hypertension (hypotension if patient is dehydrated or hypovolemic)

(3) Intracranial hypertension (this effect is lessened if it is given over 5–10 minutes rather than as a rapid push)
(4) Increased salivation

d. Excretion: Renal. Prolonged effect in patients with renal failure; consider vecuronium.

2. Vecuronium
   a. Dose: 0.1–0.2 mg/kg IV; repeat whenever patient begins to move.
   b. Duration of action: 25–40 minutes.
   c. No significant cardiovascular side effects.
   d. Excretion: primarily hepatic.

E. Obtain postintubation chest radiograph

1. Check ETT position. NOTE:
   a. Flexion of neck moves ETT tip closer to carina.
   b. Extension of neck moves ETT tip away from carina.

F. Suction ETT

1. Obtain ETT aspirate for culture if needed.
2. Instill normal saline solution without preservatives into ETT to thin secretions and facilitate their removal.

G. Aerosolized bronchodilators

Patients with intubated airways frequently develop reactive bronchospasm to ETT, ventilation, and suctioning. Use bronchodilator up to q1h as needed.

1. Metaproterenol: 200–600 μg/kg (0.2–0.6 mg/kg) per treatment. Add normal saline solution to 1–5 mL volume.
2. Terbutaline: 100–300 μg/kg (0.1–0.3 mg/kg) per treatment, maximum 3 mg. Add normal saline solution to 1–5 mL volume.
3. Albuterol: 50–200 μg/kg (0.05–0.2 mg/kg) per treatment. Add normal saline solution to 1–5 mL volume.

H. Management of blood gas values

1. P_{CO_2} is inversely proportional to minute ventilation: Minute ventilation = RR × TV.
   a. To decrease P_{CO_2} value: Increase TV, RR, or both.
   b. To increase P_{CO_2} value: Decrease TV if chest movement is excessive, decrease RR, or decrease both.
2. P_{O_2} values can be increased by the following maneuvers:
   a. Increase F_{IO_2} value.
   b. Increase TV to higher end of volume range to recruit more alveoli: Increase TV toward 15 mL/kg on vol-

ume ventilator or increase chest movement/peak pressure using pressure ventilator or manual ventilation.

c. Increase positive end-expiratory pressure (PEEP) when significant atelectasis, edema, or infiltrates are present.

d. Increase inspiratory time.

e. Other measures to consider in the patient with persistently low Po_2 values:

   (1) Hyperventilation, alkalosis to decrease pulmonary vascular resistance.

   (2) Sedation of agitated patient; consider neuromuscular relaxant.

   (3) Diuretic (furosemide) for pulmonary edema, suspicion of extra lung water.

IX. Upper Airway Obstruction

Upper airway obstruction (UAO) is largely a pediatric problem and a fairly common problem because of the small caliber of the pediatric airway. The clinical findings that identify the problem at the level of the upper airway are listed.

Stridor is a low-pitched sound heard during the *inspiratory* phase of respiration.

The phase of respiration during which airway sounds are most prominent is an important distinction to make in airway disease:

1. Noise more prominent during the inspiratory phase indicates upper (extrathoracic) airway pathologic conditions because the extrathoracic airway narrows further during inspiration.
2. Noise more prominent during the expiratory phase indicates lower (intrathoracic) airway pathologic conditions because the intrathoracic airway narrows more during expiration (e.g., wheezing in asthma; see p. 41).

   The inspiratory phase may be prolonged and becomes more pronounced as upper airway narrowing progresses.

   The patient may have a harsh, barking cough.

   Common causes (in order) of stridor include:

   1. Viral croup (largyngotracheobronchitis): most common
   2. Epiglottitis
   3. Bacterial tracheitis (membranous croup)

4. Less common causes
    a. Retropharyngeal abscess
    b. Laryngeal papillomas
    c. Laryngomalacia
    d. Soft tissue bleeding
    e. Vocal cord paralysis (primary or secondary to increased intracranial pressure, e.g., from hydrocephalus)
    f. Burns (thermal, chemical)
    g. Foreign body
    h. Compression by masses

One of the first questions that arises when the child with stridor is evaluated is whether or not the child has epiglottitis because epiglottitis is a medical emergency for which urgent intubation is needed. The three major infectious types of upper airway obstruction are reviewed because they are the most commonly encountered causes of stridor (Table 2–3).

A. Viral croup (laryngotracheobronchitis)

Viral croup is the most commonly seen cause of stridor. The subglottic airway is narrowed by this infection. It typically affects young children aged 6 months to 3 years, but older children who have abnormally narrow airways (most commonly from previous intubation) are being seen in increasing numbers. The typical course begins with an upper respiratory tract infection (URTI) of 1 or more days, followed by the development of a barking cough and stridor. There is associated fever but usually no toxicity. Stridor may be mild to severe. A small percentage of children require hospitalization.

B. Epiglottitis

Epiglottitis is a medical emergency. Once stridor develops, complete airway obstruction frequently develops within 6 to 12 hours. The etiology is most commonly *Haemophilus influenzae*, and most children have blood and epiglottis cultures positive for this organism. Children affected are usually 1 to 10 years old; infants as young as 6 months and adults occasionally develop this disease.

Most children have little or no preceding illness. Fever and toxicity develop abruptly, accompanied by complaints of a sore throat in children who can speak, then difficulty

TABLE 2–3.

Features of Diseases Frequently Causing Stridor

	Croup	Epiglottitis	Bacterial Tracheitis
Age	6 mo–3 yr	6 mo–adult	1–10 yrs
Etiology	Viral	*Haemophilus influenzae:* sepsis.	*Staphylococcus aureus,* group A *Streptococcus, H. influenzae, Streptococcus pneumoniae:* localized.
Prior illness	URTI,* possible stridor up to several days	Frequently none; rapid onset; older child may first complain of sore throat	URTI, possible stridor up to several days
Signs and symptoms and course	Stridor, barky cough, usually nontoxic; usually self-limited illness of several days' duration	Stridor, toxic; classic appearance: tripod stance, protruding jaw, drooling, anxious; complete airway obstruction common 6–12 hr after stridor appears	Stridor, toxic; may develop sudden change in picture: from severe to minimal stridor and vice versa
Lateral neck film	Subgottic narrowing	Wide epiglottis, thick aryepiglottic folds, obliterated valleculae	Subglottic narrowing; may also see ragged mucosal edge, linear or stippled densities in air column
Need for intubation	1%–5% of patients hospitalized	Virtually all transported patients	≥50% of patients at varying time in course; the ETT in many intubated airways may become obstructed with thick pus.
Other therapy	Cool mist; racemic epinephrine aerosols; ?corticosteroids	Antibiotics	Antibiotics

*URTI = upper respiratory tract infection.

swallowing, and refusal to eat. Drooling occurs when dysphagia is severe.

Stridor appears after the dysphagia and is the usual symptom that precipitates the medical visit. Airway obstruction can progress rapidly as the epiglottis and arytenoids swell. Characteristically the child assumes a sitting position with head forward (tripod stance), chin jutting forward, mouth open, drooling. The child is frequently anxious and apprehensive. Stridor is present, a barky cough may or may not be present, and the voice is frequently muffled.

Manipulating the mouth, attempting to visualize the airway, or making the patient lie down may precipitate airway closure and arrest. When the diagnosis is established, these children need intubation of their airway and IV antibiotics for the associated sepsis. Pneumonia and otitis media are commonly found in association with epiglottitis.

C. Bacterial tracheitis (membranous croup)

Bacterial tracheitis is the least common of the three major infectious causes of stridor. Affected children are 1 to 10 years of age. The airway is narrowed in the subglottic region as in viral croup, but the bacterial infection produces toxicity and a high incidence of severe airway obstruction more reminiscent of epiglottitis.

It is postulated that these children initially have a viral airway infection that becomes secondarily infected by bacteria. The most commonly identified pathogen is coagulase-positive *Staphylococcus,* but other common pyogenic pathogens are also found. The bacterial infection is localized and frequently extends to produce simultaneous bronchitis and pneumonitis. Blood cultures are usually negative, although the children are typically toxic in appearance. Mucopurulent secretions and airway membranes, which are characteristic of this disease, frequently occlude the airway.

These children therefore usually have a preceding URTI, sometimes stridor, followed by toxicity and significant stridor after the bacterial infection is established. Bacterial tracheitis must be suspected in the child with croup who is toxic. The white blood cell count is usually high with a left shift. The classic findings of bacterial tracheitis on lateral neck film are subglottic narrowing with speckled or linear densities in the air column, which represent the secretions and membranes found in this disease; ragged mucosa also suggests bacterial tracheitis. The absence of these densities, however, does not rule out bacterial tracheitis. If the diagnosis is strongly suspected, confirmation must be obtained by direct visualization of the airway with the patient under anesthesia. Subglottic narrowing with purulent material and/or membranes confirms the diagnosis.

Clinically some children have a very labile airway picture usually seen only in bacterial tracheitis; the child may look well, then suddenly develop marked stridor and distress, usually after coughing or taking a deep breath. It is thought that dislodged mucus or membranes have obstructed the airway. Subsequent coughing may then clear the airway so that the child again looks well. There are other instances when the mucus cannot be dislodged so an airway tube must be inserted.

Racemic epinephrine treatments can be helpful. Antibiotics that cover usual childhood pathogens plus coagulase-positive *Staphylococcus* need to be provided. Fifty percent or more of the patients reported require intubation. The need for an airway is not consistently emergent as in epiglottitis, but severe obstruction can develop suddenly, and the patient who is not intubated needs very close monitoring. One must also know that many of the patients with intubated airways still develop obstruction from the thick mucus or membranes, which occlude the ETTs. Many of these patients require ventilation in addition to intubation because of coexisting pneumonia.

D. Management of UAO

It is important to follow several key principles when one is working with the child with moderate to severe stridor:

1. Keep disturbances to a minimum; limit handling to essential interventions. The disturbed patient will develop increased stridor and respiratory difficulties and may decompensate.
2. Do not make the patient in moderate to severe distress lie down. If the patient has epiglottitis, this maneuver may precipitate complete airway obstruction and arrest.
3. Do not look into or insert instruments into the mouth, especially if epiglottitis is suspected. This will upset the patient and may precipitate airway closure.
4. A physician experienced with intubation should have

airway equipment available and accompany this patient to the radiology department, operating room (OR), and so forth.

Because each disease that causes stridor has its specific management, one ideally wants to establish the diagnosis for therapeutic reasons. **However, the approach to the child with stridor should first assess the severity of the airway obstruction, because this will determine the most prudent and expeditious course to pursue in evaluation and treatment of the patient.**

For these purposes, patients can be placed into one of three categories of severity of obstruction:

1. Mild: audible inspiratory stridor but with minimal or no retractions; good air movement; no obvious discomfort.
2. Moderate: inspiratory stridor; prolonged inspiratory phase; moderate retractions; good to fair air movement; normal neurologic status. Patients are in distress but are compensated. This group can be subdivided into:
   a. Patients who are cooperative (usually older patients).
   b. Patients who are incapable of being cooperative (usually because they are young).
3. Severe: marked inspiratory stridor; prolonged inspiratory phase; marked retractions; diminished to poor air movement; air hunger, anxiety, agitation; decreased responsiveness to stimuli or decreased level of consciousness; poor color (cyanosis and/or pallor). When most severe: moribund, prearrest state.

E. Guidelines for evaluation and therapy

1. *Severe distress: Respiratory failure: Patient is barely able to move air, is tiring, is in prearrest state.*
   a. *Child's airway needs to be intubated emergently!* The decision to intubate must be made on clinical criteria rather than waiting for results of x-ray studies or laboratory tests (see p. 39).
      (1) To be done in the emergency department, ward, or wherever patient is located.
      (2) To be done in the OR if patient is stable enough to withstand the trip safely.
   b. Patient needs tracheostomy or cricothyrotomy if intubation cannot be performed.
2. *Severe or moderate distress in patient incapable of cooperating:* Patient is distressed but not in respiratory failure.

a. Keep patient comfortable, minimize disturbances.
   (1) Keep patient in upright position.
      (a) Do not put patient in supine position!
   (2) Provide supplemental oxygen in manner patient will tolerate.
      (a) Blow oxygen over patient's face if this is the only means he or she will tolerate.
   (3) Keep patient in parent's arms or lap if this will calm and quiet the patient.
   (4) Leave the patient alone except to do essential tasks.
      (a) Do not look into the patient's mouth.
      (b) Do not take a lateral neck x-ray film.
      (c) Avoid further patient disturbances (i.e., defer starting IV line, doing blood work at this time unless patient appears to be near or in respiratory failure and therefore needs IV access immediately along with intubation).
   (5) An empiric trial of racemic epinephrine aerosol can be tried if time is available and if this does not unduly disturb the patient.
      (a) 0.25 mL in infant <6 months, 0.50 mL in child >6 months. Add 4–5 mL of normal saline solution, aerosolize, blow over patient's face (not by intermittent positive-pressure breathing [IPPB]).
      (b) Monitor heart rate and rhythm during treatment.
      (c) Dose frequency: q4–6h in mild cases, up to every 30 minutes for severe croup in emergency setting.

b. Call the physician who will manage the airway (e.g., anesthesiologist, surgeon, ear-nose-throat physician).
   (1) Take patient to the OR.
      (a) Visualization of the airway and intubation, if necessary, should be done in a controlled environment with the patient anesthetized.
      (b) *Avoid awake intubation* unless the patient is moribund.
   (2) Recommended OR management
      (a) Provide halothane by mask with patient in sitting position
      (b) Follow with bag and mask ventilation, which

is usually very effective once the child is asleep unless the airway is extremely narrow.

(c) Visualize the airway; establish working diagnosis.

(d) Start IV line; do blood work as possible at this time.

c. Airway management after diagnosis is established by airway visualization

(1) *Epiglottitis* or *severe airway narrowing*

(a) Intubate the airway. *Do not delay the decision to intubate or intubation itself while waiting for the transport team* (see p. 39).

(2) *Viral croup with adequate airway*

(a) Racemic epinephrine aerosol treatment (see p. 37 for dose).

(b) Dexamethasone: 0.5–1.0 mg/kg/day in 4 divided doses. Controversial.

(c) Consider furosemide: 0.5–1.0 mg/kg IV: Well-hydrated patients with severe retractions can develop pulmonary edema (ranging in degree from not being visible on radiograph to florid pulmonary edema that worsens respiratory distress from croup). Excellent improvement may follow in some patients.

(3) *Bacterial tracheitis* (narrowed subglottic space plus mucopurulent secretions or membranes in airway)

(a) *Airway compromised:* Intubate (see p. 39). NOTE: Caretakers must be aware of the high risk of ETT becoming obstructed from thick secretions or dislodged membranes.

(b) *Airway adequate:* Use same measures as for viral croup.

(c) Obtain sample for culture.

(d) Start antibiotic: semisynthetic penicillin plus a broad-spectrum cephalosporin.

3. *Mild distress* or *moderate distress in older cooperative patient*

a. Provide supplemental oxygen as tolerated: nasal cannulas, mask, or blowby.

b. May empirically try racemic epinephrine aerosol by blowby.

c. Lateral neck film for diagnosis.
   (1) Epiglottitis
      (a) Elective intubation in OR (see p. 39).
      (b) CBC, blood culture (after intubation).
      (c) Antibiotics: cephalosporin.
   (2) Viral croup
      (a) Racemic epinephrine aerosol treatment as needed.
         (i) Dose: See p. 37.
   (3) Bacterial tracheitis
      (a) Diagnosis
         (i) Diagnostic findings: subglottic narrowing, debris in airway or ragged mucosa.
         (ii) Subglottic narrowing without debris or ragged mucosa does not rule out bacterial tracheitis. If it is still suspected, diagnosis is made by visualization of the airway in OR.
      (b) Therapy
         (i) Admit patient; observe carefully.
         (ii) Start antibiotics: semisynthetic penicillin plus chloramphenicol or second-generation cephalosporin.
         (iii) Use racemic epinephrine aerosol therapy as for viral croup.

X. Airway Management of UAO

NOTE: Intubation should ideally be performed in the controlled setting of the *OR* with the patient under anesthesia. Intubation with the patient awake should be avoided. The exception to this rule is the child who is moribund and needs immediate intubation.

A. Child in OR.

1. Child is given halothane by mask in sitting position and is then put to sleep.
2. Bag and mask ventilation is provided.
3. Airway is visualized and evaluated.

B. Intubation for UAO

1. ETT
   a. Smaller than usual size by ≥ 1 mm.
   b. Uncuffed ETT.
   c. *Nasal-length* ETT to assure good stability of position.

2. Intubate airway orally initially.
   a. Switch to nasal route after oral intubation, if possible.
      (1) Nasal tube is more stable than oral tube.
         (a) Less likely to be occluded by teeth/jaws.
         (b) Less likely to be accidentally dislodged.
3. Perform needle cricothyrotomy or tracheostomy if intubation cannot be accomplished.
4. Provide Fio_2 100%.
5. Ventilate as needed. Many patients require no ventilatory support.
6. Insert NG tube and empty stomach contents; leave to gravity drainage.

C. **Maintenance of ETT**

1. Restrain patient: limb and head restraints.
   a. *Elbow restraints* are particularly useful in this situation.
2. Sedate patient.
   a. MS: 0.1 mg/kg IV q1–2h prn. Provides pain relief, sedation.
   b. Add a benzodiazepine if MS is not sufficient to sedate patient.
      (1) Diazepam: 0.1 mg/kg IV q1h prn.
      (2) Lorazepam: 0.05–0.1 mg/kg IV q4–6h prn.
      (3) Midazolam: 0.05–0.1 mg/kg IV q1h prn.
      (4) Chloral hydrate: 30–50 mg/kg NG q4–6h prn. Excellent hypnotic; excellent addition to MS, and very useful for transport.
3. If sedation is not sufficient to calm the patient and ETT maintenance is threatened, a neuromuscular relaxant and ventilatory support should be considered to maintain the airway.
   a. Pancuronium: 0.1–0.2 mg/kg IV prn movement.
   b. Or vecuronium: 0.1–0.2 mg/kg IV prn movement.
   c. Provide sedation with muscle relaxant: MS and/or a benzodiazepine.
   d. Refer to p. 29.
4. Ventilatory support
   a. Not needed if patient breathes well.
   b. Ventilatory support needed if:
      (1) Patient's respiratory efforts are decreased:
         (a) From fatigue, severe illness.

(b) From heavy sedation.
(c) From neuromuscular relaxant.

c. Refer to p. 27.

5. Obtain blood work.
   a. CBC count.
   b. Blood culture as needed.
   c. Other blood work as needed.
6. Start IV line and other therapy.
   a. Antibiotics for (suspected) epiglottitis or bacterial tracheitis.

XI. Lower Airway Obstruction

Lower airway disease, for the present discussion, refers to the intrathoracic airways. Lower airway problems are most commonly seen in patients with asthma and bronchiolitis and patients with bronchopulmonary dysplasia whose problems largely arise from their small airways. Other less frequently seen causes of lower airway disease include aspiration, chemical inhalation injuries, foreign bodies, and cystic fibrosis.

The intrathoracic airways decrease in caliber during the expiratory phase of respiration. This phenomenon explains the hallmark findings of lower airway disease: with pathologic narrowing of the intrathoracic airways, greater difficulty is encountered moving air during the expiratory than the inspiratory phase, hence, the prominence of findings during the expiratory phase of respiration. The characteristic findings are:

Respiratory noise that is more prominent during the expiratory phase. Typical findings are wheezing, which arises from the small airways, and rhonchi, which arise from larger intrathoracic airways. When obstruction is severe, grunting may be heard during the expiratory phase as the patient actively attempts to expel air.

Prolonged expiratory phase as it takes a longer time to move air out of than into the lungs. The more severe the obstruction, the longer the expiratory phase. When incomplete emptying of the lungs takes place, air trapping results and hyperinflation is seen on radiograph as well as clinically.

Asthma is the most commonly seen lower airway disease seen in pediatrics; therefore, much of the following discussion focuses on asthma, but the principles presented apply to any lower airway problem.

Understanding the pathophysiology of lower airway obstruction is of critical importance, especially when one is treating the asthmatic patient in respiratory failure: ventilator settings must take into account the pathophysiologic state to be effective. The following warnings about ventilation of the patient with lower airway obstruction must be heeded:

Asthmatic patients are among the most difficult and hazardous patients to ventilate. A high rate of morbidity and mortality is associated with the ventilation of asthmatics. Ventilator setting requirements for asthmatics are very different from those required for respiratory failure from other causes. The general rules used to manage respiratory failure do not work in this situation and, when used, may cause harm to the patient. The principles of ventilation in patients with asthma are reviewed at the end of this section.

For these reasons, status asthmaticus must be treated aggressively to avert respiratory failure. It is important to be familiar with asthma because the incidence of asthma and the mortality rate from it are both rising in spite of the major advances in the pharmacologic agents used to treat it.

A. Assessment of asthma

1. Clinical assessment
   a. Parameters to monitor
      (1) Color: normal to cyanosis.
      (2) Inspiratory breath sounds: normal to unequal to decreased or absent.
      (3) Expiratory wheezing: none to severe with prolonged expiratory phase.
         (a) Latter is associated with visible chest hyperaeration.
      (4) Use of accessory muscles: none to marked.
      (5) Level of consciousness: normal to depressed/agitated to coma.
2. Blood gas assessment of asthma
   a. Oxygen: Patient with status asthmaticus always has some degree of hypoxemia.
   b. Carbon dioxide: This is an excellent indicator of the amount of air exchange that is occurring, a very im-

portant parameter that gauges the severity of an asthmatic attack.

(1) Mild: P_{CO_2} 20–35 mm Hg.
(2) Moderate: P_{CO_2} 36–45 mm Hg.
(3) Severe, impending respiratory failure: P_{CO_2} 46–59 mm Hg.
(4) Respiratory failure: $P_{CO_2} \geq 60$ mm Hg.

A transcutaneous monitor for CO_2 may be useful to monitor response to therapy.

3. Chest X-ray studies in asthma
   a. Hyperaeration: seen in varying degrees, very marked in severe asthma.
   b. Chest x-ray findings that worsen the clinical picture substantially:
      (1) Pneumomediastinum, subcutaneous emphysema: Patients with these findings are usually very ill clinically. Usual but very aggressive medical therapy and close monitoring are needed.
      (2) Pneumothorax: Patient is usually very ill clinically; needs to have air evacuated, generally by chest tube rather than simple needle aspiration.
      (3) Atelectasis: Usually secondary to mucous plugs. Patient is again very ill clinically. Usual but very aggressive medical therapy is needed.

B. Therapy of asthma

The child in status asthmaticus needs to have all modalities of therapy used to prevent respiratory failure.

1. **Specific therapy**
   a. Oxygen: All patients with status asthmaticus are hypoxemic and need oxygen.
      (1) Provide oxygen: Use appropriate method of administration (see p. 14).
      (2) Use pulse oximeter to monitor oxygen level: Aim for O_2 saturation $\geq 90\%$ ($P_{O_2} \geq 60$ mm Hg).
   b. Aerosolized β-adrenergic agents: preferred route of administration.
      (1) Administer via blowby, not IPPB.
      (2) Use newer β_2 agents:
         (a) Albuterol: 0.05–0.20 mg/kg, maximum dose 4 mg, plus normal saline solution to 5 mL volume.
         (b) Terbutaline: 0.10–0.30 mg/kg (maximum

dose 3 mg) plus normal saline solution to 5 mL volume.

(c) Metaproterenol: 0.20–0.60 mg/kg, maximum dose 15 mg, plus normal saline solution to 5 mL volume.

(d) Isoetharine (Bronkosol): 0.10–0.20 mg/kg, maximum dose 5 mg, plus normal saline solution to 5 mL volume.

These newer β_2 agents are provided q4–6h in the stable situation. With a moderately ill child, they are given q1–2h prn. In impending or actual respiratory failure, they may be given as frequently as q15–30 minutes as long as toxicity (cardiac) is not present. In the most severe cases, the medication can be administered with increased frequency because the smooth muscles are not as responsive to medications as usual, and the intensely constricted airways allow little medication to reach them.

c. Older β_1- or β_2-adrenergic agent: aerosolized Isoproterenol.

(1) Dose: 0.25 mL in infants, 0.5 mL in older children; add normal saline solution to 5 mL volume.

(2) Monitor heart rate and rhythm for excessive tachycardia and dysrhythmias.

This is a very potent bronchodilator: When the newer β_2 agents fail to provide satisfactory improvement, isoproterenol may provide dramatic, although short duration, improvement. If this occurs, follow isoproterenol treatment with a β_2 aerosol, which can now reach the smaller airways and provide more sustained bronchodilatation. Isoproterenol treatments can be used whenever the patient's airways become very tight again.

d. Subcutaneous β-adrenergic agents: These may be useful when aerosolized administration of β-adrenergic agents fail to produce bronchodilatation.

(1) Epinephrine 1:1,000 solution.

(a) Dose: 0.01 mL/kg SC, maximum dose 0.4 mL, q 20–30 minutes × 3 doses prn

(b) Disadvantages: painful; nonselective adrenergic drug with multiple side effects (tachycardia, emesis, pallor, jitteriness).

(2) Terbutaline

(a) Dose for children <12 years: 0.005–0.01 mg/kg SC, maximum dose 0.30 mg, q 15–20 minutes × 3 doses prn

(b) Dose for children ≥12 years to adults: 0.25 mg/dose, repeated prn × 1 dose. Total dose of 0.5 mg should not be exceeded in a 4-hour period.

e. Anticholinergic aerosols

Consider anticholinergic aerosol when β-adrenergic drugs fail to produce desired response. They may be very helpful in some patients and tried empirically. They are generally less effective in children than in adults. Consider them when a child is already on anticholinergic therapy.

(1) Atropine: 0.01–0.04 mg/kg aerosol. May give this alone with normal saline solution or add it to the β-adrenergic drug simultaneously.

(2) Ipatroprium bromide: 1–2 puffs (metered dose inhalant).

f. Theophylline: Use in emergency situation.

(1) Background pharmacologic information:

(a) Theophylline levels

(i) Desired level in status asthmaticus: 10–20 μg/mL.

(ii) Aim for higher end of range for severe attack.

(b) Signs, symptoms of theophylline toxicity: Generally begin at levels ≥20 μg/mL.

(i) GI: nausea, vomiting. Hematemesis at higher levels.

(ii) CNS: irritability, sleeplessness, jitteriness. Seizures at higher levels.

(iii) Cardiac arrhythmias: not common; usually occurs at high levels.

(c) Theophylline and aminophylline: relationship between bolus dose and serum level.

(i) Aminophylline: a theophylline salt; 85% of its weight is theophylline.

(ii) *Guideline: Effect of a bolus dose on serum theophylline level (STL):*
1 mg/kg theophylline increases STL by 2 μg/mL.
1 mg/kg aminophylline increases STL by 1.6 μg/mL. For practical reasons, most people think of theophylline and aminophylline as equivalent (i.e., 1 mg/kg of either raises STL by 2 μg/mL).

(2) Dosage guidelines:
  (a) *Infants ≤12 months of age metabolize theophylline more slowly than older children and adults and have decreased dosage needs.* Daily mg/kg dose = 8 + age in months.
  (b) Older children: 20–28 mg/kg/day, or 0.9–1.2 mg/kg/hour. Children ≥9 years require doses at the lower end of the given range.

(3) Management for the patient in status asthmaticus
  (a) For the patient not taking any theophylline preparation:
    (i) Loading dose: 7–8 mg/kg aminophylline IV over 20 minutes to get to therapeutic levels.
    (ii) Follow immediately with aminophylline drip at 1 mg/kg/hour.
  (b) For the patient taking theophylline with an unknown serum level: Draw serum theophylline level.
    (i) For the patient on moderate-dose theophylline therapy or one who is known to run lower levels routinely:
      (a) Provide 3–4 mg/kg aminophylline bolus over 20 minutes.
      (b) Follow immediately with aminophylline drip at 1 mg/kg/hour.
      (c) When STL becomes available, adjust dose.
    (ii) For the patient on high-dose theophylline therapy or one who is suspected of having a high serum theophylline level:
      (a) Start aminophylline drip at 1 mg/kg/hour to maintain serum level.

(b) When STL becomes available, adjust dose.

(4) Acute correction of low serum theophylline level:
Select desired STL = X.
Actual STL = Y.
X − Y = desired rise in STL.
1 mg/kg theophylline raises STL by 2 μg/mL, therefore:
(X − Y) ÷ 2 = # mg/kg theophylline bolus needed to acutely achieve desired STL.
Interrupt theophylline drip to administer this bolus over 10–20 minutes; resume theophylline drip after bolus is infused.

Example: Desired STL = 18 = X.
Actual STL = 8 = Y.
Desired rise in STL = X − Y = 18 − 8 = 10.
(X − Y)/2 = 10/2 = 5.
Therefore, administer 5 mg/kg theophylline bolus over 20 minutes.

g. Corticosteroids

(1) Very important role in the control of inflammation, mucous production.

(2) Methyl-prednisolone (Solu-Medrol): 1–2 mg/kg IV q6h.

2. **Adjunctive therapy**

a. Fluid therapy

(1) Dehydrated patient: may be dehydrated secondary to multiple factors, including emesis, decreased intake, increased insensible losses, and diuresis from theophylline.

(a) Provide volume expander: 10–20 mL/kg normal saline solution or lactated Ringer's solution as needed to restore circulation and assure lung perfusion.

(2) Well-hydrated or overhydrated patient

In the patient with moderate to severe respiratory distress (significant retractions), pulmonary edema secondary to increased negative intrathoracic pressure has been seen; the pulmonary edema increases respiratory work, degree of illness.

The pulmonary edema ranges in degree from not being visible on chest x-ray film (but visible on microscopic sections) to overt pulmonary edema on chest x-ray film. Diuretics may be very helpful in these cases.

Therefore, furosemide, 0.25–0.50 mg/kg IV, should be provided for the patient with pulmonary edema and considered for the hydrated patient who remains in significant distress.

(3) "Maintenance" fluid administration rate

Because of the recognized risk of pulmonary edema associated with status asthmaticus, excessive fluid hydration should be avoided.

Recommended fluid administration when circulation is adequate is near maintenance rate.

b. Therapy for fever
   (1) Increases metabolic needs, oxygen needs, carbon dioxide production, and respiratory needs.
   (2) Reduce fever with antipyretic: acetaminophen, 10–15 mg/kg.
      (c) Antibiotics therapy: for associated bacterial infections.

3. **Evaluation and monitoring**
   a. Blood gases
      (1) Obtain ABG values: increasing Pco_2 values and falling pH values are important signs of worsening asthma. When supplemental oxygen is provided, significant hypoxemia is not a common indicator of respiratory failure in asthma.
      (2) Capillary blood gases from a warmed extremity can closely approximate arterial pH and Pco_2 of the patient and provide good assessment of the baseline state because they usually cause less patient agitation than do arterial punctures.
   b. Pulse oximetry
      (1) Use continuous pulse oximetry.
      (2) Aim for O_2 saturation ≥90%.
   c. Chest x-ray film
      (1) Look for associated problems: air leaks, atelectasis, pneumonia, pulmonary edema.
         (a) Pneumonia, pulmonary edema, pneumothorax are to be treated.
         (b) Pneumomediastinum, atelectasis/mucous plugging: No specific therapy is needed, but

aggressive general therapy and close patient monitoring are required because the patients are usually very ill clinically.

d. Electrolyte concentrations, CBC count
e. Theophylline level: Obtain theophylline level on patient already receiving it.
f. ECG monitoring: Indicated for the child in status asthmaticus.

4. **Isoproterenol infusion for impending respiratory failure:**
   a. Indications
      (1) Impending respiratory failure: Pco_2 40–60 mm Hg, absence of improvement with other therapy.
      (2) Respiratory failure: difficulty with ventilation, need for additional medical measures.
   b. Effects
      (1) Heart: The first effects seen at very low doses are tachycardia and increased myocardial contractility. High doses can produce arrhythmias.
      (2) Blood vessels: vasodilatation.
         (a) Systemic: Hypotension may occur.
         (b) Pulmonary: Po_2 level may fall secondary to increased ventilation/perfusion mismatch.
      (3) Airways: bronchodilatation occurs at higher doses. The half-life is 4–5 minutes: effects disappear quickly after the infusion is stopped.
   c. Cautions
      (1) Major risks associated with its use
         (a) Cardiac arrhythmias, myocardial ischemia.
         (b) Hypotension from vasodilatation.
         (c) Tremendous rebound bronchospasm if isoproterenol infusion is inadvertently slowed or IV line stops working.

         Isoproterenol infusion must therefore be used cautiously and monitored closely. Its use is generally reserved for the PICU setting, but it occasionally needs to be used in the emergency department and transport situation.
   d. Equipment needs
      (1) Two reliable IV lines in case the IV line with the isoproterenol IV line stops functioning.

(2) Reliable IV pump to control isoproterenol infusion.
(3) Cardiac monitor.
(4) Blood pressure equipment or monitor.
(5) An arterial line for frequent blood gas measurement is desirable. A transcutaneous monitor to monitor transcutaneous P_{CO_2} levels may be helpful.

e. Isoproterenol infusion preparation for asthma: A more concentrated solution is prepared than is used for cardiac purposes because the doses required for bronchodilatation usually greatly exceed those needed for cardiac purposes. Instructions for preparation follow (Table 2–4).
   (1) Prepare 100 mL of solution in a burette (Volutrol): X mg isoproterenol = weight (kg) × 0.24. Place this amount of isoproterenol in the burette.
   (2) Add enough IV fluid (e.g., D5–¼NS or D5–½NS solution) to the burette to make 100 mL of solution.
   (3) Resulting concentration for the patient's weight: *1 mL/hour = 0.04 μg/kg/min.*

f. Isoproterenol infusion dose: 0.10–2.0 μg/kg/min; use the dose that produces acceptable air movement, P_{CO_2} value, and pH value.
   (1) **Start at about 0.1 μg/kg/min = 2–3 mL/hour. Do not start at a higher dose! Doses should be raised in increments of 0.10 μg/kg/min (2–3 mL/hour).**
   (2) First response to isoproterenol: tachycardia, increased cardiac impulse. The initial cardiac response to the β effects diminish over time so the dose can be incrementally raised to levels that produce bronchodilatation. Starting at a high dose without a chance for cardiac accommodation to occur can produce malignant arrhythmias.
   (3) If hypotension develops, provide 10–20 mL/kg push of lactated Ringer's solution or normal saline solution.
   (4) If O_2 saturation drops, increase F_{IO_2} level.

TABLE 2–4.
Isoproterenol (Isuprel) (Concentrated) Drip

Preparation of 100 mL concentrated isoproterenol drip in burette (Volutrol):
1. Start with nearly empty burette
2. Add appropriate mg of isoproterenol; fill with IV fluid to 100 mL. Milligrams isoproterenol = weight (kg) × 0.24 mg/kg.
3. Shake solution; run solution through tubing, then attach to IV line.

Patient Weight (kg)	Isoproterenol (mg)	Isoproterenol* (mL)
3.0	0.72	3.60
5.0	1.20	6.00
7.5	1.80	9.00
10.0	2.40	12.0
12.5	3.00	15.0
15.0	3.60	18.0
17.5	4.20	21.0
20.0	4.80	24.0
25.0	6.00	30.0
30.0	7.20	36.0
35.0	8.4	42.0
40.0	9.6	48.0
45.0	10.8	54.0
50.0	12.0	60.0
55.0	13.2	66.0
60.0	14.4	72.0
65.0	15.6	78.0
70.0	16.8	84.0

*Concentration of stock isoproterenol = 0.2 mg/mL.

Isoproterenol drip concentration and dose:
1. Concentration: 1 mL/hr rate = 0.04 μg/kg/min.
2. Usual dose = 0.05–1.0 μg/kg/min = 1.25–25 mL/hr rate.
3. Start at 0.05–0.1 μg/kg/min = 1.25–2.5 mL/hr; titrate dose. (NOTE: The volume of stock isoproterenol needed is huge, especially for large patients. For this reason, one may choose to use the less concentrated preparation initially. See Appendix.)

(5) Check ABG values after 20 minutes: If pH still <7.30 and cardiac status is stable, increase isoproterenol infusion rate by 0.10 μg/kg/min increment (2–3 mL). Check ABG values after 20 minutes. Repeat this process until satisfactory pH and P_{CO_2} values are achieved.

(6) Stop raising isoproterenol dose when:

(a) Satisfactory pH is achieved. The same dose must usually be maintained for many hours or even days before the child is ready to have the infusion rate weaned; it may have to be raised if more respiratory difficulty develops subsequently.

(b) Heart rate exceeds 200–220 beats/min in young children and 150–180 beats/min in school-aged children. Stop or slow down infusion rate.

(c) Arrhythmias develop. Stop infusion; watch patient very carefully.

(d) Chest pain develops: may be secondary to myocardial ischemia; must be differentiated from pain from lungs, respiratory muscles, gastrointestinal distress. Stop or slow down infusion rate.

g. Concurrent therapy: Continue aerosol therapy as needed during this time; watch for cardiac arrhythmias.

(1) Theophylline: Some suggest discontinuing theophylline when high-dose isoproterenol infusion is being administered to reduce cardiac complications. If the isoproterenol dose is low (which may be the case when frequent aerosols are also being provided), it seems safe to continue the theophylline.

5. **Mechanical ventilation for respiratory failure**

As mentioned earlier, asthmatic patients are among the most difficult to ventilate, and ventilation is associated with high morbidity and mortality. The principles of ventilation are very different from those used for ventilation of other respiratory problems.

The intensely narrowed small intrathoracic airways create a unique problem. Great difficulty is encountered in moving air through them in both directions, but the problem is most pronounced during the expiratory phase when the intrathoracic airways narrow even further. The expiratory phase is thus very prolonged. However, emptying of the lungs is incomplete before the patient takes another breath to try to correct hypoxemia and acidosis.

The result is air trapping, hyperaeration, and, if severe, air leaks.

Because the exhaled air does not empty out completely, only a small portion of the freshly inhaled gas reaches the alveoli before marked lung distention occurs. Therefore, a large portion of the fresh air gets only as far as the airways, so an increased percentage of ventilation is dead space ventilation.

The best way to obtain effective gas exchange is to allow sufficient exhalation of the old air so that inspired fresh air can reach the alveoli before full lung distention occurs. When mechanical ventilation is used on these patients, this is achieved by paralyzing the patients to control respirations and by using low RRs with long expiratory time. Only then can sufficient amounts of fresh gas reach the alveoli and increase alveolar minute ventilation. In these patients, paradoxically, increasing the RR above a critical number only shortens the expiratory time, increases dead space ventilation, decreases alveolar effective ventilation (raises P_{CO_2} and lowers pH and P_{O_2} values), and increases air trapping and the risk of pneumothorax and other major air leak problems.

Because the airways are so constricted, the inflating pressures required to move air into the alveoli are great, frequently exceeding 80 to 100 mm Hg pressure acutely. These patients are usually struggling to breathe, and their muscle efforts plus airway reactivity to noxious stimuli make mechanical ventilation even more difficult. These factors may produce multiple problems during and immediately after intubation: inability to ventilate/oxygenate patients with subsequent cardiac arrest; tension pneumothorax and other severe air leaks; and severe trauma to the upper airway during intubation. For these reasons asthmatic patients who require intubation should receive sedation and neuromuscular relaxants before intubation (as the circumstances allow).

C. **Key recommendations for the intubation and ventilation of patients in status asthmaticus (or who have other intrathoracic airway obstruction)**

1. The asthmatic patient will usually derive great benefit from a neuromuscular relaxant and sedation for intubation and initial ventilation.

2. Two key principles for safe and effective ventilation of asthmatic patients or those with other intrathoracic airway obstruction:
   a. Low RR
   b. Long expiratory time
3. Intubation: Paralyze and sedate the patient to prevent intense struggling, which causes more bronchoconstriction, hypoxia, acidosis, and air leaks and to decrease the chance of a cardiac arrest (see Appendix).
   a. Muscle relaxant for intubation:
      (1) Succinylcholine, 1–2 mg/kg IV.
         (a) Precede with atropine, 0.01 mg/kg, to decrease chance of bradycardia.

      or

      (2) Vecuronium or pancuronium bromide, 0.1 mg/kg IV.
   b. Sedation for intubation:
      (1) MS: 0.1 mg/kg IV or
      (2) Ketamine: 1–2 mg/kg IV.
   c. ETT: Use appropriate size ETT with a good seal because of poor lung compliance; airway of asthmatic patient cannot be ventilated if there is a large leak around the ETT.
4. Ventilation
   a. Continue neuromuscular paralysis after intubation.
      (1) Vecuronium or pancuronium bromide: 0.1 mg/kg IV prn movement.
      (2) Continue sedation:
         (a) MS: 0.1 mg IV q1–2h.
         (b) Benzodiazepine (diazepam, lorazepam, or midazolam) is a recommended addition (see p. 29).
   b. Ventilator settings
      (1) Delivered TV: 15–20 mL/kg. High TVs are generally more effective in asthmatic patients when provided at a low RR.
   c. Low RR: suggested initial rate:
      (1) 20/min for young children.
      (2) 15/min for teenagers.
      (3) Adjust RR and TV according to blood gases; RRs will not usually be higher than suggested values, may be a bit lower.

d. Inspiratory time: Should be normal or slightly longer than usual (airways are narrow, TVs are larger). Suggest 0.5–1.0 seconds.
e. Expiratory time: *Long expiratory time is crucial* to allow air to leave lungs and fresh air to reach alveoli; also vital to minimizing air trapping, air leaks.
f. PEEP: Zero; more recent studies suggest low PEEP (3–4 mm Hg pressure) may be helpful. Either can be tried.
   (1) Conventional teaching: Alveoli are already overdistended and use of PEEP retards emptying of lungs. More recent studies suggest that low PEEP may help keep distal bronchioles open and thereby facilitate emptying of air.
g. Peak inflating pressure (PIP): Anticipate high PIP because the airways are so constricted, resistance to air flow so great.
h. Blood gases: Aim for:
   (1) Po_2: ≥80 mm Hg; use Fio_2 100% during stabilization.
   (2) pH: about ≥7.3. In this situation, slightly lower than optimum pH values are acceptable because the risk of barotrauma is great if the airways are intensely constricted and poorly responsive to therapy.
   (3) Pco_2: 30s to 40s mm Hg or even low 50s mm Hg as long as pH value is in the 7.3 range.
   NOTE: some patients may have such severe bronchoconstriction that mechanical ventilators will be unable to ventilate the patient. When this occurs, manual bag and mask ventilation will have to be provided until the child has improved to the point where he or she can be placed on a ventilator; on occasion this may take several hours.

5. Concurrent therapy
   a. Hypotension: May occur after neuromuscular relaxant is provided. Treat with 10–20 mL/kg lactated Ringer's solution or normal saline solution to restore circulation and perfusion to lungs.
   b. Stress ulcers, gastritis: high risk. Provide antacids.
   c. Concurrent asthma therapy:
      (1) Theophylline

(2) β-Adrenergic aerosols through the ETT
(3) Isoproterenol infusion: optional
(4) Corticosteroids
(5) Anticholinergic aerosols through the ETT: optional

6. Complications
   a. Air leaks
      (1) Pneumothorax: Place chest tube.
      (2) Pneumoperitoneum, pneumopericardium: Monitor closely; patient may occasionally need to be drained.
      (3) Pneumomediastinum, subcutaneous emphysema: Monitor closely.
   b. Mucous plugs, atelectasis: Atelectasis is common; occasionally huge bronchial casts may be mobilized and need to be removed by vigorous suctioning combined with external rib cage compressions (artificial cough maneuver) during the expiratory phase.
   c. Profound air trapping, difficulty emptying lungs: Compress the rib cage during the expiratory phase; compressions enhance exhalation, emptying of the lungs.

CARDIOVASCULAR SYSTEM 3

The primary function of the cardiovascular system is to deliver oxygen to the cells. The measure used to gauge the adequacy of cardiovascular function is *cardiac output,* where cardiac output = stroke volume × heart rate. Because cardiac output can be measured only through invasive equipment, cardiac output is assumed to be adequate if heart rate and blood pressure values are acceptable. Figure 3–1 shows the normal cardiovascular state.

Pediatric cardiovascular problems fall into seven broad categories, which are covered in this chapter:

1. Shock
   Failure of the cardiovascular system to deliver an adequate amount of oxygen to the cells is the metabolic definition of shock. The clinical recognition of, etiologies of, and management of shock are covered.
2. Congestive heart failure (CHF)
   Prolonged cardiac strain (i.e., excess cardiac work) to maintain adequate cardiac output produces cardiac fatigue. The compensatory mechanisms invoked to help the heart maintain adequate output produce the syndrome of CHF. The etiologies of CHF are many. Cardiac output is borderline in CHF, and the situation may deteriorate into shock.
3. Dysrhythmias
   Pediatric dysrhythmias are uncommon. Most fall into a small number of categories.
4. Hypertension
   Treatment of potentially life-threatening hypertensive emergencies is addressed.
5. Anaphylactic shock
6. Pericarditis
   Recognition and emergency treatment are addressed in this rare but serious disorder.

7. Congenital heart disease
   Problems unique to pediatrics that arise from congenital cardiac problems are reviewed for the emergency situation.

I. Shock

Shock is cardiovascular failure. Metabolically, it is defined as cardiac output inadequate to meet the body's oxygen needs. At the cellular level, anaerobic metabolism ensues, and the results are (1) lactic acid production, which is reflected in increasing metabolic acidosis, and (2) cell dysfunction, which progresses to cell damage and eventual death if left uncorrected.

Clinically, the classic picture associated with shock is tachycardia, hypotension, cool and mottled extremities, and oliguria. However, the classic picture constitutes the *decompensated* state of cardiovascular failure, and to wait for this constellation of signs to appear before recognizing and treating shock is to wait too long.

Before shock is reviewed, an overview of pediatric shock and the major principles that should be gleaned from the section follow.

A. Hypotension is a late sign of shock

Initially, systemic vascular resistance increases as stroke volume decreases so that blood pressure is maintained even though cardiac output is decreased. Therefore, it is important to recognize the early signs of circulatory insufficiency to institute early therapy and avoid the major difficulties that arise after decompensation takes place.

B. Pediatric shock

In children, shock most commonly is hypovolemic in origin; therefore, fluid therapy constitutes correct therapy for most pediatric patients. However, a significant number of pediatric shock patients have cardiogenic shock and require inotropes rather than fluids for therapy; these patients must be recognized so that appropriate therapy will be provided.

C. Differentiating hypovolemic from cardiogenic shock

Usually this can be accomplished in the emergency setting using readily available information. Many times a brief history and physical examination will suffice. For example, the dehydrated-appearing shocky infant with a 2-day history of gastroenteritis is likely to have hypovolemic shock. When the cause of shock is not readily apparent from the history, the following parameters can usually be used to differentiate the two different classes of shock: the presence or absence of a gallop, jugular venous distention, and hepatosplenomegaly; and the heart size and pulmonary vascularity on chest x-ray film.

D. Inotrope therapy

There are times when children require and safely tolerate inotrope doses far higher than those recommended and far greater than those adults can tolerate. This most commonly occurs in severe septic shock and in some severe cardiomyopathies. In these situations very high inotrope doses are required to achieve the desired cardiac responses because the heart fails to respond to usual doses. These patients derive great benefit when the high doses are able to produce the desired response, and many eventually do well. To stop raising doses when the usual recommended maximum dose is reached when the patient remains shocky results in a poor outcome.

E. Empiric trial of therapy when the presence of shock is not certain

When one is not certain if early shock is present but suspects hypovolemia is present, an empiric trial of a 20 mL/kg bolus of lactated Ringer's or normal saline solution rarely harms the patient and more frequently helps the patient. Similarly, if one is suspect but is not certain of the presence of cardiac dysfunction, an empiric trial of low-to-moderate dose inotrope infusion is unlikely to harm the patient who does not need it; it will, however, provide tremendous benefit for the patient who does have cardiac dysfunction.

F. Shock, in general, is far more disruptive of organ function than respiratory failure

Profound multisystem organ failure (MSOF) or dysfunction is the frequent aftermath of shock, especially after septic shock, cardiogenic shock, and severe hypovolemic shock. Complete care includes postshock resuscitation care, which is very complex when MSOF is present.

G. Progression of events in shock

The initiating event is ongoing hemorrhage that produces progressively decreasing blood volume and stroke volume:

Case illustration

1. Cardiovascular responses in order of development
   a. Tachycardia: first response. Tachycardia is the compensatory response to *maintain* cardiac output.
   b. Redistribution of blood flow: Adequate cardiac output can no longer be maintained while pressure is maintained by increased systemic vascular resistance. Blood flow to the brain, heart, and respiratory muscles is protected at the expense of blood flow to the skin, skeletal muscles, and splanchnic bed. Clinical findings:
      (1) Cool, mottled/pale, clammy extremities.
      (2) Weakness: secondary to decreased muscle strength.
      (3) Oliguria.
      (4) Altered mental status: nonspecific restlessness, agitation.
      (5) Normotension: increased vascular resistance maintains BP; diminished distal pulse amplitude.
   c. **Hypotension: a late development.** A *decompensated state* with very low cardiac output. Rapid downward course follows.
2. Metabolic changes
   a. Metabolic acidosis secondary to lactic acid production.
      (1) Early shock: normal to high pH values secondary to respiratory compensation.
      (2) Late shock: uncompensated with low pH and variable partial pressure of carbon dioxide (Pco_2) values.
3. Organ dysfunction and damage
   a. Global involvement: Degree of damage is related to the severity of shock.
      (1) Early shock: Findings are limited to laboratory value abnormalities.
      (2) Late shock: Clinical organ dysfunction becomes apparent. At its worst, MSOF is the result: MSOF does not reverse itself when circulation is restored; it persists for hours to days after circulation is restored, is a tremendously difficult state to treat, and is associated with high morbidity and mortality.

b. Individual organ system dysfunction and damage: mild, severe.
   (1) Renal system: oliguria, associated renal metabolic abnormalities; acute tubular necrosis, anuria.
   (2) Gastrointestinal tract
      (a) Ileus; bleeding, mucosal slough, necrosis.
      (b) Liver: abnormal liver function test results; hepatic failure.
   (3) Hematologic system: coagulopathy, thrombocytopenia, anemia; overt disseminated intravascular coagulation.
   (4) Central nervous system (CNS): decreasing level of consciousness to coma; cerebral atrophy.
   (5) Cardiovascular system
      (a) Capillary leaks: early shock.
      (b) Ischemic myocardial damage: late shock.
   (6) Lungs: dysfunction, pulmonary edema; adult respiratory distress syndrome.
   (7) Metabolic: acidosis, hypoglycemia, hypocalcemia.
   (8) Muscles: profound weakness; atrophy.
   (9) Skin: desquamation; necrosis.

H. Clinical shock states

1. *Early shock:* Initial findings are subtle. Because hypotension is a late sign, findings of decreased stroke volume (decreased pulse amplitude) and increased systemic vascular resistance (perfusion changes to skin, muscles) must be sought.
   a. Tachycardia, frequently unexplained.
   b. Absence of hypotension: In more advanced state distal pulses may be decreased in amplitude.
   c. Tachypnea: Grunting respirations in the absence of pneumonia suggests shock.
   d. Cool, mottled, clammy extremities.
   e. Oliguria: mild.
   f. Subtle CNS changes: restlessness, agitation.
   g. Laboratory findings: mild metabolic acidosis; normal to high pH secondary to respiratory compensation.
2. *Classic shock:* decompensated state.
   a. Tachycardia.
   b. Hypotension, weak pulses.
   c. Tachypnea, sometimes hyperpnea: Grunting may be present.

   d. Cool, clammy extremities; cyanotic to pale.
   e. Oliguria.
   f. Depressed level of consciousness and responsiveness.
   g. Diaphoresis: suggests cardiogenic rather than hypovolemic etiology.
   h. Laboratory findings: significant metabolic acidosis; pH near normal value.
3. *Late shock:* moribund, prearrest state.
   a. Tachycardia; bradycardia heralds impending arrest.
   b. Profound hypotension; thready to absent pulses.
   c. Tachypnea, sometimes hyperpnea; falling respirations herald impending arrest.
   d. Cold extremities; blue to white.
   e. Profoundly depressed level of consciousness; coma in severe shock.
   f. Laboratory findings: severe uncompensated metabolic acidosis: low pH; multiple abnormal laboratory values reflect multisystem organ injury.

I. Guide to pediatric BP values

Pediatric blood pressure values are lower than adult values and are age related. A guideline to acceptable BP values by age is provided. (Many children will have BP values higher than those that follow; values 20% to 30% higher than listed are within acceptable range; values approximately 20% lower than listed are worrisome.)

1. Neonate, infant: Systolic BP 60–70 mm Hg.
2. Children 1–2 years of age: Systolic BP 70–80 mm Hg.
3. Children $\geq$ 2 years of age
   a. Systolic BP = 80 + (2 $\times$ age in years).
   b. Diastolic BP is usually ⅔ systolic value.

J. Etiology and classification of shock

The clinical picture of shock is fairly uniform. However, the etiology of shock varies, as does its therapy. It is therefore important to know the different categories of shock, how to clinically distinguish them, then how to provide appropriate therapy.

Because cardiac output = heart rate $\times$ stroke volume, anything that decreases heart rate and/or stroke volume can cause shock.

1. *Causes of decreased cardiac output*
   a. Heart rate disturbances
      (1) Bradycardia
      (2) Other dysrhythmias

b. Decreased stroke volume, the result of:
   (1) Hypovolemia (decreased intravascular volume)
      (a) Absolute: fluid deficit.
      (b) Relative: abnormal vessel tone (e.g., vasodilatation).
   (2) Decreased cardiac contractility

2. *Classification of shock and appropriate therapy*
   a. Hypovolemic shock: fluid deficit (Fig 3–2):
      (1) Therapy: fluids (i.e., volume expander).
   b. Cardiogenic shock: decreased cardiac contractility (Fig 3–3):
      (1) Therapy: inotropic agents.
   c. Distributive shock: abnormal vessel tone, abnormal distribution of blood flow; includes septic shock.
      (1) Therapy: vasoactive agents and/or fluids for abnormal vasodilatation.

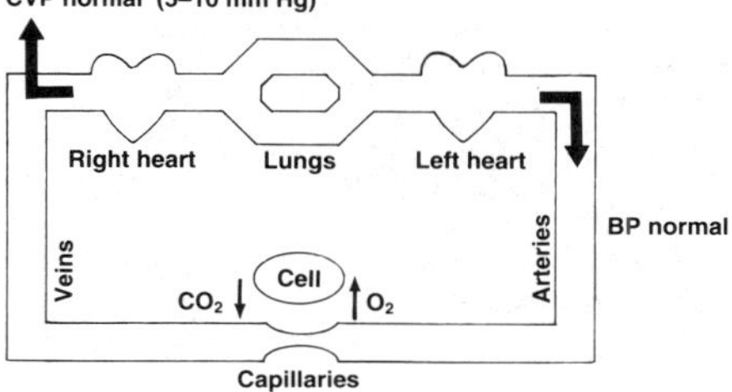

FIG 3–1.
Normal Cardiovascular State.

A. Cardiovascular system is composed of three components:
1. Heart: the pump.
2. Blood vessels: system of pipes, which are elastic in nature.
3. Blood: circulating medium that fills system and delivers oxygen.

B. Function of cardiovascular system is to deliver a sufficient amount of blood (i.e., oxygen) to the cells, represented in the diagram by the arrow moving in clockwise direction through the series of blood vessels.

C. Pressure measurements in cardiovascular system:
1. Arteries: systemic blood pressure.
2. Central venous pressure *(CVP):* measure of pressure in and distention of the right atrium, central inferior vena cava and superior vena cava.

FIG 3–2.
Hypovolemic shock.

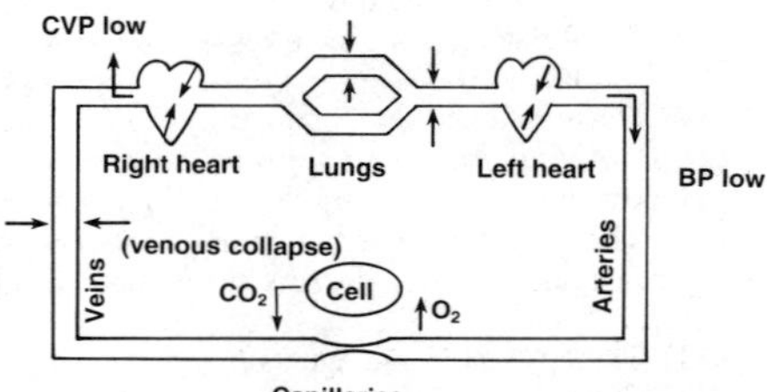

Hypovolemia: Vascular volume is low and size of cardiovascular structures decreases.

A. **Clinical picture: Shock plus findings of venous collapse.**
   1. Superior vena cava: jugular venous collapse.
   2. Inferior vena cava: normal to small liver and spleen.

B. **Central venous pressure** *(CVP)* low.

C. **Chest x-ray film:**
   1. Small heart.
   2. Diminished pulmonary vasculature.

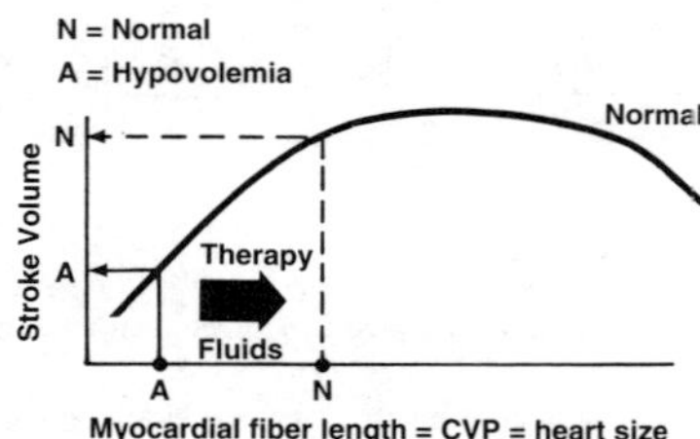

Frank-Starling curve.
Myocardial fiber length = CVP = heart size.

A. **Heart functions on normal Frank-Starling curve.**

B. **Low stroke volume is secondary to diminished myocardial fiber stretch, hypovolemia.**

C. ***Therapy:*** Restore intravascular volume to move from point *A* (hypovolemia) to point *N* (normal).

FIG 3–3.
Cardiovascular shock.

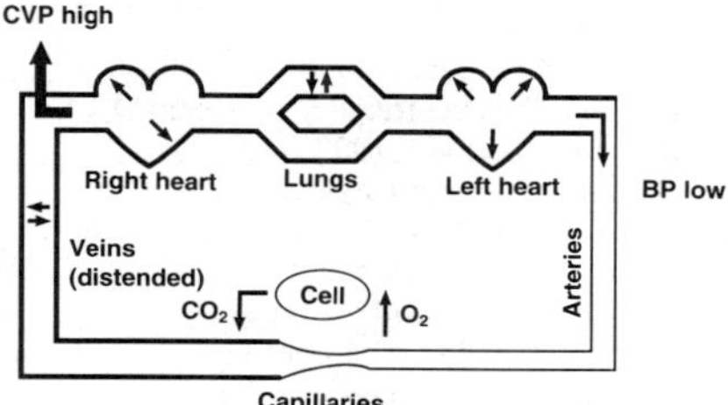

Cardiac dysfunction: Heart fails to pump sufficient volume of blood forward; blood backs up in counterclockwise direction to produce distention of these cardiovascular structures.

A. Clinical picture: Shock plus findings of vascular engorgement.
1. Cardiac enlargement; may hear gallop rhythm.
2. Pulmonary vascular congestion; may produce rales, rhonchi, wheezing when severe.
3. Superior vena cava: Jugular venous distention.
4. Inferior vena cava: Hepatosplenomegaly.

B. Central venous pressure elevated.

C. Chest x-ray film:
1. Heart enlarged.
2. Pulmonary vascular engorgement, which when marked can produce pulmonary edema, pleural effusion.

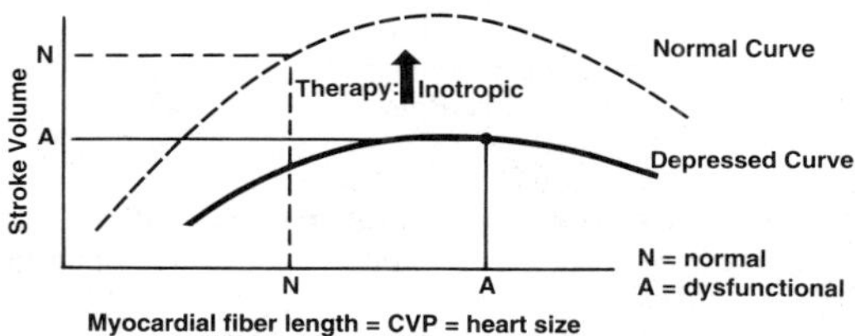

Frank-Starling curve

Myocardial fiber length = CVP = heart size.

A. Heart functions on depressed Frank-Starling curve.

B. ***Therapy:*** Provide inotropic agents to move Frank-Starling curve up to normal.

d. Obstructive shock: pericardial tamponade, tension pneumothorax, massive pulmonary embolus.
   (1) Therapy: surgical intervention.

K. Therapy of shock

1. **Initial stabilizing measures**
   a. Oxygen: Provide fractional concentration of oxygen in inspired gas (Fio_2) 100%.
      (1) Intubate, ventilate as needed.
   b. Patient position: supine; may elevate legs.
      (1) Avoid Trendelenburg position; it increases diaphragmatic work to breathe.
   c. Start intravenous (IV) line: butterfly, plastic catheter, cutdown, intraosseous, anything.
   d. Obtain laboratory work only if does not consume excessive time and delay urgently needed therapy.
      (1) Complete blood cell count (CBC), electrolyte values, glucose level, rapid glucose test, calcium level
      (2) Arterial blood gas (ABG) values or capillary blood gas (CBG) values.
      (3) As indicated: blood culture; prothrombin time/partial thromboplastin time; type and crossmatch; toxicology screen; possibly blood urea nitrogen (BUN), creatinine, aspartate aminotransferase, and alanine aminotransferase levels.
   e. Insert indwelling bladder catheter.
   f. Assess type of shock: The two *functional* categories of shock are hypovolemic and cardiogenic.
      (1) History and physical examination.
      (2) Parameters that help identify type of shock:
         (a) Presence or absence of jugular venous distention, hepatosplenomegaly, gallop.
         (b) Chest x-ray studies: heart size, pulmonary vascularity.
2. **Specific therapy for restoration of circulation**
   a. *Hypovolemic shock:* Therapy = fluids (plasma volume expanders).
      (1) *Push* plasma volume expanders until satisfactory blood pressure, pulses return.
         (a) Fluid choices
            (i) *Crystalloids:* normal saline and lactated Ringer's solutions. Avoid 5% dextrose in

normal saline (D_5NS) solution or 5% dextrose in lactated Ringer's (D_5 LR) solution. Ten mL/kg D_5NS has the same amount of glucose as 1 mL/kg 50% dextrose solution, which raises serum glucose levels by 250 mg/dL. Inadvertent use of D_5NS solution or D_5LR solution pushes will produce iatrogenic hyperglycemia, followed by osmotic diuresis, which will aggravate existing fluid deficit.

(ii) *Colloids:* 5% albumin, fresh frozen plasma (FFP), blood.

(b) Fluid volumes for shock

(i) Shock secondary to hypovolemia requires a *minimum* 20 mL/kg push.

(ii) Severe volume depletion: 40–60 mL/kg in additional increments of 10–20 mL/kg pushes may be required to restore vascular volume.

(iii) In the presence of very active ongoing losses (e.g., gastrointestinal losses, hemorrhage), even greater volumes than those previously listed may be required to maintain vascular volume.

(2) Clinical signs of positive response to volume push: decreased heart rate, improved pulses, improved perfusion, improved responsiveness/level of consciousness, increased urine output, improved blood pressure.

(3) Stop volume pushes.

(a) When desired clinical improvement is achieved.

(b) If clinical signs of improvement fail to appear, reevaluate the patient and reassess type of shock (clinically and by chest x-ray studies).

(c) If clinical signs of volume overload develop (hepatosplenomegaly, jugular venous distention, gallop, rales, or wheezes), proceed to inotropes (see below).

(4) Use chest x-ray studies and central venous pressure (CVP) to evaluate therapy. In the emergency and transport setting, use of chest x-ray studies alone frequently suffices.
   (a) Continue with more volume pushes when circulation remains unsatisfactory if:
      (i) Chest x-ray studies show small heart and diminished pulmonary markings, or
      (ii) CVP is $<5-10$ mm Hg.
   (b) Proceed with inotropes when circulation remains unsatisfactory if:
      (i) Chest x-ray studies show large heart, pulmonary vascular congestion/pulmonary edema/pleural effusion, or
      (ii) CVP is $> 10-15$ mm Hg.

b. *Cardiogenic shock:* Emergency management therapy: inotropic agents. (*Inotropes* are agents that increase myocardial contractility.) In the emergency setting inotrope use is usually limited to the basic few that will accomplish the basic goals.
   (1) Inotropes for hypotension with tachycardia: Select an agent with minimal chronotropic properties. (*Chronotrope* is an agent that increases heart rate.) See Appendix II–3 for pediatric drip preparations and uses.
      (a) *Dopamine:* has dose-related extracardiac effects.
         (i) Usual dose: 1–30 μg/kg/min.
            (a) Titrate dose: Use the dose that produces the desired effects.
            (b) Prepare solution appropriate for patient weight (see Appendix II–3, A).
         (ii) Dose-related extracardiac effects:
            (a) 2–5 μg/kg/min: primarily dopaminergic (i.e., increased renal and splanchnic blood flow); little inotropic effect.
            (b) 5–10 μg/kg/min: β (inotropic) effects and dopaminergic effects.
            (c) 10–20 μg/kg/min: primarily β (inotropic) effects with increasing α (vasoconstrictor) effects.

(d) 20–30 μg/kg/min: β effects, increasing α effects, which may offset gains in improved myocardial contractility.

(iii) Recommendation: Start at 5–10 μg/kg/min, rapidly titrate dose upward (q2–3min) prn. Decrease dose if overshoot occurs.

(b) *Dobutamine:* pure β effects.

(i) Usual dose: 2–20 μg/kg/min.

(a) Titrate the dose that produces the desired result.

(b) Prepare solution appropriate for patient weight (see Appendix II–3, B).

(ii) β_1 drug without α or dopaminergic properties.

(a) Generally has little effect on heart rate at usual doses; high doses will produce tachycardia.

(iii) Recommendation: Start at 5–10 μg/kg/min, rapidly titrate as needed.

(2) Inotropes for hypotension with normal or low heart rate: Use an agent with both inotropic and chronotropic properties.

(a) Isoproterenol (Isuprel): mixed β effects.

(i) Usual dose: 0.05–1.0 μg/kg/min.

(a) Titrate the dose: Use the dose that produces the desired result.

(b) Prepare solution appropriate for patient weight (see Appendix II–3, C).

(ii) Pure β drug with mixed β properties:

(a) Chronotropic activity: produces tachycardia. Some patients are exquisitely sensitive to this property; therefore, it must be started at a low dose and raised cautiously. Chronotropic effects appear before inotropic effects do in responsive hearts and can produce dysrhythmias. The heart usually accomodates quickly to the chronotropic properties to allow the dose to be raised further for inotropic needs.

(b) Inotropic properties.
(c) Smooth muscle relaxation: Vasodilatation and bronchodilatation occur at higher doses.

(iii) Recommendation: Start at 0.05–0.10 μg/kg/min; titrate. If tachycardia is pronounced but acceptable, wait awhile; tachycardia may lessen to allow further increase in dose as needed.

(b) Epinephrine: mixed α and β effects; potent α effects.

(i) Usual dose: 0.05–1.0 μg/kg/min.
(a) Titrate the dose: Use the dose that produces the desired result.
(b) Prepare solution appropriate for patient weight (see Appendix II–3, D).

(ii) Most commonly used when previously listed inotrope infusions at high doses and in combination fail to produce desired cardiac response.
(a) Has potent inotropic, chronotropic, and vasoconstrictor (produces hypertension and pallor) properties in the responsive patient.

(iii) Recommendation: Start at 0.05–0.10 μg/kg/min; titrate dose.

(c) Additional inotrope infusion drugs: Infrequent use during stabilization; use only after recommendation by referral center.

(i) Norepinephrine (levarterenol): β_1 (cardiac) effects plus potent α activity.
(a) Usual dose: 0.05–1.0 μg/kg/min; start at 0.05–0.1 μg/kg/min.
(b) For preparation see Appendix II–3, F.

(ii) Amrinone: noncatecholamine inotrope with vasodilator properties.
(a) Loading dose: 0.75 mg/kg IV over 2–3 minutes. Follow with continuous infusion at 5–10 μg/kg/min; titrate dose.
(b) Preparation of infusion: Do not prepare the infusion in dextrose-containing solutions. The drug, however, is

compatible with all of the other inotropes and can be in contact with other infusions that contain dextrose as long as the infusions are freely running. The infusion should be prepared in the same manner as dopamine and dobutamine, using the "rule of 6" (see Appendix II–3, A).

(3) Therapeutic options when an inotrope infusion at high dose fails to produce the desired hemodynamic changes

(a) Add a second, third inotrope as needed: First inotrope may be insufficient for the heart with severe disease.

(i) Inotropic effects of the different drugs are additive.

(ii) All of the drips may run into the same IV site because they are compatible.

(b) The usual recommended maximum doses may need to be exceeded as long as there are not toxic side effects (e.g., dysrhythmias).

(i) The myocardium is sometimes not responsive to usual doses and needs greater stimulation to elicit the desired response.

(ii) This situation most commonly occurs in florid septic shock: Some patients exhibit poor response to usual inotrope doses but respond well to massive doses of one or many inotropes (and have excellent eventual outcomes).

(c) When usual therapeutic measures—preload and inotrope therapy—fail to produce the desired cardiovascular response, *afterload reduction* therapy may improve the limited cardiac output of the profoundly weakened myocardium. (Consult pediatric regional center.)

(i) Sodium nitroprusside: vasodilator, anti-α-agent. For preparation, see Table II–3, H.

(a) Dose: 0.5–7.0 μg/kg/min.

(b) Recommendation: Start at 0.5 μg/kg/min. Wait a minimum of 5–10 min-

utes before increasing the dose by another 0.5 μg/kg/min.

(4) The different inotropes can be combined to achieve the desired result.

(a) ***Example:*** patient with bradycardia and hypotension.

(i) Start with isoproterenol; heart rate rapidly increases to tachycardic range at low dose, but blood pressure remains low.

(ii) Maintain low-dose isoproterenol infusion for heart rate effects. Start either dopamine or dobutamine infusion for inotropic effects to achieve desired blood pressure and pulses.

c. Septic shock

(1) Septic shock is secondary to endotoxin or exotoxin release.

(2) Although classified as distributive shock, therapy involves fluids and inotropes.

(3) Clinical effects of toxin release and therapy:

(a) Early (mild) shock: capillary leaks, change in blood vessel tone.

(i) Frequently responds to volume expanders alone if recognized and treated early.

(b) Classic shock: capillary leaks plus myocardial depression from toxin.

(i) Both volume expanders and inotropes are needed to restore circulation.

(ii) Significant organ dysfunction is present.

(c) Severe shock: very resistant to usual therapy, fulminant downhill course, frequent association with widespread purpura and disseminated intravascular coagulation. Massive capillary leaks and profound myocardial depression develop over the first few hours.

(i) Massive volumes of plasma volume expanders are required during the resuscitation phase and beyond.

(ii) High-dose intropes, frequently greatly exceeding usual maximum doses, and multiple inotropes are commonly required to restore circulation.

(iii) Widespread organ failure is present.

(4) Patients with septic shock may experience major cardiovascular deterioration in the first 12 hours or so after presentation. The administration of antibiotics does not prevent further cardiovascular deterioration. In fact, there is speculation that some patients experience further deterioration in this period from increased endotoxin release that occurs when bacteria are lysed by the antibiotics.

(5) Prompt recognition and aggressive treatment of septic shock is critical. Delays in therapy allow shock to progress with escalating rapidity and make correction more difficult.

3. **Adjunctive therapy for restoration of circulation**
   a. Correct negative inotropic conditions
      (1) Hypoxia: Provide oxygen; ventilate as needed.
      (2) Acidosis: Aim to get pH to 7.35 to 7.4 range.
         (a) Ventilator for respiratory acidosis.
         (b) Sodium bicarbonate, 1–2 mEq/kg IV per dose, to correct metabolic acidosis determined from blood gas value. Be sure that the patient is adequately ventilated before giving $NaHCO_3$.
      (3) Hypoglycemia: Follow glucose levels frequently; hypoglycemia commonly develops. It may be present when the patient is admitted or may not appear for 6–24 hours (even when initial glucose level is high).
         (a) Therapy of hypoglycemia
            (i) 1–2 mL/kg D_{25} solution in infants.
            (ii) 1 mL/kg D_{50} solution in older children.
            (iii) Increase dextrose concentration in IV solution.
      (4) Hypocalcemia: commonly seen during and after shock. May not develop until 24 hours after shock. Calcium is a very important inotrope; hypocalcemia depresses cardiac contractility, especially when cardiovascular dysfunction is present.
         (a) Therapy of hypocalcemia: 10% calcium gluconate (100 mg/mL) IV over 5–10 minutes. (Do not push rapidly: Bradycardia, cardiac

tetany, and standstill will result. Monitor electrocardiogram [ECG] during infusion.)

(i) Neonates, young infants: 100–150 mg/kg/dose.

(ii) Older infants, toddlers: 50–100 mg/kg/dose.

(iii) Older children, adolescents: 20–50 mg/kg/dose, maximum dose 2 g.

b. Treat underlying problem (e.g., sepsis, diabetic ketoacidosis).

c. Fever: Reduce fever to reduce oxygen needs.

(1) Antipyretics.

(2) Expose skin by removing clothing and coverings.

d. Place indwelling bladder catheter to monitor urine output.

(1) Expected urine volumes *after* circulation is restored:

(a) Infants: 1–2 mL/kg/hour.

(b) Toddlers, young children: 1 mL/kg/hour.

(c) Adolescents: 0.5–1.0 mL/kg/hour.

(2) If oliguria or anuria persists *after* circulation is restored, consider giving a diuretic to restore urine output.

(a) Furosemide: 0.5–1.0 mg/kg IV, or

(b) Mannitol: 0.5–1.0 gm/kg IV.

Massive diuresis may follow at times. If this occurs and circulation worsens, a push of plasma volume expander will be needed to restore circulating volume and circulation.

e. Hematologic abnormalities

(1) Coagulopathy: commonly observed.

(a) For very abnormal coagulation values or clinical bleeding:

(i) FFP: 10 mL/kg IV.

FFP dose may have to be increased to 20 mL/kg or repeated frequently when active consumption is present.

(2) Thrombocytopenia: commonly observed.

(a) One may choose to treat a platelet count <20–50,000 when associated with bleeding.

(b) 1 unit of platelets/7 kg of patient weight will raise the platelet count by 50–100,000.
   (i) Platelet rise will be less when active bleeding and consumption are present.

(3) Anemia: commonly observed.
   (a) In *stable* state (euvolemia, equilibrated hematocrit [Hct] value, absence of active bleeding/hemolysis), 1 mL/kg of packed red blood cells (PRBCs) will raise Hct by 1.

f. Corticosteroids: controversial, of possible benefit.
   (1) For suspected adrenal hemorrhage: 1 mg/kg hydrocortisone q6h will more than suffice.
   (2) For septic shock: of possible value. Recommended corticosteroid doses vary widely.
      (a) Dexamethasone: 0.25–1.0 mg/kg IV initially.
      (b) Methylprednisolone: 1–30 mg/kg IV initially.
      NOTE: A management summary of shock is presented in Appendix I–4.

4. **Further cardiovascular injury from shock: effects on therapy**

The cardiovascular system frequently sustains damage from shock that causes recurrent shock and complicates its correction. The extent and severity of damage to the cardiovascular system are related to the severity of shock.

The first injury to the cardiovascular system that arises from shock is to the capillary. Mild to moderate shock is sufficient to produce capillary leaks, which, when large enough, produce hypovolemia; severe shock can produce massive capillary leaks, edema, and profound hypovolemia. The more severe the insult, the larger the leaks and the longer the duration of the problem. Capillary leaks may not peak for 12 to 48 hours and may be ongoing for 24 to 72 hours. Therefore, recurrent shock secondary to hypovolemia is common after the initial correction, and one must be prepared to provide volume expanders appropriately.

Severe shock, in addition to injuring the capillaries, can produce an ischemic injury to the myocardium; the injury impairs myocardial contractility. Like capillary leaks, the myocardial injury response will not peak until many hours after the insult, so myocardial dysfunction may not be apparent until several hours after the initial shock episode. Inotrope therapy will be needed when myocardial dysfunction is significant, and inotrope support may need to be increased for the first 12 to 48 hours until the inflammatory response peaks. Use of clinical parameters mentioned earlier and a chest x-ray film may help differentiate the cause of recurring shock.

In summary:

a. The patient who has been treated for shock may lapse into shock again from capillary leaks (hypovolemia), myocardial dysfunction (cardiogenic), or both.
b. The patient with severe hypovolemic shock may subsequently require inotropes because of ischemic myocardial damage; the patient with cardiogenic shock may subsequently require plasma volume expanders because of capillary leaks.

5. **Postshock (Postresuscitation) Care**

Care of the child with shock does not end with restoration of circulation. There are frequently many aftereffects of shock, namely, multiorgan injury, which become the focus of the next stage of therapy of shock (see p. 95).

II. Congestive Heart Failure

Congestive heart failure is a *syndrome* in which the heart is encountering significant difficulty providing the cardiac output necessary to meet the body's oxygen needs. The extra work that has been demanded of the heart over a period of time causes cardiac fatigue and weakness. The compensatory responses that have been invoked to help the heart maintain cardiac output produce the signs recognized as CHF. Cardiac output is borderline in CHF, and with further deterioration the patient may lapse into shock.

Although concern focuses on the heart in CHF, it is important to emphasize that CHF is the end result of a problem that caused the heart to work excessively. The dilated, failing heart is only the *final common pathway* for a diverse number of problems: Many of the primary problems are cardiac in origin, but many others are noncardiac in nature. It is important to search for and identify the primary problem when one is caring for the patient with CHF, because the primary problem frequently needs urgent therapy, too. Examples are presented to illustrate and reinforce this point.

Examples: *Common clinical findings of patient with CHF:* History: not eating well; irritable, lethargic, tachypneic, diaphoretic with exertion. Physical examination: pale, tachypneic, tachycardic; cool clammy skin, diaphoretic at times; irritable and/or tired; gallop on auscultation; hepatomegaly, jugular venous distention, occasional edema; rales or wheezes commonly found on auscultation. Chest x-ray film: cardiomegaly; increased pulmonary vasculature or pulmonary edema.

Case 1: 2-month-old boy. Clinical findings as just described. Physical examination: grade 3/6 systolic ejection murmur, gallop. Chest x-ray film: as described. Echocardiogram: moderate-sized ventricular septal defect (VSD). Therapy: furosemide and digoxin. Diagnosis: CHF secondary to left-to-right shunting from VSD. (Primary problem: cardiac.)

Case 2: 20-month-old girl. Clinical findings as just described. Treated with oxygen, diuretics. Vital signs consistent with CHF, but BP 200/120. Treated with diazoxide, followed by hydralazine and furosemide. Later found to have nephritis, renal failure, which eventually led to a renal transplant. Diagnosis: CHF secondary to malignant hypertension, which was secondary to a primary renal disease.

Case 3: 8-month-old. Clinical findings as just described, plus pallor. Laboratory work: blood appeared serosanguinous. Hemoglobin (Hgb) = 3 g. The child required emergency partial exchange transfusion in addition to diuretics and oxygen. Diagnosis: CHF secondary to severe anemia, which was secondary to a macrobiotic diet.

A. Causes of congestive heart failure

1. Excess volume load
   a. Cardiac lesions
      (1) Left-to-right shunts (e.g., VSD, patent ductus arteriosus, atriovenous canal).
      (2) Valvular regurgitation.
   b. Arteriovenous fistulas.
   c. Severe anemia.
   d. Hypervolemia.
      (1) Excess fluid intake or administration.
      (2) Inadequate fluid excretion.
         (a) Oliguria, anuria.
         (b) Syndrome of inappropriate antidiuretic hormone (SIADH)

2. Excess pressure load
   a. Systemic vascular system
      (1) Structural (e.g., aortic stenosis, coarctation of the aorta).
      (2) Functional: hypertension.
   b. Pulmonary vascular system
      (1) Structural: as pulmonary stenosis, advanced pulmonary hypertension.
      (2) Functional: pulmonary hypertension.
         (a) Primary pulmonary hypertension.
         (b) Secondary to hypoxia, hypoventilation (e.g., Ondine's curse), severe upper airway obstruction (e.g., adenoidal hypertrophy).
3. Myocardial problems
   a. Cardiomyopathy
   b. Myocarditis
   c. Myocardial ischemia
      (1) Anomalous coronary artery, cardiac thrombosis in Kawasaki disease.
   d. Metabolic disorders
      (1) Hypoglycemia, hypocalcemia, hypophosphatemia.
      (2) Acidemia.
   e. Dysrthythmias (e.g., supraventricular tachycardia, congenital heart block).
4. Excess myocardial demand:
   a. Thyrotoxicosis.
   b. Fever.

B. Pathophysiology

The heart is unable to contract well, stroke volume is diminished, and the cardiac chambers increase in volume. The signs and symptoms of CHF are secondary to the compensatory mechanisms that arise.

1. *Dilatation of the Heart:* This occurs largely because of diminished forward flow. The increased muscle stretch produced by cardiac enlargement increases cardiac contractility on the Frank-Starling curve. When the descending limb of the curve is reached, however, contractility decreases.
2. *Increased sympathetic nervous system activity: Increased sympathetic activity arises from the increased atrial and venous stretch receptor stimulation and the decreased blood and pulse pressures detected by the baroreceptors.*

The effects are:

a. Increased α activity: Diminished blood flow to the limbs, splanchnic bed and kidneys because of vasocontriction. The clinical result is pale, cool extremities with decreased pulses, and decreased urine output.
b. Increased β activity: Increased heart rate and myocardial contractility result.
c. Fluid retention: Fluid retention is the result of diminished renal blood flow. This stimulates increased aldosterone and antidiuretic hormone secretion which produce sodium and water retention. When significant, soft tissue edema and pulmonary edema are seen.

C. Clinical picture

A characteristic clinical picture of CHF exists in spite of the great variety of problems that may have caused it. The characteristic picture of CHF follows.

1. *History, presenting complaints*
   a. Pallor.
   b. Rapid breathing.
   c. Sweating with exertion.
   d. Malaise, irritability.
   e. Decreased appetite.
2. *Physical findings*
   a. Tachycardia, tachypnea.
   b. Pallor.
   c. Pale/mottled, cool extremities.
   d. Diaphoretic with stress, although body is cool, clammy to touch.
   e. May have rales, wheezes.
   f. May have gallop.
   g. May have jugular venous distention, hepatosplenomegaly.
   h. May have edema.
   i. Pulses may be diminished to palpation, hypotension may occur.
   j. Findings specific for underlying cause (e.g., murmur in VSD, profound pallor in severe anemia).
3. *Chest X-ray findings*
   a. Increased heart size.
   b. Pulmonary vasculature congestion to pulmonary edema.

D. Approach to and management of congestive heart failure

1. Nonspecific therapeutic measures
   a. Administer oxygen, fractional concentration of oxygen in inspired gas (Fio_2) 100%.
   b. Position of comfort: supine, head elevated.
   c. Diuretic: furosemide, 0.5–1.0 mg/kg IV or IM.
   d. Antipyretic for fever:
      (1) Acetominophen, 10–15 mg/kg.
      (2) Ibuprofen, 5–10 mg/kg.
   e. Sedation for agitation: morphine sulfate, 0.1 mg/kg IV or IM.
      (1) Watch blood pressure, respirations; be prepared to intubate if hypoventilation develops.
   f. Fluids: restricted amount.
   g. Consider:
      (1) Inotrope for significant cardiac dysfunction (cardiac dysfunction may be either primary or secondary in etiology).
         (a) Digoxin: see doses on p. 81.
         (b) Inotrope infusion (e.g., dobutamine or dopamine) if cardiac function is very poor or if shock develops. See inotrope infusion preparation in Appendix II–3.
      (2) Bronchodilator for wheezing.
         (a) Aerosolized beta-adrenergic drug. (see p. 30).
         (b) Aminophylline, 5–7 mg/kg IV bolus
2. Patient examination
   a. Obtain vital signs.
   b. Perform physical examination to look for underlying causes of CHF.
3. Laboratory tests
   a. Chest x-ray film.
   b. CBC count.
   c. Electrolyte values.
   d. Glucose levels: Hypoglycemia is common, especially in infants.
   e. Blood gas determinations.
   f. Consider:
      (1) BUN and creatinine levels.
      (2) ECG.

4. Specific therapy for identified primary cause
   a. Primary cardiac problem: inotrope therapy
      (1) Digoxin.
         (a) Administration of total digitalizing dose (TDD):
            (i) Give one half of the TDD initially.
            (ii) Complete digitalization by giving one fourth of the TDD 8 hours and 16 hours after the first dose.
         (b) TDD
            (i) Premature infant: 20 μg/kg po or 15 μg/kg IV/IM.
            (ii) Term infant: 30 μg/kg po or 20 μg/kg IV/IM.
            (iii) <2 years of age: 40–50 μg/kg po or 30–40 μg/kg IV/IM.
            (iv) 2–10 years of age: 30–40 μg/kg po or 20–30 μg/kg IV/IM.
            (v) >10 years of age: 0.75–1.25 *mg* po or 0.75–1.25 *mg* IV/IM.
         (c) Excretion: Digoxin is renally excreted; use with caution in renal failure.
         (d) Contraindication: contraindicated for patients with ventricular dysrhythmias.
         (e) Cardioversion or calcium infusion in patients on digoxin therapy may cause ventricular fibrillation. Pretreatment with lidocaine, 1 mg/kg IV, may prevent ventricular fibrillation.
         (f) For the patient already taking digoxin: Obtain serum digoxin level. Therapeutic level is 0.8–2.0 μg/L. (NOTE: A serum level obtained less than 8–10 hours after a dose of digoxin may be spuriously high; consult pediatric cardiologist for this problem.)
      (2) Inotrope infusion if cardiac function is very poor or if shock develops.
         (a) See the section on cardiogenic shock (p. 68) and Appendix II–3 for preparation and administration of inotrope infusions.
   b. Dysrhythmias: antiarrhythmic agents and maneuvers (see p. 83)

c. Hypertension: antihypertensives (see p. 87).
d. Pulmonary hypertension secondary to hypoxemia and hypoventilation: oxygen, airway/ventilation
   (1) Oxygen for hypoxemia.
   (2) Intubation for upper airway obstruction.
   (3) Intubation and ventilation for hypoventilation and hypoxemia.
e. Severe anemia: cautious transfusion
   (1) Partial exchange transfusion for anemic patient with CHF (see p. 226).
   (2) Furosemide and transfusion given cautiously (1–2 mL/kg/hour of PRBCs) to patient with low Hgb level but no or minimal CHF.
   (3) In most cases where Hgb level is very low (e.g., ≤4 g), raising the Hgb level to 6–7 g is sufficient for the emergent situation if no other major problems coexist.
f. Volume overload in oliguric or anuric patient
   (1) Morphine sulfate, 0.1 mg/kg IV or IM. Watch respirations.
   (2) Phlebotomy can relieve fluid overload when diuresis is not possible.
      (a) Withdraw 5 mL/kg blood, monitor response.
      (b) Repeat increments as needed; may need 10–20 mL/kg withdrawal to relieve overload.
      (c) If anemia results from phlebotomy, a partial exchange transfusion may be necessary.
         (i) ***Example:*** Withdraw 5 mL/kg blood; infuse 2.5 mL/kg PRBCs. Repeat process until net desired blood volume (fluid) is removed.
g. Abnormal metabolic states: Provide replacement.
   (1) Hypoglycemia
      (a) Neonates, young infants: 1–2 mL/kg D_{10} solution.
      (b) Older infants, toddlers: 1–2 mL/kg D_{25} solution.
      (c) Older children: 1 mL/kg D_{50} solution.
   (2) Hypocalcemia: calcium gluconate, slow IV push over 10 minutes.
      (a) Neonates, young infants: 100–150 mg/kg.
      (b) Infants, toddlers: 50–100 mg/kg.

(c) Children, adolescents: 20–50 mg/kg, maximum dose 2 g.

III. Dysrhythmias

Always obtain a 12-lead ECG for documentation and diagnosis of dysrhythmias.

A. Bradydysrhythmias

1. Significant bradycardia is indicated by:
   a. Heart rate: <80 in neonates, <50 in infants, and <40 in older children *with*
   b. Hemodynamic instability: decreased BP, poor perfusion.
2. Sinus bradycardia, heart block
   a. Do not treat immediately if the patient is hemodynamically stable.
      (1) Consider other treatable causes of bradycardia (i.e., increased intracranial pressure). The majority of cases of pediatric bradycardia are not primary (i.e., the low heart rate is related to an underlying cause, e.g., respiratory failure or hypoxia). Treatment of the underlying etiology is required in these situations.
   b. Therapy of symptomatic bradycardia
      (1) *Provide oxygen; assist ventilation if needed.*
      (2) Atropine: 0.02 mg/kg IV. (Minimum dose 0.1 mg, maximum dose 1.0 mg.)
      (3) Isoproterenol infusion: 0.05–1.00 μg/kg/min (see Appendix II–3).

B. Tachydysrhythmias

1. Narrow complex: supraventricular tachycardia (SVT), atrial flutter: QRS duration <0.1 second in children, <0.12 second in adolescents and adults. Absent P waves in SVT.
   a. If hemodynamically *stable:*
      (1) Vagal maneuvers: ice bag to entire face for 15–20 seconds; rectal probe; gag; unilateral carotid massage or Valsalva's maneuver. Do not compress orbits.
      (2) Drug therapy: Discuss drug considerations and doses first with pediatric cardiologist.
         (a) Digoxin: 0.02 mg/kg IV. (See p. 81 for digitalization guidelines.) If cardioversion is sub-

sequently required, the risk of dysrhythmias is increased by the presence of digoxin in the system.

(b) Verapamil: 0.05 mg/kg IV. Repeat once if needed.
   (i) Do not give verapamil to infants.
   (ii) Contraindicated in CHF and shock.
   (iii) Use IV calcium to treat hypotension, bradycardia that may follow its use.

(c) Propanolol: 0.05–0.1 mg/kg IV. Do not use both verapamil and propanolol.

(d) Adenosine
   (i) New drug: effective in SVT, including Wolff-Parkinson-White syndrome; not effective in atrial flutter, atrial fibrillation.
   (ii) Dose. Adults: 6 mg IV; if not effective in 1–2 minutes, 12 mg IV; may repeat once. Children: 1–6 mg IV has been used effectively; 50 μg/kg initially; may double dose twice, to 200 μg/kg, if initial dose is not successful.
   (iii) *Must be given as very rapid IV push,* followed by saline push to be effective. The faster the rate of administration and the closer to the heart it is administered, the more effective a given dose will be. (Drug is rapidly metabolized and disappears from circulation almost immediately.)
   (iv) Side effects: very short acting; include dyspnea, facial flushing, and chest pain; occasional transient dysrhythmias, primarily bradycardia. Bradycardia usually resolves spontaneously within 15–30 seconds.
   (v) Drug competes with theophylline for receptors. Therefore, patients receiving theophylline may require higher than usual doses for effectiveness.

b. If hemodynamically *unstable* (i.e., shock, significant CHF):
   (1) Sedation is recommended: midazolam or diazepam.
   (2) Intubate or prepare for rapid airway management.
   (3) Give *synchronized* DC countershock 0.5 j/kg. Double dose and repeat if needed. Synchronized mode may not work secondary to rapid rate; in that case use unsynchronized mode with the awareness that other arrhythmias may result and require treatment.
   (4) Consider digitalization after SVT is resolved.
   (5) Remember that the patient who was in shock initially will need close monitoring for postshock complications.

2. Always assume ventricular tachycardia unless proved otherwise.
   a. If hemodynamically *stable:*
      (1) Lidocaine: 1 mg/kg IV, followed by infusion at 20–50 μg/kg/min (see Appendix II–3, for lidocaine infusion preparation.)
      (2) Bretylium: 5 mg/kg. May repeat at 10 mg/kg.
         (a) May induce nausea, vomiting, or hypotension (treat hypotension with volume expansion).
         (b) May worsen dysrhythmias in digitalized patient.
      (3) Consider procainamide:
         (a) Dose
            (i) Loading dose: 3–10 mg/kg IV over 10–30 minutes; maximum dose 200 mg.
            (ii) Follow with continuous infusion: 2–5 mg/kg/hour; maximum daily dose 2 g. (Dilute with 5% aqueous dextrose solution to concentration <100 mg procainamide/mL.)
         (b) May induce hypotension (treat with volume expansion).
   b. If hemodynamically *unstable:*
      (1) Synchronized cardioversion 1.0 j/kg. Double dose and repeat if needed.

(2) Then load with lidocaine, 1.0 mg/kg IV, and start infusion as earlier.
(3) Bretylium (as above).

IV. Hypertension

A strict definition of hypertension:

1. >2 standard deviations above the mean for age and sex.
2. Requirement of three measurements in nonstressful circumstances (rarely practical in the emergency setting).

Measurements must be taken by a cuff of appropriate size (i.e., one half to two thirds the length of the upper arm with the inflatable bladder encircling the arm). Discussion here will be limited to evaluation and treatment of hypertensive emergencies.

A. Hypertensive emergencies

1. Malignant hypertension
   a. Definition:
      (1) <10 years of age: systolic BP > 160 mm Hg or diastolic BP > 105 mm Hg.
      (2) >10 years of age: systolic BP > 170 mm Hg or diastolic BP > 110 mm Hg.
   b. End-organ damage present. Findings may include:
      (1) Retinal artery spasm, papilledema, or hemorrhages and exudates on fundoscopy.
      (2) Murmur, CHF, facial palsy or hematuria.
      (3) Hypertensive encephalopathy (see later).
2. Accelerated hypertension
   a. Acute rise in systolic BP or diastolic BP on existing hypertension.
   b. May have end-organ damage: murmur, CHF, facial palsy, or hematuria.
3. Hypertensive encephalopathy
   a. Medical emergency that can cause death or permanent disability if not treated immediately.
   b. Diagnosis confirmed by rapid improvement in signs and symptoms when BP is lowered.
   c. Signs and symptoms
      (1) Hypertension
      (2) Headache
      (3) Visual changes

(4) Nausea, vomiting
(5) Altered mental status
(6) Seizures

B. Underlying causes of hypertension

1. Renal: glomerulonephritis, hemolytic-uremic syndrome, pyelonephritis, obstruction, vascular disease.
2. Cardiac: coarctation of the aorta.
3. Neurologic: infection, drugs, tumor, cerebral edema with impending herniation (see p. 420 for identification, therapy of increased intracranial pressure).
4. Endocrine: pheochromocytoma, Cushing's syndrome, corticosteroid therapy, hyperthyroidism.
5. Toxins, poisons.
6. Primary (essential) hypertension.

C. Upper limits of normal BP

1. ≤2 years: systolic BP 110, diastolic BP 65.
2. 3–6 years: systolic BP 120, diastolic BP 70.
3. 7–10 years: systolic BP 130, diastolic BP 75.
4. 11–15 years: systolic BP 140, diastolic BP 80.

D. Treatment

For severe, symptomatic hypertension, the BP should be lowered before proceeding with an investigation of the underlying cause. Hypertensive encephalopathy is a medical emergency and must be treated immediately. Short-acting IV antihypertensives are the treatment of choice for acute hypertensive emergencies.

The goal of antihypertensive therapy in hypertensive emergencies is to lower the BP but not to the normal range.

Lowering the BP to normal in hypertensive emergencies is contraindicated: A rapid drop in BP to normal is likely to produce tissue ischemia. In children, this is likely to be manifested clinically as shock (in spite of normal to slightly elevated BP values), encephalopathy, hypoventilation, apnea. To avoid both the clinical disasters of hypertensive emergencies and excessive BP correction, a reasonable goal is to acutely lower the mean arterial BP by 20% to 25%. (Mean arterial BP will be read out on many automated BP machines or can be calculated. Mean arterial blood pressure = [(2 × diastolic BP) + Systolic BP]/3).

1. Diazoxide: 3–5 mg/kg IV.
   a. Onset of action: minutes.
   b. Administer by *rapid* IV infusion (15–30 seconds) because of rapid protein binding.

   c. Causes salt and water retention, hyperglycemia; may cause tachycardia.
   d. See no. 5.
2. Hydralazine: 0.1–0.5 mg/kg IV (maximum dose 20 mg).
   a. Onset of action: 15–30 minutes.
   b. Administer by IV infusion over several minutes.
   c. May cause tachycardia, headache, vomiting, flushing, salt and water retention.
   d. May repeat dose in 20–30 minutes as needed. Consider alternative medications after 2–3 doses.
   e. See no. 5.
3. Captopril: ≤2 months: 0.05–0.1 mg/kg po; >2 months: 0.1–0.3 mg/kg po.
   a. Useful for patients with existing renal hypertension in an accelerated or malignant phase.
   b. Onset of action: 1 hour.
   c. Administer orally.
   d. If initial dose is ineffective, double the dose in 1–2 hours.
   e. See no. 5.
4. Nitroprusside: Start at 0.5 μg/kg/min.
   a. Instantaneous action, uniformly effective; requires infusion pump and continuous monitoring for hypotension.
   b. May increase q10–15min to maximum dose of 8.0 μg/kg/min.
   c. See Appendix II–3, for preparation.
   d. See no. 5.
5. Vascular volume status and fluid therapy: critical adjunct to antihypertensive therapy.
   a. The fluid needs of the patient with hypertensive crisis varies. Clinical evaluation is required to determine these needs. Two usual considerations are presented.
   b. After the BP is lowered, patients with hypertensive crises, unlike the patient with moderate hypertension, may be volume depleted: some may have had a pressure-driven diuresis; vasodilatation increases vascular capacity. These patients may need plasma volume expanders (see p. 6) to restore circulation.
   c. Other patients may show signs of fluid overload, CHF. These patients will need diuretics, especially because some of the antihypertensive agents have salt- and water-retaining effects.

E. Initial diagnostic studies

1. Urinalysis, serum BUN level, and creatinine clearance.
2. CBC and platelet count.
3. Chest x-ray film.
4. ECG.
5. Electrolyte values; consider toxicology screen.

V. Anaphylactic Shock

Systemic anaphylactic shock can be the result of multiple causes, including food, medications, insect bites, and environmental substances. A wide range of problems can result, some of which are life threatening. The life-threatening problems caused by anaphylactic shock are:

1. *Respiratory problems:* usually related to airway narrowing, both upper and lower airways.
2. *Cardiovascular problems:* shock secondary to loss of vascular tone and increased vascular permeability.

Numerous interventions may be needed in treating anaphylactic shock, but the key pharmacologic agent is epinephrine. It alone can begin to correct the life-threatening respiratory and cardiovascular manifestations of anaphylaxis. Epinephrine's usefulness lies in its adrenergic properties, which counter the anaphylactic responses that produce the life-threatening problems.

1. α Effects: vasoconstriction.
   a. Decreases laryngeal hyperemia, edema; important for upper airway.
   b. Restores vascular tone; helps restore blood pressure, circulation.
2. β Effects
   a. Bronchodilatation: important for lower airways.
   b. Inotropic property: improves myocardial contractility.

Epinephrine (and oxygen) are therefore the first-priority medications in anaphylaxis. Other medications, if needed, are provided secondarily.

A. Clinical picture

1. Life-threatening problems
   a. Respiratory problems
      (1) Laryngeal edema: stridor; loss of voice.
      (2) Bronchospasm, bronchial edema: wheezing.

b. Cardiovascular problems
   (1) Hypotension secondary to:
      (a) Vasodilatation: loss of vascular tone.
      (b) Increased capillary permeability.
   (2) Dysrhythmias.

2. Other problems
   a. Skin: urticaria, flushing; angioneurotic edema.
   b. GI tract: nausea, vomiting, diarrhea, cramping.

B. Therapy

1. Immediate therapy.
   a. Oxygen; assisted ventilation if needed.
   b. Discontinue administration of inciting agent when applicable.
      (1) Place tourniquet proximal to injection site or bite.
   c. Epinephrine: administer to the patient with:
      (1) Shock: Epinephrine 1:10,000 solution, 0.1 ml/kg IV.
         (a) Use ETT route if the airway is intubated and the patient has no IV access.
      (2) Adequate cardiovascular status: Epinephrine 1:1,000 solution, 0.01 mL/kg SQ. Maximum dose 0.4–0.5 mL SQ.
      (3) Repeat epinephrine dose q10–20min prn for respiratory or cardiovascular symptoms. Monitor heart rate, rhythm, and BP.
2. Additional therapy
   a. Respiratory system
      (1) Bronchospasm
         (a) Aerosolized β-sympathomimetic agent (albuterol, metaproterenol, or terbutaline). See p. 30.
         (b) Aminophylline, 5–7 mg/kg IV over 20 minutes, in addition to aerosol. May choose to follow loading dose with aminophylline drip or intermittent bolus doses of aminophylline. See pp. 46.
      (2) Stridor: aerosolized racemic epinephrine, 0.25–0.5 mL, plus 3–5 mL NS solution. See p. 37.
   b. Cardiovascular system
      (1) Hypotension: If epinephrine bolus injection is not sufficient to restore and maintain circulation, use:
         (a) Plasma volume expander: NS or LR solution, 20 mL/kg IV push; repeat as needed.

(b) Epinephrine drip: Start at 0.1 μg/kg/min, and titrate dose. See p. 83 for preparation.

(2) Dysrhythmias: See p. 83.

c. Other therapy

(1) Diphenhydramine for urticaria: 1–2 mg/kg IV or po.

(2) Hydrocortisone: 5–7 mg/kg IV for a moderate to severe anaphylactic reaction.

(3) Intervention to decrease absorption of inciting agent from a bite or injection.

(a) Epinephrine: 1:1,000 solution 0.01 mL/kg into site of injection or bite. Maximum dose 0.3 mL. Given in addition to previously administered epinephrine.

VI. Pericarditis

A. Causes

Infection, rheumatologic disorders, trauma, malignancies, postpericardiotomy syndrome.

B. Diagnosis

History of etiology: chest pain; signs of CHF; friction rub; pulsus paradoxus (>10 mm Hg); ECG with decreased voltage, elevated ST segments, and/or diffuse T-wave inversions; enlarged heart on chest x-ray film if effusion is present. When tamponade develops: distant heart sounds, distended jugular veins, decreased pulse amplitude and pulse pressure, classic signs of shock.

C. Treatment

1. Oxygen: Assure adequate ventilation.
2. If patient is hemodynamically unstable from apparent effusion, consider therapeutic pericardiocentesis (see p. 348). Save sterile specimen for laboratory studies.
3. If infectious etiology is suspected, obtain blood cultures and begin antibiotics to cover *Staphylococcus aureus, Haemophilus influenzae, Neisseria meningitidis,* and *Streptococcus pneumoniae* (anti-*Staphylococcus* drug and broad-spectrum cephalosporin).
4. Fluids: Treat or prevent dehydration; adequate hydration is important. The use of diuretics is contraindicated in the patient suspected of having pericardial tamponade: good cardiac chamber dilatation is needed for optimal cardiac function; the cardiac chambers are decreased from exter-

nal compression, and diuretics will further decrease their size and cardiac function.

5. Cardiogenic shock: Myocardial dysfunction commonly accompanies bacterial pericarditis. Florid cardiogenic shock may develop at any time, and one must be prepared to provide intrope infusions (see p. 68 and Appendix II–3).
6. Postpericardiotomy syndrome: seen with increasing frequency as more cardiac surgery is performed. It is an inflammatory response associated with fever, malaise, and classic signs and symptoms of pericarditis. It most commonly develops 1 to 4 weeks after cardiac surgery. Pericardial effusions vary in amount and can occasionally be large enough to produce tamponade and require pericardiocentesis. Corticosteroids are given to treat this disease.

VII. Congenital Heart Disease

A. Neonatal (<4 weeks) cyanotic congenital heart disease

1. Specific diagnosis of underlying anatomy is not necessary.
2. Exclude other causes of cyanosis in the newborn (airway obstruction, primary pulmonary disease) by history, physical examination, chest radiograph, ECG, and hyperoxia test.
   a. Hyperoxia test: Measure Po_2 directly in Fio_2 100% by ABG or transcutaneous monitor (not by pulse oximetry because 100% oxygen saturation may occur with Po_2 of 80 mm Hg). Note whether measurement is preductal or postductal.
      (1) Po_2 <100 mm Hg: possible cyanotic heart disease.
      (2) Po_2 100–200 mm Hg: possible heart disease with complete mixing and increased pulmonary blood flow.
      (3) Po_2 > 250 mm Hg: heart disease unlikely.
3. If respiratory distress is moderate to severe, intubate and assist ventilation. Aside from improving respiratory status, this will decrease metabolic needs.
4. If perfusion is poor:
   a. Give 10 mL/kg volume expander, NS solution or 5% albumin.

   b. Follow, if needed, by dopamine, 5–20 μg/kg/min (see Appendix II–3).
5. Along with other initial studies, check glucose level and four extremity BP values with neonatal-size cuff.
6. Consider prostaglandin E1 (PGE1) infusion (consult pediatric cardiologist first, if possible) if:
   a. Po_2 <30–40 mm Hg and/or oxygen saturation <70% in Fio_2 100%.
   b. Femoral pulses are diminished or absent with poor perfusion.
   c. Metabolic acidosis (pH <7.3) persists with good ventilation and volume/inotropic support.
7. PGE1 administration
   a. Start PGE1 infusion at 0.05 μg/kg/min (Table 3–2).
      (1) Dose range: 0.01–0.20 μg/kg/min.
      (2) May increase dose in increments of 0.05 μg/kg/min if the clinical response is inadequate.
   b. Side effects of PGE1
      (1) Apnea: Patients being transported on doses of PGE1 should have intubation considered (in con-

TABLE 3–2.
Prostaglandin E1 Infusion Preparation: Weight Specific

Patient Wt (kg)	PGE1 (μg)	PGE1 (mL)
2.0	120	0.24
2.5	150	0.30
3.0	180	0.36
3.5	210	0.42
4.0	240	0.48
4.5	270	0.54
5.0	300	0.60

Preparation and Administration of Weight-Specific PGE1 Drip:
1. PGE1 stock solution: 500 μg PGE1/mL.
2. Prepare 100 mL of PGE1 solution:
   a. Start with nearly empty Volutrol.
   b. Add appropriate μg of PGE1; fill with IV fluid to 100 mL. μg of PGE1 = weight (kg) × 60 μg/kg.
   c. Shake solution; run through tubing, then attach to IV line.
3. PGE1 drip concentration and dose:
   a. Concentration: 1 mL/hour rate = 0.01 μg/kg/min.
   b. Usual dose: 0.05–0.10 μg/kg/min = 5–10 mL/hour rate.
   c. Start at 0.05 μg/kg/min = 5 mL/hour; titrate dose.

junction with receiving institution) prior to transport.

(2) Fever: In the initial work-up of a cyanotic newborn, a sepsis work-up has usually been performed, and the patient is usually receiving antibiotic therapy. If the patient is not receiving antibiotics and develops a fever when given PGE1, appropriate cultures should be obtained and antibiotics given as for any other neonate with fever.

(3) Vasodilatation: Treat hypotension with a 10 mL/kg bolus of volume expanders; repeat as needed.

(4) Seizures: Treat seizures with phenobarbital, 10–20 mg/kg IV.

POSTRESUSCITATION CARE 4

Critical care does not end with the reversal of life-threatening conditions such as shock, respiratory failure, and cardiopulmonary arrest. Life-threatening problems frequently produce widespread hypoxic and other injuries that become the next set of problems that need addressing after the primary destructive force has been corrected and has departed. It is similar to the situation one faces after a hurricane: The hurricane and its destructive forces have passed, but one is left to face the aftermath. The aftermath—a constellation of problems that arises from the primary insult—constitute the *postresuscitation injuries or state,* the next medical stage in the continuum of critical care.

The injury to the cells and tissues initiates an inflammatory response that typically takes 1 to 3 days to peak and a longer period to fully subside. As inflammation mounts, organ function declines. The severity of injury ranges from mild disturbances limited to transient laboratory value abnormalities without clinical expression—typically transaminase, glucose, blood urea nitrogen (BUN), and creatinine levels, prothrombin time (PT), and partial thromboplastin time (PTT)—to profound multisystem organ failure (MSOF).

Because the inflammatory response takes several days to peak after major insults, postresuscitation organ damage and dysfunction may not be apparent immediately after primary resuscitation. The damage and dysfunction may not become apparent until several hours after resuscitation, and organ dysfunction may not reach its nadir for several days. An apparently stable state immediately after resuscitation does not assure future stability.

The factor that most clearly predicts the magnitude of postresuscitation problems is the severity of the initial insult. The more severe the initial insult, the sooner the damage will become apparent, the greater the inflammatory response (injury) will be, and the longer period it will take to peak (2–3 days rather than 12–24 hours). The patient with severe injury (e.g., severe shock) is likely to manifest global postresuscitation injuries very early (sometimes during the primary resuscitation phase), develop galloping organ and metabolic dysfunction that progresses to MSOF; the patient may not reach the nadir of illness during this phase for another 2 to 3 days.

Other factors that increase the likelihood of sustaining significant injury and having significant postresuscitation problems include the patient's age (young patients, especially infants), nature of the initial insult (asphyxia, septic shock, cardiogenic shock, and multiple trauma tend to produce far more tissue injury than isolated respiratory failure, isolated hypovolemic shock), the child with preexisting debilitation, and inadequate treatment of the primary problem.

When MSOF or dysfunction arises, care requirements equal the complexity and difficulty of critical care resuscitation. Because of these considerations, the child who is successfully resuscitated may require transport to a tertiary care pediatric center for several days of observation and therapy. Awareness, monitoring, and treatment of problems that can arise during the postresuscitation period provide the patient with the best chances for minimal morbidity and intact survival.

Key principles that guide postresuscitation care follow:

1. Adequate oxygen delivery must be maintained. Primary focus remains on the respiratory and cardiovascular systems.
2. Measures that reduce the body's metabolic expenditure should be used, especially after significant injuries. In the postresuscitation state, the body's metabolic needs are increased, whereas the body's ability to deliver oxygen is reduced (muscle weakness, reduced respiratory and cardiovascular function). Metabolic (oxygen)–sparing measures that help maintain positive oxygen balance may significantly reduce patient morbidity and improve patient outcome.
3. One must be aware of postresuscitation responses and injuries. They should be anticipated with appropriate monitoring, and appropriate intervention must be provided as needed.

I. Common Pediatric Postresuscitation Problems

A fairly comprehensive list of postresuscitation problems is presented at the end of this chapter; the list is most applicable to the child who has sustained a major primary insult.

More commonly, the child has sustained milder insults such as isolated respiratory failure, shock that is corrected fairly easily, sepsis that is not overwhelming, or multiple trauma without system failure. These children do develop illness-associated or postresuscitation problems, but a limited number of them. A list of *commonly seen problems* after mild to moderate insults follow. They are usually discovered in the first few hours after resuscitation, and it is important to stress that their incidence is increased in young infants. It is important to identify these problems; if they are left unrecognized and untreated, the consequences are potentially severe. These common responses should be anticipated in all children who have had critical illnesses and resuscitation.

A. Hypoglycemia

Hypoglycemia is commonly seen after a significant insult. Glucose stores are used; gluconeogenesis is impaired, then hypoglycemia results. It is most common in infants: The younger the infant, the greater the likelihood that hypoglycemia will develop in the postresuscitation period. It also commonly follows significant insults (e.g., shock). It is important to note that *hyperglycemia* is commonly the initial stress response, only to be followed by hypoglycemia at a later time. Serial glucose monitoring (bedside methods, e.g., Dextrostix or Chemstrips, are adequate) is therefore important in the postresuscitation state. Hypoglycemia commonly develops in the first 6 to 12 hours after hyperglycemia but may be seen initially in overwhelming illness.

B. Capillary leaks

Capillary damage resulting in capillary leaks is very common after mild to moderate insults. Fluid losses from the vascular compartment may amount to volumes large enough to show up as circulatory compromise in the first 6 to 24 hours; the losses will be evident sooner in the child whose primary problem was shock or dehydration. Therefore, one must commonly provide plasma volume expander pushes to restore circulation in the postresuscitation period even though the child initially was not dehydrated and even though the primary insult was not cardiovascular in origin. After severe insults, capillary leaks are massive (children develop gross edema), recurrent hypovolemic shock common, and the volume replacement needs are likewise massive.

C. Hypocalcemia

Hypocalcemia is less commonly seen than hyperglycemia, hypoglycemia, or capillary leaks in the postresuscitation period. It is more likely to follow moderate to severe insults, usually appearing at a later time (e.g., 12–24 hours after resuscitation). In more severe illness (especially after septic or cardiogenic shock, asphyxia) and in young infants, however, it may appear sooner. Calcium values can fall to very low levels. There is, however, disagreement about the need to treat low values that are without clinical findings. The situation is very different when circulation is impaired. Hypocalcemia can adversely affect myocardial contractility. Volume and inotrope therapy fail to restore circulation in the face of hypocalcemia. In this situation, correction of hypocalcemia is crucial. One must therefore be aware of hypocalcemia, appropriately monitor calcium values, and treat hypocalcemia when it coexists with circulatory impairment.

II. Postresuscitation Problems and Care

A. Respiratory system

1. Assure good partial pressure of oxygen (Po_2) value: Provide supplemental fraction of inspired oxygen (Fio_2), continue to use Fio_2 100% until the child is in a pediatric intensive care unit (PICU).
2. Provide *controlled ventilation* for the patient who has required mechanical ventilatory support until the child is in the controlled setting of a PICU. Rationale:
   a. To assure good ventilation, oxygenation (see p. 28). Blood gas goals:
      (1) $Po_2 \geq 90$–100 mm Hg in the patient with previously normal Po_2 values; $Po_2 \geq$ usual values in a child with baseline hypoxemia.
      (2) pH 7.35–7.59.
      (3) Partial pressure of carbon dioxide (Pco_2) value to achieve desired pH (pH as low as 20 mm Hg is safe).
   b. To decrease energy expenditure (oxygen needs).

3. Postresuscitation pulmonary problems
   a. Pulmonary dysfunction: impaired gas exchange, deteriorating blood gas values secondary to pulmonary capillary leaks, cell damage.
   b. Pulmonary edema; adult respiratory distress syndrome, which may develop 2–3 days after a severe insult.

B. Cardiovascular system

1. Maintain good cardiac output.
2. Shock (recurrent) commonly develops secondary to hypoxic-ischemic injury in the first 6–12 hours; may recur for up to 72 hours.
3. Secondary shock may be caused by:
   a. Capillary leaks: common injury (the most common cause of shock in postresuscitation period).
      (1) May be an ongoing problem for up to 48–72 hours; leaks may be *massive* after severe insults.
      (2) Therapy: plasma volume expanders, 10–20 mL/kg boluses as often as needed (see p. 66).
   b. Myocardial ischemia: far less common cause; usually seen only after profound hypoxic-ischemic insult.
      (1) May take 6–12 hours after insult to become apparent; when present, myocardial inflammation and dysfunction may worsen for 48–72 hours before stabilizing and reversing.
      (2) Therapy: inotrope infusions (see p. 68); also consider calcium (see p. 73).

C. Metabolic disturbances

1. Glucose levels: variable findings that may be biphasic; hypoglycemia is of concern.
   a. Hyperglycemia: the common initial acute stress response; needs no therapy because it gradually corrects itself.
      (1) Hyperglycemia may produce large osmotic diuresis, which causes hypovolemia and shock when extensive. Osmotic diuresis in no way reflects the adequacy of circulation.
   b. Hypoglycemia: commonly seen in the first 6–24 hours after insult; may be profound, especially in infants and after severe shock.
      (1) Monitor glucose levels serially (bedside test is adequate).

(2) When hypoglycemia is present: Give glucose (dextrose) bolus (see p. 73); increase intravenous (IV) concentration of dextrose.

2. Calcium: hypocalcemia
   a. Hypocalcemia commonly develops in the first 12–24 hours after insult, occasionally earlier. Calcium levels may fall progressively over several days after a severe initial insult.
   b. Hypocalcemia can produce severe myocardial depression.
   c. Therapy of hypocalcemia: Views differ.
      (1) In the absence of symptoms (i.e., absence of cardiac symptoms, especially circulatory compromise), therapy may not be needed.
      (2) In the presence of circulatory compromise, provide calcium gluconate or calcium chloride IV. (see p. 73).
3. Metabolic acidosis
   a. Correct etiology of metabolic acidosis.
   b. Specific therapy: Sodium bicarbonate, 1 mEq/kg IV; repeat as necessary according to blood gas and electrolyte values.

D. Renal dysfunction

1. Abnormal renal metabolic values: common, even in the absence of oliguria.
   a. Elevated BUN and creatinine levels are most common.
   b. Elevated uric acid, phosphate, and potassium levels are seen when more severe dysfunction is present.
   c. Therapy: Maintain good oxygenation and cardiac output.
2. Oliguria, anuria: seen after profound shock, asphyxia.
   a. Renal metabolic abnormalities are more severe.
   b. If oliguria or anuria persists *after* circulation is restored, attempt to initiate urine output with:
      (1) Furosemide: 1 mg/kg IV; increase dose if needed, or use:
      (2) Mannitol:
      0.5–1.0 g/kg IV.

E. Hematologic system

1. Anemia: common secondary to both marrow suppression and decreased red blood cell (RBC) life span.
   a. Give packed RBC (PRBC) transfusion as indicated: 10 mL/kg PRBC transfusion will raise hematocrit (Hct)

value by 10 in euvolemic patient; Hct rise will be less in a patient who is hypovolemic, is actively bleeding, or is hemolyzing RBCs (see p. 225).

2. Thrombocytopenia: common after a major insult; platelet count may continue to drop for as long as 1 week after a severe insult.
   a. Give platelet transfusion as needed (see p. 228).
3. Coagulopathy: Prolonged PT and PTT are common for the first 24–48 hours after insult.
   a. If prolongation is not marked, if no clinical bleeding is present, and if the patient's underlying problem is being corrected, the PT and PTT will usually correct on their own in 48 hours.
   b. For very prolonged PT, PTT, disseminated intravascular coagulation, or clinical bleeding (see p. 229), supply:
      (1) fresh frozen plasma: 10 mL/kg IV; 20 mL/kg for active bleeding; repeat as needed.
      (2) Other factor therapy as indicated (see p. 229).

F. Liver

1. Elevated transaminase levels are common; nonspecific finding.
2. More severe insult: function is impaired (i.e., find hypoglycemia, hypoalbuminemia, coagulopathy, hypofibrinogenemia).

G. Gastrointestinal (GI) tract

1. Ileus: present in all moderately to severely ill patients.
   a. Keep patient npo until acute problems resolve.
2. GI bleeding, sloughing of intestinal mucosa, and necrosis occur after severe shock.
   a. Antacids, H_2 blockers for bleeding, stress (see pp. 366, 370, 391).

H. Central nervous system

1. Level of consciousness is depressed to the point of coma in severe cases; will last for at least 1–2 days.
   a. With severe hypoxic insult, cell death will result in eventual atrophy.
2. Seizures: Treat with anticonvulsants in usual manner (see p. 127).

I. Muscles

1. *Profound muscle weakness* accompanies severe illness! Weakness is most profound after shock, where it may take several weeks for strength to return.

a. Important consideration: intubation, mechanical ventilation to assure good blood gas levels and to reduce metabolic expenditure (oxygen needs).

J. Limited energy availability and oxygen delivery capability

1. Use measures that reduce energy/oxygen needs to maintain balance in favor of supply.
2. Temperature regulation: Aim for euthermia.
   a. Reduce fever to decrease energy needs: antipyretics; minimal coverings.
   b. Provide warmth for hypothermic patient.
3. Sedate the agitated, thrashing patient to minimize energy needs.
   a. Before using sedation, be certain that:
      (1) The patient is not hypoxic.
      (2) The airway is intubated, ventilated.
   b. Sedation: see p. 29.

5

CENTRAL NERVOUS SYSTEM

I. Central Nervous System Problems

Critical central nervous system (CNS) problems in children commonly produce significant discomfort in initial care providers, perhaps increasingly so as we continue to witness those who survive critical illness or injury with neurologic damage.

The sources of discomfort are genuine. Significant neurologic problems are very complex medical problems. Difficulties frequently inherent in the settings of the initial encounter and transport—diagnostic limitations that render therapeutic decisions difficult (e.g., lack of computed axial tomography [CAT] scan, intracranial pressure [ICP] monitoring, subspecialists to interpret findings); limited therapeutic capabilities, specifically the inability to perform neurosurgical procedures without a neurosurgeon—add to the anxiety that already exists in neurologic emergencies and heighten the concern that as a result, neurologic outcome will be compromised.

For the initial encounter and transport settings, two important conditions must be recognized: (1) diagnostic and therapeutic capabilities will frequently be limited; and (2) within these limits remain critical decisions to be made, critical actions to be taken that can still dramatically affect neurologic outcome. It is especially important to recognize that many of these critical interventions are not specifically directed to a neurologic problem or to the neurologic system. The interventions instead provide conditions crucial to maintaining neurologic viability and survival where this potential exists.

Example: The child with multiple trauma in need of neurosurgery must receive the critical respiratory and cardiovascular support that supplies the brain with oxygen and keeps the brain viable until neurosurgery can be performed. These interventions are the responsibility of the initial responders and transport teams that care for the patient with neurologic problems.

The focus of this chapter is the recognition of impending neurologic compromise, the understanding of interventions that support brain viability, and the presentation of problems where specific therapy exists.

II. The Brain: Overview and Approach to Therapy

The principles of emergency medicine clearly operate during neurologic emergencies. In first-encounter and transport settings, a sense of control is often absent, diagnosis frequently lacks the desired precision, and therapeutic capabilities may be limited. One must then do the best that one can do. In this setting, this entails making knowledgeable assessments based on available information and knowedgeable decisions about therapy, largely in anticipatory manner. Therapy is directed toward likely etiologies of the problem and control of secondary problems that can potentially arise.

This approach, based on physiologic and pathophysiologic principles of the brain and brain injuries, is especially useful in pediatric neurologic emergencies. On this framework the information and therapeutic capabilities at hand are used to formulate (1) the best assessment possible and (2) a therapeutic plan based on both the findings and the anticipation of significant problems likely to be associated with the brain injury or disease.

With this goal in mind, the following overview of the brain and organization of therapy is presented before proceeding with specific CNS problems and their treatment.

1. Basic CNS needs: oxygen and glucose.
2. Primary and secondary brain injury.
3. Brain responses to injury.
4. Intervention in brain injury: priorities in therapy.
5. Clinical assessment of CNS function in the emergency setting.

A. **Basic CNS needs: oxygen and glucose**

The brain's two most critical needs are *oxygen* and *glucose*. Oxygen, by far, is the most important need and is the focus of this section.

Constant oxygen delivery to the brain is imperative for intact function and integrity. Within 10 seconds of oxygen delivery being cut off to the brain (e.g., by tying the carotid arteries), unconsciousness ensues. With continued hypoxia, CNS dysfunction progresses to CNS damage: after 4 to 6 minutes, irreversible cortical brain damage develops, followed several minutes later by irreversible damage to the brain stem.

Uninterrupted oxygen delivery is even more crucial when brain injury is present. Lesser than usual amounts of hypoxia may render reversibly damaged cells irreversibly damaged. Maintenance of adequate oxygen delivery is a crucial determinant in maintaining the viability of cells that sustain a nonlethal (and potentially reversible) primary injury and is a key means of minimizing the extent of irreversible brain damage.

Oxygen delivery to the brain is therefore the concern of first priority in CNS disease/injury and takes precedence over the specific therapy for the primary CNS disorder when the latter exists. This critical need coincides well with the cardinal principle of critical disease and injury: focus first on the respiratory and cardiovascular systems to assure oxygen delivery to the body.

B. **Primary and secondary brain injury**

Brain injury may be one of two types. The first, termed *primary injury,* is the result of an insult to the brain that can be traumatic, infectious, metabolic, toxic, or hypoxic in origin. The primary insult may be treatable, either specifically or supportively; the inflicted injury may be reversible if the damage from the primary insult is not too severe. The injury is untreatable when the inflicted damage is severe enough to cause cell or organ death.

The brain's response to the injury can produce conditions that cause further injury to the brain. Injury arising from these conditions is termed *secondary injury*. Secondary injury can extend the primary CNS damage in two ways: (1) increase the severity of the injury by making existing injury worse, as well as by converting an initially reversible injury to an irreversible injury; and (2) increase the area of CNS injury by damaging cells that were spared the primary insult.

The irreversible brain damage already present initially cannot be changed. Further damage, especially irreversible damage, however, can hopefully be prevented. This is the goal of therapy. Means of accomplishing this include providing specific therapy (in situations where such therapy exists) to halt the primary process and its infliction of further damage and controlling the brain's responses to injury to prevent or minimize the development of secondary injury.

C. Brain responses to injury

The brain can be injured in many ways. Its responses to injury, however, are uniform.

It is important to note that the severity of the initial injury determines the magnitude of the injury response in both its severity and duration. The more severe the primary injury, the more intense (clinically apparent) the injury response (inflammation, CNS dysfunction), the more rapidly it appears, and the longer it lasts (up to >1 week in cases of severe CNS injury). Therefore, the spectrum of brain responses to injury is wide, and the management of the injury responses is guided by the intensity of the injury responses.

1. Altered function (clinical)
   a. *Altered level of consciousness:* Altered level of consciousness is usually readily apparent. Assessment of the level of consciousness is important, because it provides the guidelines for therapy and serves as a barometer for the course of injury and of response to therapy. Critically low levels of brain function indicate impending CNS catastrophe and the need for aggressive intervention.
   b. *Seizures.* Seizures are common after CNS injury and disease. Seizures need appropriate therapy, as well as investigation into their etiology. Prolonged seizures increase metabolic needs and can, of themselves, produce CNS damage.
   c. *Altered respiratory function:* Altered respiratory function, specifically transient hypoventilation or apnea, is a fairly frequent occurrence in children

with acute CNS problems. It is most commonly observed with seizures or immediately after head trauma and is most commonly observed in infants and young children. This can produce significant hypoxemia, hypercarbia, and acidosis, all of which alter blood flow and oxygen delivery to the brain. Mechanical ventilatory support may be an important intervention during this period. In the majority of cases, the hypoventilation is transient and lasts for several minutes to several hours.

d. *Loss of autoregulation:* Autoregulation is the phenomenon by which the amount of blood flow to the brain is regulated and protected over a wide range of blood pressures. With significant brain injury, autoregulation is lost. Blood (oxygen) flow to the brain is no longer protected and becomes dependent on *cerebral perfusion pressure* (CPP). Cerebral perfusion pressure is determined by the difference between mean arterial pressure (MAP) and intracranial pressure (ICP), the two variables that must be regulated in this situation.

   It is prudent to assume that autoregulation is deranged or absent after moderate to severe head injury (i.e., a Glasgow Coma Scale of ≤8; see p. 437). Efforts to maintain MAP and to control ICP become the additional critical factors in maintaining oxygen delivery to the brain.

e. *Cerebral swelling:* Cerebral swelling or *cerebral edema* is a nonspecific response to injury. Sufficient cerebral swelling can produce *ICP elevation,* which, when of sufficient magnitude, can cause further damage to the brain in two ways: (1) by decreasing blood flow (oxygen delivery) to the brain; and (2) by pressure phenomena, the extreme cases being brain herniation.

f. *Syndrome of inappropriate antidiuretic hormone* (SIADH): SIADH is a nonspecific response to brain injury. When it is coupled with an excessive amount of fluid administration, water retention results. The consequences of significant water retention are hyponatremia with neuronal dysfunction (decreased level of consciousness, seizures) and further cerebral swelling, which exacerbates ICP problems.

D. **Intervention in brain injury: priorities in therapy**

For organizational purposes, therapy of brain injury can be divided into three broad areas of concern and approached accordingly. They are presented in order of priority and in the order in which therapy should proceed.

1. Oxygen delivery to the brain.
2. Specific therapy for the primary process, when such therapy exists.
3. Control of and compensation for brain injury responses: prevention and minimizing of secondary injury.

Adherence to this scheme permits one to put order into observations of a chaotic situation—a child with an actively bleeding scalp laceration, decorticate posturing, blood and emesis in the nostrils and mouth, labored breathing—then proceed with therapy in an organized and effective manner.

A working guide on the order in which to approach therapy follows. NOTE: Some aspects of care fall into more than one subdivision and are artificially assigned to one area.

1. Restore and maintain oxygen delivery to the brain
   - a. Respiratory system: Maintain good partial pressure of oxygen (Po_2).
     - a. Intubate, ventilate as needed.
   - b. Cardiovascular system: Maintain cardiac output.
     - a. Provide volume expanders, inotropes as needed.
   - c. CPP: an additional requirement to meet when significant brain injury exists.
     - a. Maintain MAP.
     - b. Lower suspected elevated ICP.
     - (1) Osmotic diuretics, hyperventilation, sedation, neuromuscular relaxants, other measures as needed.
2. Provide specific therapy (when such therapy exists)
   - a. Neurosurgical problem: *Get the patient to neurosurgery as quickly as possible* after rapid, essential stabilization.
   - b. Other specific therapy
     - a. Antibiotics for infection, anticonvulsants for seizures, correction of primary metabolic imbalances.

3. Prevent secondary brain injury
   a. Maintain oxygen delivery to brain (as earlier).
   b. Maintain glucose level.
   c. Limit fluid administration *after* circulation is restored.
   d. Treat seizures (i.e., secondary seizures).
   e. Decrease oxygen and energy needs.
      1. Temperature control: euthermia.
      2. Decrease excessive activity: Use sedation, control ventilation in the patient with intubation and ventilation.
   f. Maintain metabolic balance, especially sodium.
4. Monitor the patient
   a. Vital signs.
   b. Neurologic status.

E. Clinical assessment of CNS function in the emergency setting

Assessment of CNS function is an important measure that guides the choice of initial stabilization therapy. Ongoing monitoring of the patient's clinical neurologic status provides an important indicator of the success of the stabilization process or the need for more aggressive intervention.

Clinical assessment tools include:

1. Complete neurologic examination.
2. Glasgow Coma Scale: adult and infant scales (see Appendix II–4, p. 437).
3. Signs of increased ICP and herniation (see Appendix I–8, p. 420).

The Glasgow Coma Scales and signs of increased ICP are used in both the initial assessment to determine needed intervention and the serial monitoring of the patient's clinical course.

III. Oxygen Delivery to the Injured Brain

A. Cerebral perfusion pressure (CPP)

After moderate to severe CNS injury (Glasgow Coma Scale score ≤ 8), *autoregulation,* the important regulator of blood/oxygen flow to the brain, may be impaired or lost.

When autoregulation fails to operate, cerebral blood flow (i.e., oxygen delivery to the brain) becomes dependent on one additional condition: *CPP,* where

$$\text{CPP} = \text{MAP} - \text{ICP}$$

$$\text{MAP} = \frac{\text{Systolic BP} + (2 \times \text{Diastolic BP})}{3}$$

$$\text{Normal ICP} = 10 \text{ mm Hg.}$$

An example illustrating the calculation of CPP is presented. Assume that the patient is an adult who has had a head injury, has lost autoregulation, but retains normal blood pressure (BP) and ICP values:

$$\text{BP} = 120/80.\ \text{MAP} = 93 \text{ mm Hg.}$$

$$\text{ICP} = 8 \text{ mm Hg.}$$

$$\text{CPP} = \text{MAP} - \text{ICP} = 93 - 8 = 85 \text{ mm Hg.}$$

An adult study demonstrates the critical importance of maintaining CPP in the patient with brain injury:

1. CPP >50 mm Hg: Normal brain function and integrity are maintained.
2. CPP 40–50 mm Hg: Inadequate blood flow to brain results in the unconscious state.
3. CPP <40 mm Hg: Grossly inadequate blood flow to the brain produces brain damage, eventual brain death.

The critical importance of maintaining adequate CPP when significant brain injury exists is clear. To protect oxygen delivery to the brain after significant brain injury, four conditions must be met: (1) adequate respiratory function, (2) cardiovascular function, (3) hemoglobin value, and (4) CCP.

Comments on CPP, MAP, ICP, their interrelationships, and their clinical importance in clinical management follow.

1. CPP will be optimal when normal MAP and ICP are maintained. NOTE: Lowest acceptable CPP values for infants are not established but are probably less than 50

mm Hg because their baseline MAP values are lower than those for adults.

2. CPP will be decreased when any of the following conditions exists:
   a. MAP is low.
   b. ICP is high.
   c. Worst condition: low MAP and high ICP.
3. Relative contributions of MAP and ICP to CPP:
   a. MAP, by virtue of its greater numerical value, is a greater determinant of CPP than is ICP.
   b. Early in the course of disease or injury, MAP is likely to have greater variability in value than ICP and consequent greater effect on CPP.
   c. *MAP is the variable that takes first priority in regulation and management of CPP;* this coincides with the ABCs of resuscitation.
4. MAP:
   a. Low MAP must be corrected immediately. Therapy:
      (1) Plasma volume expanders for hypovolemia.
      (2) Inotropic agents for myocardial dysfunction.
   b. When ICP is (suspected to be) high, it is more imperative than usual to maintain good, if not slightly high, MAP to preserve CPP > 50 mm Hg.
   c. Because the injured brain has little reserve, small hypoxic insults (i.e., MAP drops) may be sufficient to convert a reversible injury to an irreversible injury. It is important to strive to maintain *consistently* adequate MAP.
5. ICP:
   a. Deleterious consequences of elevated ICP:
      (1) Hypoxic brain damage from decreased CPP and decreased oxygen delivery to the brain.
      (2) Tissue damage from high pressure (e.g., third nerve compression, herniation syndromes).
   b. Because ICP changes are generally less rapid and of lesser magnitude than MAP changes in the emergency situation, ICP therapy, although important, is second to MAP in priority in this equation.

B. Requirements

One should assume that autoregulation of blood flow to the brain is lost or impaired after moderate to severe brain injury. Adequate oxygen delivery to the brain is then best assured by meeting the following conditions (i.e. assuring *satisfactory*):

1. Respiratory function
2. Cardiovascular function
3. Hemoglobin value
4. CPP
   a. MAP
   b. ICP

IV. Fluids in Brain Injury

A. Their role in CPP

Fluid administration has a critical role in the management of brain injury or disease. Their role, however, needs clarification. Teachings have focused primarily on the need to limit fluid administration because of SIADH, cerebral edema, and ICP concerns. In fact, this principle is so well indoctrinated that it is common to find it strictly adhered to without consideration of other needs, sometimes to the patient's detriment.

Example: The multiply injured child with decorticate posturing, bilateral femur fractures, tachycardia, and poor peripheral perfusion needs a bolus of plasma volume expanders (PVEs) to restore circulation, MAP, and CPP (i.e., oxygen delivery to the brain). Adherence to fluid restriction would aggravate the circulatory compromise, which is secondary to hypovolemia (blood loss in femur fractures) and result in lower MAP, CPP, and oxygen delivery to an already obviously injured brain.

Therefore, no one rule alone serves to treat brain injury. There are, instead, two distinct roles of fluids in brain injury, both of which play important roles in determining CPP:

1. *Emergency fluids:* Fluids that restore circulation compromised by hypovolemia. They affect MAP in CPP equation.
2. *Maintenance fluids:* Fluids for ongoing needs. They affect ICP in the CPP equation.

Emergency fluids: The universal rules of resuscitation apply to brain injury: First restore/maintain oxygen delivery (i.e., respiratory function, cardiovascular function, hemoglobin value, and CCP for the injured brain). When cardiovascular function is compromised from hypovolemia—hemorrhage, dehydration—fluid, in the form of *PVEs,* must be given rapidly to restore circulation. This restores/maintains the MAP, which is critical in the equation that determines CPP (CPP = MAP − ICP) and oxygen delivery to the injured brain. Any time circulation again shows signs of compromise secondary to hypovolemia (e.g., from ongoing bleeding, capillary leaks, or other fluid losses), PVEs must be given to restore circulation, MAP. *The need to provide volume expanders to restore circulation (MAP) takes precedence over other fluid concerns.*

Maintenance fluids: After circulation is restored/assured, fluid (i.e., *usual maintenance solution*) is usually administered in limited *("restricted")* volume because of the frequent incidence of SIADH after head injury. SIADH's primary effect is increased water absorption by the kidneys, which is manifested clinically by decreased urine (water) output. Fluid administration is therefore decreased by an amount equal to an anticipated decrease in urine output to avoid excessive water retention. Excessive water retention can have especially deleterious consequences in brain injury: exacerbation of cerebral swelling, which can increase ICP, decrease CPP (i.e., decrease oxygen delivery to the brain), and decrease serum sodium, with associated neuronal dysfunction. Cerebral swelling of significance caused by water retention occurs over time—hours to days. Therefore, restriction of ongoing fluids takes second precedence to the urgent need to give plasma volume expanders when circulatory compromise secondary to hypovolemia exists. Excessive water retention is usually avoided by administering usual maintenance fluids at 50% to full maintenance rate (not more); subsequent input adjustments are made according to monitoring (input and output totals, electrolytes, weights).

When circulation is compromised secondary to hypovolemia, plasma volume expanders must be given rapidly to restore circulation as is done in any other situation: 10–20 mL/kg lactated Ringer's (LR) or normal saline (NS) solution in nonhypotensive shock, 20 mL/kg LR or NS solution in hypotensive shock with repeated doses until circulation and BP are restored; blood products are given as needed. *After* circulation is restored, usual fluids are provided at a limited rate.

B. Management

1. **Restore, maintain circulation, MAP** (i.e., treat hypovolemia).
   a. If circulation is compromised secondary to hypovolemia:
      (1) PVE: LR or NS solution.
         (a) Blood, fresh frozen plasma, or 5% albumin: usually needed only after large hemorrhage.
      (2) Volume: Begin with 20 mL/kg of PVEs.
         (a) Reassess circulation; repeat 10–20 mL/kg boluses as needed.
         (b) Patient with decompensated shock (i.e., hypotension) may require massive volumes of PVEs to restore circulation.
2. **Limit fluid volume after circulation (MAP) is restored.**
   a. Suggested therapy for first 24–48 hours
      (1) Fluids: Usual maintenance solution.
         (a) May choose increased NaCl content over usual amount (e.g., ½ NS solution).
      (2) Rate (volume): 50%–75% of usual maintenance rate. Specifically recommend avoiding greater than maintenance rate.
      (3) Monitor input/output, electrolyte levels, patient weight to guide further therapy.
3. **Treat recurring episodes of circulatory compromise, BP drops that subsequently occur.**
   a. If circulation worsens during the course of therapy (decreased perfusion to overt hypotension) and is secondary to hypovolemia (ongoing bleeding capillary leaks, osmotic diuretics), circulation and MAP must be restored to maintain CPP.
      (1) Provide PVE push (see earlier).
      (2) Return to ongoing maintenance fluid regimen after circulation is again restored.

V. Intracranial Pressure

One of the many unique aspects of the brain is its architecture: It is the only organ enveloped by bone, the cranium. Although protective of its inner contents, the bony encasement creates problems when the volume of the intracranial contents increases acutely: the noncompressible intracranial contents expanding against the nondistensible cranium raise the pressure in the cranium. Increased ICP is the result.

Significantly elevated ICP is deleterious to the brain in two ways. First, CPP is decreased when ICP is significantly elevated; oxygen delivery to the brain is decreased at critically low CPP values, and hypoxic injury to the brain results. Second, high ICP, of itself, can injure the brain. ***Examples:*** High ICP can compress the third cranial nerve and cause loss of pupillary constriction; high ICP can produce brain herniation syndromes. For these reasons, control of ICP is one of the goals of treatment of brain injury.

Figure 5–1 is the idealized curve that shows the relationship between intracranial volume (ICV) and ICP. NOTE:

1. When the ICV is low, increases in ICV initially produce little rise in ICP (points *A* to *B*). The explanation for this observation is the initial displacement of CSF from the intracranial to extracranial space (i.e., the subarachnoid space around the spinal cord). Therefore, the normal brain can accomodate a degree of ICV increase without developing a significant rise in ICP.

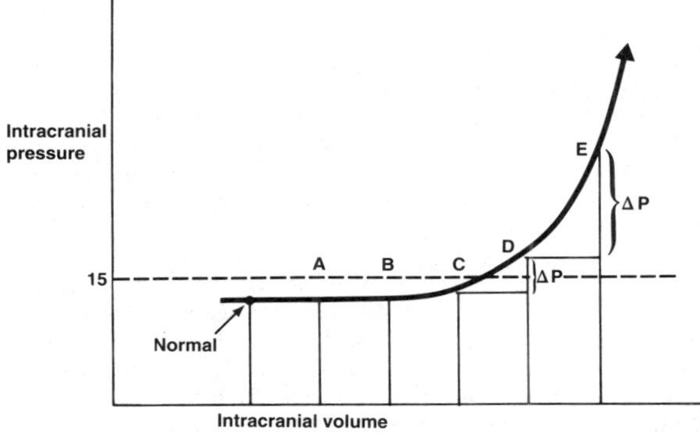

FIG 5–1.
Idealized curve of relationship between intracranial volume and intracranial pressure.

2. As the ICV progressively increases, cerebrospinal fluid (CSF) is no longer displaced, and successive increments in ICV produce correspondingly greater rises in ICP (points *C* to *D*). The increasing ICP rise is explained by the decreasing intracranial compliance.
3. When the ICV and ICP are very high (e.g., at point *D* on the graph), the slope is very steep so that small changes in ICV in either direction will produce large ICP changes in the corresponding direction. Therefore the patient with high ICP will derive great benefit from measures that decrease ICV by even small amounts and, conversely, suffer greatly from further increases in ICV, again by even small amounts.

Before we proceed with recommendations for ICP management, a closer examination of ICP and its genesis follows. Two fundamental principles with which to begin are:

1. Increased ICP is the result of increased ICV.
2. *Reduction of ICP is achieved by decreasing ICV.*

The second principle is especially important. Although discussions usually focus on measures that decrease ICP, *therapeutic measures are better viewed as measures that decrease ICV.* When such measures are effective, ICV is decreased, and ICP reduction follows. Selection of an intervention that will decrease the size of the component in the cranium that is increased in volume will most effectively reduce ICV and ICP. An overview of the intracranial contents follows. Table 5–1 summarizes the intracranial components, their pathologic states, and therapy that reduces the volume of that component.

There are normally three major intracranial components. By volume they are the brain (90%), *intravascular* blood (5%), and CSF (5%). The respective pathologic conditions are cerebral edema; hyperemia, venous congestion; and hydrocephalus. At times, a fourth component is pathologically present and will be termed "foreign body."

Cerebral swelling (edema) is the result of brain injury and varies in intensity from mild to massive and fulminant. It is an injury response (i.e., an inflammatory response) and will run its

TABLE 5–1.

Intracranial Contents: Relationship to ICP

Intracranial Contents (% of ICV)	Pathologic States: Increased Volume	Therapeutic Interventions That Reduce Specific Intracranial Compartment Volumes
1. **Brain** (90%)	Cerebral edema	Fluid restriction Adequate Na^+ input for: Normal/increased serum Na^+ Normal/increased serum osmolality Diuretic: furosemide Osmotic diuretic: mannitol; glycerol Corticosteroids: for peritumor or periabscess edema [Hypothermia] [Barbiturate coma]
2. **Intravascular Blood** (5%)	Arterial system: hyperemia	Normalize ABG values: Correct low PO_2, high PCO_2, low pH Hyperventilation to induce vasoconstriction: low PCO_2, high pH
	Venous system: venous congestion	Measures to facilitate drainage: Elevation of head Midline head position Avoid/stop Valsalva's activity: sedation; neuromuscular relaxant Minimum PEEP to maintain adequate oxygen Relieve obstruction (e.g., SVC obstruction)
3. **CSF** (5%)	Hydrocephalus	Remove CSF: tap, drain, or shunt
4. **Foreign body**	Tumor, abscess, hematoma, bullet, etc.	Surgical removal of foreign body

course once initiated. Interventions are employed to modify the degree of swelling by either (1) preventing further swelling: fluid restriction, providing adequate Na^+ to maintain normal to high serum Na^+ and osmolality, corticosteroids in certain conditions (effective in peritumor and periabscess edema); or (2) reducing existing swelling: diuretics. Two of the listed modalities, induced hypothermia and barbiturate coma, do not affect swelling per se but decrease brain metabolism and thereby aid this problem indirectly; they are not indicated for use in the stabilization or transport phases.

Intravascular blood volume can be increased in two ways: the *arterial and venous systems*. The *arterial vessels* are affected by oxygenation and ventilation. They dilate whenever there is hypoxemia, hypercarbia, and/or acidosis (i.e., hypoventilation); correction of all of these conditions restores arterial vessel size to normal, once again underscoring the need to attend to the respiratory system. The arterial vessels can be reduced further in size to a volume below normal while still providing adequate oxygen delivery with hyperventilation. The P_{CO_2} is lowered to levels as low as 20 mm Hg, and the pH is raised correspondingly (up to 7.59). Hyperventilation is employed to reduce intravascular blood volume when brain injury and swelling are severe.

Intracranial venous congestion is seen in situations where blood return from the head to the chest is impeded. It is most severe in superior vena cava syndrome (obstruction), an uncommon occurrence. Usually its impact is far less pronounced, and simple medical measures that enhance venous drainage are used: the head is kept elevated and midline; Valsalva's maneuvers are avoided. When ICP is elevated and volume reduction of all intracranial components is important, additional measures are used to assure unimpeded blood return to the chest. They include the use of minimum positive end-expiratory pressure (PEEP) that allows adequate oxygen levels (to avoid excessive lung distention), sedation, and, if needed, neuromuscular relaxants in patients who are intubated or ventilated.

Hydrocephalus is the condition where excessive CSF is present. The problem can be corrected only by removal of CSF, an invasive procedure.

Foreign objects are significant sources of increased ICP. They include tumors, hematomas, abscesses, and penetrating objects. Surgical removal is the only acute intervention available to relieve this problem.

With this perspective, the approach to ICP problems can be organized schematically in the following manner:

1. *Prevention:* When brain injury or disease is present but is mild and without indications of elevated ICP, anticipatory measures can be used to prevent or minimize the development of increased ICP. Measures include assurance of good respiratory function; fluid restriction, provision of adequate Na^+ to minimize cerebral swelling; head elevation, and avoidance of disturbances to assure return of venous blood to the chest.
2. *Specific therapy directed at known cause of elevated ICP:* Examples include corticosteroids for peritumor or abscess edema; osmotic diuretics for diffuse cerebral edema; diuretics and extra Na^+ for cerebral edema secondary to hyponatremia; shunt tap for blocked ventriculoperitoneal shunt; or surgery to evacuate a hematoma. Included in this section is specific therapy of the underlying problem, when present, such as antibiotics for CNS infections.
3. *Compensatory therapy for elevated ICP:* When specific therapy for the known cause of increased ICP is either unavailable at the moment (neurosurgery) or insufficient to reduce the ICP to acceptable range (e.g., in severe cerebral edema), medical measures that decrease the volumes of other intracranial components should be used. Volume reductions of other intracranial components can compensate for the increased volume of the involved component. For example, osmotic diuretics to shrink the brain and controlled hyperventilation to decrease intravascular blood volume can be employed to decrease the high ICV and ICP caused by massive hydrocephalus or a large tumor until neurosurgery can be performed.

Normal ICP value is less than 10 mm Hg in units used by ICP monitoring equipment. (This corresponds to 140 mm H_2O pressure obtained by lumbar puncture using a manometer; Hg is approximately 14 times denser than water.) The generally accepted high normal ICP value is 15 mm Hg (210 mm H_2O pressure by lumbar puncture). When cardiorespiratory functions are normal, an individual can probably tolerate episodes of ICP values up to 20 mm Hg without deleterious consequences. When the ICP is monitored in the pediatric intensive care unit (PICU), efforts are made to keep the ICP less than 15 to 20 mm Hg and the

CPP more than 50 mm Hg (except in infants where an acceptable CPP is probably lower than 50 mm Hg).

In the emergency and transport situations, ICP monitoring is rarely available or indicated. ICP magnitude must therefore be inferred from clinical findings and available radiologic studies, and therapeutic decisions are based on the derived assessments. Unfortunately, there is no established correlation between clinical picture and ICP values that are mildly to moderately elevated, the area of specific concern because it is at these levels that the decision to use more aggressive treatment measures for ICP control is made.

The dilemma this situation poses is evident: No widely accepted rules exist regarding clinical findings indicative of elevated ICP, and the point at which invasive ICP control measures need to be instituted. It is therefore important to preface further discussion about these issues with the following statement:

> *It is highly recommended that the reader, after using material in this section as a resource, consult his or her tertiary pediatric center for specific recommendations regarding assessment and managment of the child suspected to have mild or moderate ICP elevation.* For reasons just given, there may be significant differences among different PICUs and transport systems over the guidelines presented here, and it is advisable to use one's regional guidelines in caring for the patient.

With this, suggestions are provided to serve as the basis on which to gauge the ICP status (low or high); guidelines for ICP management follow the assessment section.

A list of clinical findings that suggest elevated ICP (i.e., an ICP $\geq$ 20 mm Hg) and their etiology follow. The findings may, however, also be the direct result of an injury or medical problem. ***Examples:*** A large and unreactive pupil may be the direct result of a third nerve injury, a brain stem contusion, or damage from bacteria (cerebritis) and not elevated ICP. Dilated or assymmetric pupils may be a sign of an active or recent seizure (an especially important consideration in the patient receiving neuromuscular relaxants), and consideration must be given to the use of anticonvulsants along with therapy for increased ICP.

Because one cannot usually differentiate the causes with certainty in the emergency/transport situations, it is prudent to proceed with therapy that assumes elevated ICP because the latter problem is potentially treatable and reversible.

A. Findings suggestive of elevated ICP*

1. Glasgow Coma Score ≤ 8 (see p. 437).
2. Signs of brain stem dysfunction in comatose patient
   a. Eyes
      (1) Loss of pupillary constriction to light, especially in the absence of miotic drugs (e.g., narcotics)
      (2) Loss of oculocephalic, oculomotor reflexes
   b. Abnormal central respiratory patterns
   c. Abnormal motor responses to pain (incorporated into Glasgow Coma Score)
3. Acute asymmetric findings in comatose patient
   a. Pupil size, pupil reactivity
   b. Motor response, strength
4. Brain herniation syndromes (see p. 420).

B. Medical management of anticipated or mild ICP elevation

(Glasgow Coma Score ≥ 9, no acute asymmetric neurologic findings)

1. Respiratory status: Provide supplemental oxygen.
   a. Intubate, ventilate as indicated.
2. Restore, maintain circulation.
   a. Restore circulation.
      (1) PVE for hypovolemia: NS or LR solution, 10–20 mL/kg push; repeat until circulation is restored. Must restore MAP and CPP.
      (2) Inotropes for cardiac dysfunction.
3. Head position
   a. Elevate head of bed.
   b. Keep head in midline position as possible.
4. Minimize disturbances, agitation, Valsalva's maneuvers.
5. Use NG tube in obtunded, stuporous, or comatose patient.
6. Keep NPO.
7. IV fluid therapy
   a. Limit fluid volume: 50%–100% maintenance.
   b. IV solution: Use usual solution; it must contain NaCl.

---

*NOTE: Consult your regional PICU for specific recommendations about ICP assessment and subsequent therapy, especially regarding the child suspected to have mild or moderate ICP elevation.

c. Provide volume expanders for hypovolemia.
8. Other medications, where indicated:
   a. Corticosteroid (e.g., dexamethasone, 0.5–1.0 mg/kg/day in 4 divided doses, for peritumor and peri-abscess edema; controversial in meningitis).
   b. Mannitol, 0.25–1.0 gm/kg IV over 10–20 minutes (for edema seen on CAT scan or known to be present in association with metabolic problem as symptomatic water intoxication). Associated measures, warnings:
      (1) Place indwelling bladder catheter.
      (2) For brisk diuresis that causes circulatory compromise, provide LR or NS solution, 10–20 mL/kg IV bolus; repeat as needed to restore MAP, CPP.
      (3) To be used with caution when CNS bleed is present: Abrupt brain shrinkage may disrupt clot, produce increased bleeding. When, however, signs of high ICP are clinically evident (e.g., dilated pupils, posturing, impending herniation) and neurosurgery is not readily available, it must be used, with this information in mind, in the hope of buying time to get the patient to neurosurgery with a viable brain.
9. Treat fever with antipyretics; remove excess coverings.
10. Monitor vital signs, neurologic signs.
11. Treat underlying problem where therapy exists.
    a. Examples: bacterial meningitis, metabolic abnormality, seizure disorder.
12. Obtain CAT scan, if available, while waiting for transport team.

C. **Medical therapy of (suspected) increased ICP**
(For the patient with Glasgow Coma Score ≤ 8; see p. 437 for additional criteria.)
1. Use the measures previously listed in addition to the measures that follow.
2. Intubation, hyperventilation.
   a. Rapid-sequence intubation is highly desirable (see p. 413).

b. Ventilator settings
   (1) Use Fio_2 100%.
   (2) Use higher than normal respiratory rate (see p. 27).
   (3) Use usual tidal volume, 10–15 mL/kg.
   (4) Use PEEP 3–4 mm Hg. Avoid excessively high PEEP. High PEEP must be used as needed for significant pulmonary disease to attain adequate Po_2, but the minimum PEEP that keeps the alveoli adequately inflated should be used.

c. Blood gas goals
   (1) $Po_2 > 100$ mm Hg.
   (2) Pco_2 in 20 to low 30 mm Hg range. It is safe to lower Pco_2 to as low as 20 mm Hg, even high teens, without producing ischemia, hypoxia to the brain.
   (3) pH > 7.35 (up to 7.59).

3. Control of agitation
   a. Sedation for the agitated patient (see p. 26):
      (1) Narcotic (morphine sulfate or fentanyl) and/or
      (2) Benzodiazepine (midazolam, lorazepam or diazepam).
   b. Neuromuscular relaxant: especially useful in the hypertonic or posturing patient (see p. 29).
      (1) Pancuronium or vecuronium.
      (2) Must use in conjunction with sedation.
4. Mannitol:
   0.25–1.0 g/kg IV.
   a. Use with the same considerations listed on p. 122.
5. Barbiturate therapy, induced hypothermia
   a. Not indicated for the emergency department or transport setting. These modalities should be reserved for the patient in a PICU with an ICP monitor and documented ICP hypertension in spite of full therapy.
6. Specific therapy for underlying etiology when present.
   a. Neurosurgical problem: get the patient to neurosurgery as quickly as possible after rapid, essential stabilization.

7. Caveat: Development of dilated, unreactive pupils in the patient receiving a neuromuscular relaxant drug.
   a. Development of large, unreactive pupils may be a sign of herniation and must not be regarded lightly.
   b. They may also be a sign of generalized seizures, especially in the patient in whom herniation was not anticipated (e.g., the patient given a neuromuscular relaxant for ventilatory control); may have associated tachycardia, diaphoresis suggesting seizure.
   c. After appropriate evaluation for herniation, a trial of anticonvulsant therapy (e.g., a benzodiazepine) for a suspected seizure may help determine this. Pupils become smaller and reactive, heart rate usually decreases when the cause was a seizure. When this occurs, follow with a loading dose of a long-acting anticonvulsant (e.g., phenytoin or phenobarbital, 20 mg/kg IV).

VI. Status Epilepticus

A. Overview

Status epilepticus is a commonly encountered critical care problem in pediatrics. Although the control of seizures is the primary concern, several distinct medical problems that also need attention commonly exist concomitantly during an episode of status epilepticus:

1. Seizures.
2. The primary problem, if any, that caused the seizure.
3. Associated problems
   a. Respiratory: major problems.
      (1) Central hypoventilation or apnea.
      (2) Airway obstruction: nasal or upper airway.
      (3) Aspiration.
   b. Sympathetic stimulation.
      (1) Fever, tachycardia, hypertension.

A review of patients with status epilepticus at Children's Hospital Oakland[1] provides a good perspective of this problem in children:

1. Age: Most patients are young. 61% were <3 years old, 73% were <5 years old.
2. The episode of status epilepticus was the patient's initial seizure in 71% of the cases.

3. A large percentage of the patients required intubation and ventilation. Hypoventilation and apnea are fairly common in pediatric status epilepticus. (NOTE: This was a tertiary pediatric center's experience.)
4. The mortality rate from status epilepticus was 6%. Some of the deaths took place at times long after the episode of status epilepticus and were not directly caused by status epilepticus.
5. Etiology of status epilepticus differed significantly by age groups:

    a. Children < 1 year: Identifiable acute causes predominate.
        (1) Acute causes: 75%.
            (a) Meningitis: 28%.
            (b) Metabolic: 30%. Hyponatremia is a major cause; hypoglycemia and hypocalcemia are less common causes.
    b. Children 1–3 years
        (1) Acute causes: 47%.
            (a) Meningitis: 15%.
            (b) Sodium abnormalities: 13%.
        (2) Idiopathic: 32%.
    c. Children >3 years
        (1) Acute causes: 28%; numerous etiologies.
            (a) Head trauma: 8%; leading single acute cause.
        (2) Known seizure disorders: 38%.
            (a) Subtherapeutic anticonvulsant level: 25%.
        (3) Idiopathic: 13%.

Significant respiratory problems are commonly encountered in status epilepticus. The most common problem is upper airway obstruction, which can occur during the seizure, as well as in the postictal period. The tongue may obstruct the airway during the seizure. Mucus or vomitus in the nostrils of a young infant who is still an obligate nose breather can produce obstruction at the nasal level. Poor airway muscle tone in the postictal period commonly obstructs the airway and may require positioning efforts (jaw thrust), an oral airway or an endotracheal tube to restore airway patency. Aspiration of emesis or upper airway secretions is common.

After obstruction, the most pressing respiratory problem during the emergency phase is central hypoventilation or apnea, which is not uncommon in children. This may occur during the seizure or in the period that immediately follows. It can also occur in association with the administration of anticonvulsants. Hypoventilation ranges in severity from mild or moderate, where stimulation or bag-valve-mask ventilation suffices to support the patient for the transient problem, to severe, where the pH can fall to values as low as 6.9 and Pco_2 levels rise to levels greater than 100 mm Hg. Intubation and mechanical ventilation are required for the latter situation.

In the majority of situations, the hypoventilation or apnea is transient, resolving in 6 to 24 hours, unless it occurs in association with major head injuries or disease. Also, if the seizure is not associated with major head injury or disease, the presence of hypoventilation does not appear to have significant predictive value on the severity of the seizure disorder, and the patients appear to have no significant sequelae after receiving appropriate support.

Therapy of patients with status epilepticus must therefore frequently address three specific concerns: seizure control, respiratory function, and the underlying problem, when known. *The approach to therapy, in order of priority, is:*

1. Respiratory intervention to maintain oxygen delivery.
2. Control of seizures.
3. Therapy of the underlying problem.

Before therapy of status epilepticus is listed, anticonvulsant guidelines are provided:

1. The IV route is the preferred route of medication administration in status epilepticus. The IM or rectal routes can be used for certain medications when IV access is not available.
2. It is frequently recommended that a rapidly acting drug be used as the first-line anticonvulsant to stop seizures in the actively seizing patient. This should be followed by the administration of a long-acting anticonvulsant because the anticonvulsant activity of first-line drugs is usually short lived.
3. Loading doses of long-acting anticonvulsants are given to rapidly achieve therapeutic drug levels. Serum levels

higher than those routinely aimed for may need to be used when usual drug levels fail to control seizures.

4. When seizures persist, administer a loading dose of an anticonvulsant before proceeding to a second long-acting anticonvulsant. It is generally not effective to administer small doses of several anticonvulsants to the patient with status epilepticus.
5. In all instances, one must be prepared to intervene if the patient develops hypoventilation or hypotension after administration of an anticonvulsant.

B. Therapy

1. Respiratory support
   a. Provide supplemental oxygen, Fio_2 100%.
   b. Relieve upper airway obstruction (UAO).
      (1) For UAO secondary to tongue, altered airway muscle tone, mucus:
         (a) Chin lift, jaw thrust, oral airway or intubation.
         (b) Suction airway.
      (2) For nasal obstruction in young infants: Clear nostrils; intubate if clearing fails.
   c. Central hypoventilation, apnea. May find pH as low as 6.9, $Pco_2 > 100$ mm Hg; Po_2 value is usually good with supplemental Fio_2.
      (1) Bag-valve-mask ventilation until resolved.
      (2) Intubation, mechanical ventilation for marked blood gas abnormalities and/or prolonged hypoventilation.
2. Anticonvulsant therapy
   a. First-line, rapidly acting drugs to stop seizure
      (1) Lorazepam (Ativan): 0.05–0.2 mg/kg IV or IM; maximum dose 8 mg at once.
         (a) May repeat dose in 15–30min once.
         (b) Side effects: hypoventilation, apnea (less common than with diazepam); hypotension may occur.
      (2) Diazepam (Valium): 0.1–0.4 mg/kg IV; maximum dose 10 mg at once.
         (a) Repeat dose q15–20min × 2 if needed.
         (b) Side effects: hypoventilation, apnea (quite common), hypotension (less common).

b. Long-acting anticonvulsant to follow first-line drug
   (1) Phenobarbital: 20 mg/kg loading dose IV or IM. May also be used as a first-line drug.
      (a) Loading dose in neonate or small infant may need to be 30 mg/kg to produce therapeutic levels. Suggest giving 20 mg/kg, followed by 10 mg/kg.
      (b) Rate of administration: over 10–20 minutes IV.
      (c) Side effects
         (i) CNS and respiratory depression. These are not problems for the patient with an intubated airway.
         (ii) Hypotension.
      (d) For resistant status epilepticus, a total loading dose of 40–50 mg/kg in 10 mg/kg additional increments may be needed to control seizures. Be prepared to provide respiratory support when using these doses.
      (e) When phenobarbital and benzodiazepines are used concurrently, respiratory depression is potentiated and hypotension may occur. Be prepared to treat these problems.
   (2) Phenytoin (Dilantin): 20 mg/kg IV loading dose; maximum dose 1,000 mg at once. Do not use IM.
      (a) Rate of administration: 1–2 mg/kg/min (loading dose over 10–20 minutes). Faster rate can produce profound cardiac complications.
      (b) Side effect: can produce significant hypotension, dysrhythmias, especially bradydysrhythmias. Therefore, monitor heart rate, heart rhythm, BP.
      (c) Avoid interaction between phenytoin and glucose in an IV solution: Interaction rapidly produces crystalline precipitate, which completely occludes IV line. To avoid this problem, clear the IV line well with saline solution before and after administration of phenytoin.
      (d) Advantage over phenobarbital: produces little CNS and respiratory depression.

These advantages make it the anticonvulsant of choice for head trauma patients with seizures whose airways are not intubated.

c. Options for failure of a loading dose to control seizures
   (1) Proceed to a second long-acting anticonvulsant. Administer a loading dose of the second anticonvulsant. Add other anticonvulsants in similar manner as needed (e.g., diazepam, lorazepam).
   (2) Use higher than usual doses to achieve supertherapeutic drug levels when associated side effects are acceptable.
      (a) Phenobarbital is effective, relatively safe for this situation. The primary problem, hypoventilation, can be compensated for well with intubation, ventilation.
      (b) The benzodiazepines can be used in like manner. Again, mechanical respiratory support will probably be necessary.

d. Rectal anticonvulsants: generally used when IV access is not possible; may be used as additional anticonvulsant when standard measures fail to control seizures.
   (1) Rectal diazepam: Use when IV route is not available.
      (a) Dose: 0.2–0.5 mg/kg PR.
   (2) Rectal paraldehyde: Use after standard anticonvulsants fail to control seizures. Concentration: 1 g/mL.
      (a) Dose: 0.3 mL (300 mg)/kg/dose mixed 1:1 with cottonseed or olive oil. Maximum dose 5 mL.
   (3) Rectal valproate (Depakane). Concentration: 250 mg/5 mL.
      (a) Dose: 20 mg/kg PR mixed 1:1 with water.

3. Treat fever.
   a. Acetaminophen: 10–15 mg/kg NG or PR.
   b. Ibuprofen: 10–15 mg/kg NG if acetaminophen is insufficient.
   c. Remove excess coverings.

4. Diagnostic studies: considerations, suggestions
   a. History and physical examination
   b. Blood work
      (1) For initial seizure:
         (a) Electrolytes, glucose, calcium, magnesium, blood urea nitrogen (BUN), and creatinine levels, complete blood cell count (CBC), and differential.
         (b) Consider toxicology screen, aspartate aminotransferase (AST), alanine aminotransferase (ALT), and ammonia levels, and blood culture.
      (2) For known seizure disorder:
         (a) Electrolyte levels, glucose level, CBC count, anticonvulsant level; other labs as indicated.
   c. Lumbar puncture for suspected meningitis, encephalitis.
   d. CAT scan of the head for trauma, other suspected structural abnormalities.
5. Treat the underlying problem that caused the seizure.
   a. Infection, metabolic abnormality, for example.

VII. Approach to Unconscious Child

A. Etiologies of unconsciousness

1. Common etiologies
   a. Ingestion
   b. Infection: meningitis, sepsis
   c. Head trauma
   d. Seizure or postictal state
   e. Respiratory failure
   f. Shock
   g. Hypoglycemia
   h. Diabetic ketoacidosis
2. Less common etiologies
   a. Intussusception
   b. Other metabolic aberration, including Reye's syndrome
   c. Intracranial catastrophe: tumor, nontraumatic bleed

B. Immediate therapy

1. Assure airway patency; protect cervical spine in trauma.

2. Provide respiratory assistance if needed.
3. Assure adequate circulation.
4. Obtain test-strip glucose assessment; administer 0.25 g/kg glucose if needed.
5. Administer naloxone, 0.01–0.10 mg/kg IV or IM.
6. Evaluate for increased ICP (see p. 420); evaluate Glasgow Coma Score (see p. 437).

C. **Further emergent assessment and treatment**
1. Obtain history to evaluate etiology. If etiology is clear, see relevant section for evaluation and treatment.
2. If etiology is unclear:
   a. Obtain electrolytes, BUN, creatinine, ALT, AST, and NH_3 levels; serum, urine, and gastric toxicology screen (regardless of negative history for poisons in home).
   b. Consider blood cultures, lumbar puncture (only if the patient is *stable* with no evidence of increased ICP), CAT scan.
   c. Consider starting broad-spectrum antibiotics.
3. Monitor patient continuously for changes in respiratory, cardiac, and neurologic status.

REFERENCE

1. Phillips SA, Shanahan RJ: Etiology and mortality of status epilepticus in children: A recent update. *Arch Neurol* 1989; 46:74.

RENAL, METABOLIC, AND ENDOCRINE DISORDERS 6

I. Fluids and Electrolytes

A. Basic fluid and electrolyte requirements

Fluid and electrolyte administration must be tailored to meet the specific needs of children. It is worth spending time to be certain that both appropriate fluid solutions and volumes are given, because something as seemingly simple as intravenous (IV) fluid administration can, especially in children, create tremendous iatrogenic problems when administered improperly.

There are several ways in which fluid needs can be determined. A simple and widely used method based on patient weight is presented and used in this chapter. Two other basic fluid and electrolyte guidelines are provided.

1. *24-hour fluid requirements*
   a. 100 mL/kg: for first 10 kg of weight
   b. +50 mL/kg: for second 10 kg of weight
   c. +20 mL/kg: for remaining weight >20 kg
   See Appendix II–2, p. 424, with precalculated values.
2. *Fluid utilization: per 100 mL:*
   a. Evaporative (insensible)
      (1) Skin: 35
      (2) Lungs: 15
   b. Urine: 50
   c. Stool:
   d. Water of oxidation: −10

3. *Electrolyte requirements:*
   a. Sodium: 2–3 mEq/100 mL fluid
   b. Potassium: 2–3 mEq/100 mL fluid

      The electrolyte requirements translate to 20–30 mEq of Na^+ and K^+/L. IV solutions that closely meet Na^+ and K^+ requirements are *D_5 – ¼NS + 20–30 mEq of KCl/L or D_5–⅓NS + 20–30 mEq of KCl/L. These are usual maintenance IV solutions.* **Do not use plain D_5W in children!**

B. Fluid therapy

1. Fluid volume: calculate appropriate volume using the previously mentioned formula.
2. Fluid composition: Maintenance IV solutions.
   a. Essential components
      (1) Dextrose: usually 5%.
      (2) Sodium chloride: a very important constitutent of IV fluids; virtually any administered IV fluid in children should contain NaCl.
         (a) IV fluids that contain no NaCl can produce severe, symptomatic hyponatremia in children and must be avoided except in very rare situations. Specifically, 5% aqueous dextrose solution (D_5W) must not be used for maintenance: The net contents administered after the dextrose is used is free water. Therefore, *do not give plain D_5W to children.*
   b. Additional IV components
      (1) Potassium chloride is a usual additive.
      (2) Other modifications in fluid composition are made as needed.
   c. Usual maintenance IV solutions
      (1) D_5–¼NS + 20–30 mEq KCl/L.
      (2) D_5–⅓NS + 20–30 mEq KCl/L.
3. Modified fluid requirements
   a. Restricted fluid rates: Fluid volume administration is reduced for conditions where water needs are decreased; common conditions are listed. As a starting point, fluid volumes are commonly reduced to 50%–75% of the usual maintenance volume.
      (1) Syndrome of inappropriate secretion of antidiuretic hormone (SIADH) (see p. 171).

(2) Congestive heart failure, fluid overload.
(3) Renal failure with oliguria or anuria.

b. Extra fluid requirements
(1) Dehydration: Administered fluid volumes are the sum of maintenance fluid plus deficit fluid volumes (see p. 139).
(2) Special conditions (e.g., hemoglobinuria).

C. Calculation of fluid volumes

1. Calculation of maintenance fluid volumes
   a. 8 kg child

$$8 \text{ kg} \times 100 \text{ mL/kg} = 800 \text{ mL/24 hours} = 33 \text{ mL/hour}$$

   b. 15 kg child

$$\begin{array}{rl} 10 \text{ kg} \times 100 \text{ mL/kg} = & 1{,}000 \text{ mL} \\ + 5 \text{ kg} \times 50 \text{ mL/kg} = & 250 \text{ mL} \\ \hline & 1{,}250 \text{ mL/24hours} = 52 \text{ mL/hour} \end{array}$$

   c. 70 kg adult

$$\begin{array}{rl} 10 \text{ kg} \times 100 \text{ mL/kg} = & 1{,}000 \text{ mL} \\ + 10 \text{ kg} \times 50 \text{ mL/kg} = & 500 \text{ mL} \\ + 50 \text{ kg} \times 20 \text{ mL/kg} = & 1{,}000 \text{ mL} \\ \hline & 2{,}500 \text{ mL/24 hours} = 104 \text{ mL/hour} \end{array}$$

2. Calculation of restricted fluid volume: 9 kg child with bacterial meningitis. Child is to be restricted to two-thirds maintenance fluids after circulation is adequate.
   a. First calculate maintenance volume:

$$\text{Maintenance fluid volume} = 9 \text{ kg} \times 100 \text{ mL/kg} = 900 \text{ mL/24 hours}$$

   b. Next multiply maintenance volume by degree of restriction desired to obtain restricted volume:

$$\tfrac{2}{3} \text{ maintenance fluids} = \tfrac{2}{3} \times 900 \text{ mL/24 hours} = 600 \text{ mL/24 hours} = 25 \text{ mL/hour}$$

3. Calculation of extra fluid volume: 8 kg child needs 1.5 times maintenance fluids.
   a. First calculate maintenance volume:

$$\text{Maintenance fluids} = \\ 8 \text{ kg} \times 100 \text{ mL/kg} = 800 \text{ mL/24 hours}$$

   b. Multiply this volume by the amount over maintenance desired:

$$1.5 \times \text{maintenance fluids} = \\ 1.5 \times 800 \text{ mL/24 hours} = \\ 1{,}200 \text{ mL/24 hours} = 50 \text{ mL/hour}$$

D. Dehydration

Dehydration is a commonly encountered problem in pediatrics because of several factors, including the greater fluid needs of children on a weight basis, the common occurrence of gastroenteritis in young children, and the anorexia that commonly accompanies illness in young children.

Dehydration is important because it can lead to shock, severe metabolic problems, and death. Therefore, assessment of the severity of dehydration is important.

Dehydration can be assessed in two ways: (1) by weight change, when weights before and during the dehydration episode are available; and (2) by clinical assessment based on the constellation of physical findings that are commonly associated with each of the three classes of dehydration. All weight lost during the acute phase of illness (e.g., from gastroenteritis) is assumed to be the result of water loss. This water loss is termed the *fluid deficit,* which must be replaced during therapy.

Clinical assessments of dehydration are only *estimates* of the magnitude of fluid deficits but serve the important function of providing the initial assessment of the severity of dehydration on which the rehydration plan is formulated. Because the clinical assessment is only an estimate of fluid deficits, the patient must be evaluated carefully during rehydration therapy for any overestimates or underestimates of fluid deficit; plans must be reformulated when the patient does not respond to therapy in the expected manner.

Therefore, dehydration is assessed to be *mild, moderate,* or *severe*. In terms of weight loss, these categories correspond with 5%, 10%, and 15% dehydration (weight loss) in infants and young toddlers; the categories correspond with 3%, 6%, and 9% dehydration in older children and adults.

Clinical signs associated with the three categories of dehydration are provided in Table 6–1. The clinical finding of greatest threat to the patient is usually circulatory compromise. Those with moderate dehydration have clinical signs of impaired perfusion but are not hypotensive, whereas those with severe dehydration have decompensated shock (i.e., are hypotensive and moribund). In each of these situations, restoration of circulation with fluids takes first priority.

1. Assessment: Examples
   a. Dehydration assessment by weight

      Example: A 10 kg child develops recurrent emesis and anorexia; 2 days later his weight is 9 kg.

Weight loss = Fluid deficit = 10 kg − 9 kg = 1 kg

% dehydration = weight loss/usual weight = 1 kg/10 kg
= 10% dehydration
Fluid deficit = 1,000 mL

   b. Dehydration assessment based on clinical findings

      The child just described comes in and has no known previous weight. History is as described, plus the observation that he has a decreased number of wet diapers.

      Physical findings include weight 9 kg, tachycardia, normal blood pressure (BP), lethargy, decreased skin turgor, very dry mucous membranes, cool extremities, and fair pulses.

      Clinical assessment includes moderate dehydration (i.e., about 10% dehydration). Therefore, the fluid deficit is 10% of the child's weight, 0.9 kg or 900 mL.

      NOTE: Fluid therapy can be based on either the ideal (predehydration weight) or dehydrated weight. In the previous patient, the difference in the fluid deficit calculated by each method amounts to 100 mL = 0.1 kg, or 1%, of this patient's weight. This difference is a clinically insignificant value, an amount of fluid excess or deficit that one can tolerate without problems. Calculation of fluid therapy based on ideal vs. dehy-

TABLE 6–1.
Clinical Assessment of Dehydration

Clinical Parameter	Mild	Moderate	Severe
Weight loss			
Infant	5%	10%	15%
Older child	3%	6%	9%
Skin turgor	± Decreased	Decreased	Poor; tents
Mucous membranes	Dry	Very dry	Parched
Urine output	± Low	Oliguric	Oliguric/anuric
Heart rate	Mildly elevated	Elevated	Very elevated
Blood pressure	Normal	± Normal	Decreased to absent
Perfusion	± Prolonged capillary refill time	Prolonged capillary refill time	Very prolonged capillary refill time
Skin color	Pale	Gray	Mottled, blue, or white
Level of consciousness	Irritable, otherwise normal	Lethargic	Very lethargic to comatose

drated weights results in differences that do not exceed 1% to 1.5% body weight.

2. Dehydration presents two primary problems:
   a. Water loss: Problems range from dehydration to hypovolemic shock.
   b. Electrolyte losses: Electrolyte, primarily Na^+, imbalance may result. Types of dehydration are:
      (1) Isotonic (isonatremic) dehydration: Na^+ 130–150 mEq/L; 65%–75% of cases.
      (2) Hypernatremic dehydration: $Na^+ > 150$ mEq/L.
      (3) Hyponatremic dehydration: $Na^+ < 130$ mEq/L.

   Therapy of dehydration is aimed at correcting both the water and electrolyte deficits. The IV solution that most closely matches the water and electrolyte losses is selected to correct the deficits. Table 6–2 lists the water and electrolyte losses that have been observed in balance studies; the right-hand column of the table indicates the IV solution that is used to replace the deficit.

3. IV therapy

   The general approach to therapy of dehydration is the replacement of water, Na^+, and much of the K^+ deficit over 12 to 24 hours (an important exception to this general approach is hypernatremic dehydration). There are numerous ways in which this can be accomplished; no one regimen has any notable major advantages over others. A fairly simple method of rehydration is presented in this section. First, some points about rehydration that need emphasis follow.

   a. Fluid volume: Fluid volume needs for the first 24 hours of therapy must include both (1) the deficit volume and (2) the ongoing maintenance fluid needs.
   b. Fluid administration: The fluid must be administered in several phases according to patient needs. Common phases of fluid administration in rehydration are:
      (1) Emergency phase: Fluid (volume expander) is provided rapidly to restore circulating volume and circulation.
      (2) Replacement of deficit volume.
      (3) Administration of maintenance fluids: In some rehydration regimens this phase is combined with the replacement of deficit volume.

TABLE 6–2.

Water and Electrolyte Losses in Dehydration

Type of Dehydration	Losses in 10%–12% Dehydration (Amount/kg)				Replacement IV Solution for Water/Electrolyte Losses*
	Water Losses (mL)	Na^+ (mEq)	K^+ (mEq)	Cl^- (mEq)	
Isonatremic	100–120	8–10	8–10	8–10	D_5-½NS + K^+†
Hyponatremic	100–120	10–12	8–10	10–12	D_5NS + K^+†
Hypernatremic‡	100–120	2–4	0–4	2–6	D_5-¼NS + K^+† or D_5-⅓NS + K^+†

*D_5-½NS = 5% dextrose in 0.50 normal saline solution; D_5NS = 5% dextrose in normal saline solution; D_5-¼NS = 5% dextrose in 0.25 normal saline solution; D_5-⅓NS = 5% dextrose in 0.33 normal saline solution.

†Potassium deficits take more than 24 hr to be corrected because the upper concentration of K^+ is usually limited to 40 mEq/L.

‡Hypernatremic dehydration requires very special management to prevent complications.

4. **Suggested approach**

NOTE: The following approach applies to only *isonatremic* and *hyponatremic dehydration*. *Hypernatremic dehydration* requires very different therapy and is reviewed separately on p. 151.

a. Assessment
   (1) Assess severity of dehydration.
      (a) Obtain assessment by weight change or clinical picture.
      (b) Calculate fluid deficit after severity of dehydration is assessed.
   (2) Obtain laboratory work.
      (a) Electrolyte values: Na^+ value indicates the tonicity of dehydration.
      (b) Complete blood cell (CBC) count, blood urea nitrogen (BUN) level, and creatinine: Provide corroborative evidence for severity of dehydration.
      (c) Glucose level, calcium level, and other laboratory tests as indicated.

b. Fluid therapy: 24-hour plan
   (1) Emergency phase: Restore compromised circulation if present.
      (a) Provide lactated Ringer's (LR) or NS solution 20 mL/kg IV *push*.
         (i) Repeat 10–20 mL/kg pushes until circulation is restored. Up to 60 mL/kg total may be needed in severe dehydration.
      (b) LR or NS solution is used to restore circulation regardless of the type of dehydration present. Therefore, one can use either solution without worry when electrolyte values are not available.
   (2) Replacement of deficit volume: follows emergency phase
      (a) For this regimen, the deficit volume is replaced in the first 12 hours of therapy.
         (i) Calculate deficit volume (X).
         (ii) Subtract the amount of fluid given to restore the circulation (Y) from the deficit volume.

(iii) The remaining volume (X − Y) is administered IV over 12 hours. The hourly IV rate is (X − Y)/12.

(b) IV solution: Select the rehydration solution appropriate for the type of dehydration present (see Table 6–2.)

(3) Administration of maintenance fluids: to follow administration of deficit volume

(a) Calculate maintenance fluid needs.

(b) Select usual maintenance IV solution.

(i) Modify fluid composition for existing electrolyte imbalances.

(a) Modify Na^+ content according to serum Na^+ value.

(b) K^+ content will probably need to be higher than usual because the K^+ deficit usually requires more than 24 hours to be corrected.

(c) This volume is to be administered IV over 12 hours.

c. Patient monitoring during rehydration

(1) Physical assessment

(a) Vital signs: especially heart rate, BP, pulses, and perfusion.

(b) Mucous membranes, tissue turgor.

(c) Level of consciousness.

(2) Urine output.

(3) Weight.

(4) Laboratory tests

(a) Electrolyte values.

(b) CBC count, BUN level, creatinine, other tests as needed.

(5) Be prepared to modify rehydration regimen if patient response veers from expected course.

Case example: infant with 10% isotonic dehydration: A 1-year-old child has a 2-day history of diarrhea and vomiting. Weight is 10 kg, temperature 38.5°C, heart rate 160 beats/min, respiratory rate 40, and BP 90/65. He is lethargic but rouses appropriately with stimulation. Extremities are cool to touch, color is grayish, and pulses are fair. Mucous membranes are dry; skin turgor is diminished. A wet diaper reveals scant volume, very concentrated appearance. Recent weight is not known. Laboratory results are Na^+ 138, K^+ 4.2, Cl^- 105, HCO_3^- 15mEq/L; hemoglobin (Hgb) 13.5 g, hematocrit (Hct) 41%; BUN 29 mg/dL, creatinine 1.2 mg/dL; glucose 126 mg/dL.

a. Assessment: (1) moderate dehydration (i.e., 10% dehydration) with signs of early shock; (2) isotonic (isonatremic) dehydration.

b. Fluid deficit = Weight × % Dehydration = 10 Kg × 0.1 = 1 kg or 1,000 mL fluid.

c. Treatment plan

   (1) *Fluid volumes*

      (a) Deficit volume: 1,000 mL.

      (b) Maintenance volume for 10 kg: 1,000 mL.

   (2) *IV solutions*

      (a) Deficit replacement solution: 5% dextrose in 0.50 NS solution + K^+, probably 30–40 mEq KCl/L.

      (b) Maintenance solution: 5% dextrose in 0.33 NS solution + K^+ or 5% dextrose in 0.25 NS solution + K^+. K^+ will probably be 30–40 mEq/L because K^+ deficit is not likely to have been corrected by this time.

      (c) Volume expander solution: LR or NS solution will be used to restore circulating volume. In this case, assume that 20 mL/kg (i.e., 200 mL) LR solution was needed to improve circulation.

   (3) *Fluid regimen plans*

      (a) Emergency phase: 200 mL LR solution (20 mL/kg) is given as a push; adequate circulation results.

      (b) Replacement of deficit

         (i) Deficit to be replaced over 12 hours

            (a) Remaining deficit volume: 1,000 mL − 200 mL = 800 mL.

            (b) Deficit volume to be administered at rate of 800 mL/12 hours = 67 mL/hour × 12 hours.

         (ii) IV solution for isonatremic dehydration: 5% dextrose in 0.50 NS solution + KCl, probably 30–40 mEqKCl/L.

(iii) Summary of replacement therapy: 5% dextrose in 0.50 NS solution + 30–40 mEq KCl/L to run at 67 mL/hour for 12 hours.

(c) Administration of maintenance fluids

(i) 24-hour maintenance fluids are to be administered IV over next 12 hours.

(ii) Maintenance fluids for 10 kg: 1,000 mL.

(a) Maintenance fluid to be administered at a rate of 1,000 mL/12 hours: 83 mL/hour for 12 hours.

(iii) IV solution for maintenance: 5% dextrose in 0.25 or 0.33 NS solution + KCl, probably 30–40 mEq/L. Extra KCl is needed to continue to replace K^+ deficits.

(iv) Summary of administration of maintenance fluids: 5% dextrose in 0.25 or 0.33 NS solution + 30–40 mEqKCl/L to run at 83 mL/hour for 12 hours.

(d) Fluid therapy (volumes, composition) will be modified in response to patient course, follow-up laboratory values.

5. **Hyponatremic dehydration**

Approach to therapy is the same as presented in the case for isonatremic dehydration except for the following changes:

a. Deficit replacement solution is 5% dextrose in NS solution + K^+. The Na^+ concentration used for hyponatremic dehydration is greater than that used for isonatremic dehydration.

b. If hyponatremia is severe and produces significant central nervous system (CNS) symptoms, the serum Na^+ must be acutely raised (see p. 166).

6. **Hypernatremic dehydration**

Hypernatremic dehydration requires very special considerations. It is reviewed in full on p. 151.

7. **Clinical effects of Na^+ values on fluid distribution**

Dehydration presents two major problems.

The first is the fluid deficit, which, when severe, causes shock. Assessment and correction of the fluid deficit have been reviewed.

The second problem is the electrolyte status, notably the Na^+ value. The differentiation of dehydration into isonatremic, hyponatremic, and hypernatremic states has been alluded to; the deficits incurred in each type of dehydration and the replacement fluids have been reviewed. In addition to the differing Na^+ deficits, the Na^+ value is important because (1) abnormal Na^+ values affect CNS function and produce CNS problems, and (2) the Na^+ value affects fluid distribution and can alter the vascular volume status and assessment of dehydration. The effect of Na^+ values on fluid distribution is illustrated in the following diagrams.

The rules that regulate fluid distribution and explain the diagrams follow. Fluid in the body can be divided into two compartments: the intracellular and extracellular compartments, which are separated by the cell membrane. The cell membrane is semipermeable: Water can cross it freely, but most other substances are prohibited free access across it. The extracellular compartment is further subdivided into two subcompartments: the interstitial fluid and vascular subcompartments. Maintenance of the vascular compartment volume is critical to maintain good cardiac function and good cardiac output.

Fluid distribution is regulated by the following two principles:

1. The cations in each compartment differ. Na^+ is the primary cation in the extracellular fluid (ECF), K^+ is the primary cation in the intracellular fluid (ICF). The Na^+-K^+ pump in the cell membrane maintains the cation difference.

2. The osmolalities (i.e., number of particles) of the two compartments must be equal at all times. If the osmolalities are not equal, water will move across the cell membrane to equalize the osmolalities; water moves from the compartment with low osmolality to high osmolality.

Serum osmolality is normally 280–290 and can be calculated from the Na^+, glucose, and BUN values. Serum osmolality = $(2 \times Na^+)$ + glucose/18 + BUN/2.8. In a normal child with Na^+ 140 mEq/L, glucose 80 mg/dL, BUN 9 mg/dL, the serum osmolality = $(2 \times 140) + 80/18 + 9/2.8$, which is approximately 287. The greatest determinant of serum osmolality is Na^+. In the cell, K^+ is

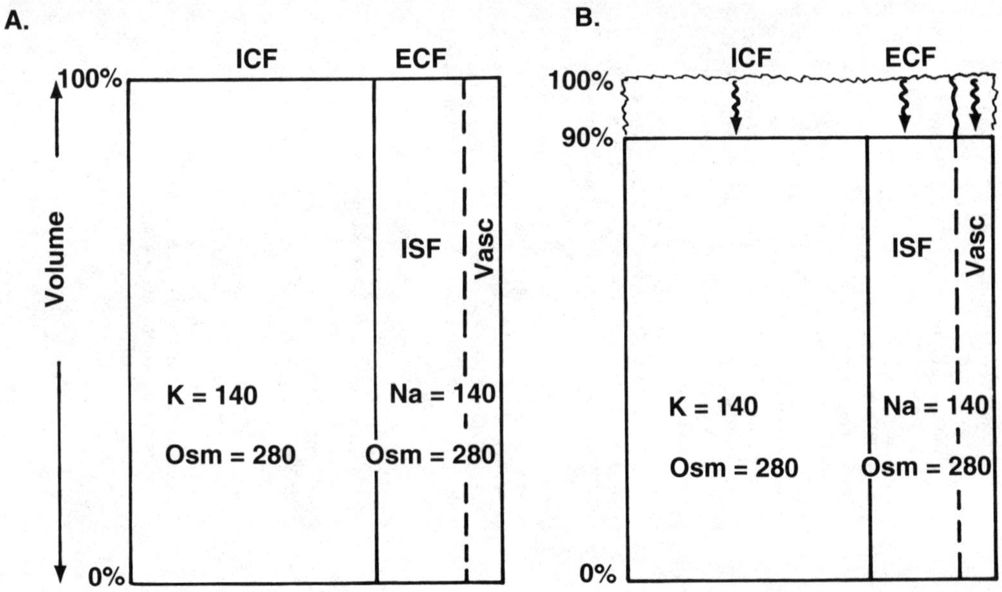

A.

ICF

ECF

100%

Volume

ISF

Vasc

K = 140

Osm = 280

Na = 140

Osm = 280

0%

B.

ICF

ECF

100%

90%

ISF

Vasc

K = 140

Osm = 280

Na = 140

Osm = 280

0%

approximately 150 mEq/L, and K^+ is the greatest determinant of intracellular osmolality. For ease of presentation, the following values will be used: normal serum Na^+ and intracellular K^+ will be 140 mEq/L; the normal serum and intracellular osmolalities will be 280 mEq/L, i.e. ($2 \times Na^+$) and ($2 \times K^+$), respectively (Fig 6–1).

In each of the diagrams, the infant has 10% dehydration. The fluid compartments are indicated. Volume status is indicated on the y-axis.

Isonatremic (isotonic) dehydration (see Fig 6–1): The fluid loss is evenly distributed among all compartments: Each compartment has lost 10% of its volume. The reduction in the vascular compartment volume is sufficient to produce clinical signs of early shock: Findings are likely to include cool extremities, gray to mottled color, increased capillary refill time, beginning appearance of diminished distal pulses, and tenting of the skin.

Hypernatremic (hypertonic) dehydration (Fig 6–2): The same amount of fluid has been lost as in the other states. However, the increased serum Na^+ increases the serum osmolality. Because the serum osmolality is greater than the intracellular osmolality, fluid moves from the in-

---

FIG 6–1.

A, normal hydration:

1. Normal water distribution:
   a. Total body water = 60% body weight.
   b. Intracellular fluid (ICF) = 40% body weight.
   c. Extracellular fluid (ECF) = 20% body weight.
   ISF = interstitial fluid; Vasc = vascular fluid.
2. Assumptions (for illustrations):
   a. ECF Na = 140.
   b. ICF K = 140.
   c. ECF Osm = 2 × Na = 280.
   d. ICF Osm = 2 × K = 280.

B, isotonic dehydration 10%:

1. Osmolalities are unchanged; therefore water losses are proportionate in all compartments.
2. Significant reduction in vascular volume produces hypovolemic shock.

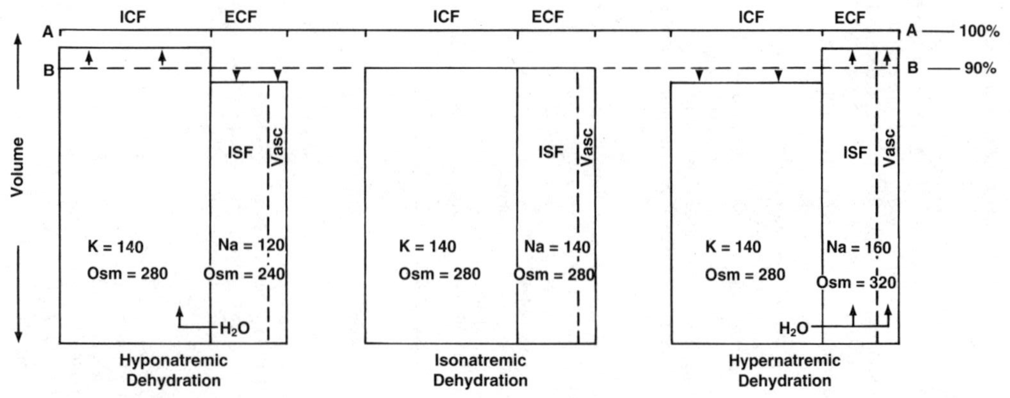
ICF
ECF
ICF
ECF
ICF
ECF
A
A — 100%
B
B — 90%
Volume
ISF
Vasc
K = 140
Osm = 280
Na = 120
Osm = 240
H₂O
ISF
Vasc
K = 140
Osm = 280
Na = 140
Osm = 280
ISF
Vasc
K = 140
Osm = 280
Na = 160
Osm = 320
H₂O
Hyponatremic Dehydration
Isonatremic Dehydration
Hypernatremic Dehydration

tracellular compartment into the extracellular compartment to equalize the osmolalites. The results of the fluid shift are two. First, a smaller portion of the fluid loss comes from the ECF; the vascular (ECF) compartment volume is relatively well preserved, hence the observation that shock is a late finding in hypernatremic dehydration and that the degree of dehydration (water loss) is frequently underestimated on clinical assessment. Second, a greater proportion of fluid is lost from the intracellular compartment. If the ICF box is taken to represent the cranium, the shrinkage of the ICF compartment represents shrinkage of the brain; the brain pulls away from the cranium, bridging vessels between the two structures are stretched, and tearing and bleeding of the bridging vessels can result. Because the brain is rich in thromboplastin, thrombosis of cerebral vessels may follow the tears. CNS symptoms originate from the effects of hypernatremia on CNS cell function, as well as from vascular insults; the latter insults may produce permanent CNS damage.

Hyponatremic (hypotonic) dehydration (see Fig 6–2): The low Na^+ level causes the serum osmolality to fall. The serum osmolality is lower than intracellular osmolality, so fluid moves from the ECF compartment into the ICF compartment. The major clinical result of the fluid shift is the reduction of the ECF compartment volume, notably the vascular compartment volume. Shock

---

FIG 6–2.

Ten percent dehydration. Effects of Na on fluid distribution.

Hyponatremic dehydration:

1. Water moves from ECF to ICF to equalize osmolalities.
2. Result: greater loss of water from vascular compartment and earlier manifestation of shock.

Isonatremic dehydration:

1. Water losses are proportionate in all compartments. No fluid shift occurs.

Hypernatremic dehydration:

1. Water moves from ICF to ECF to equalize osmolalities.
2. Result: better preservation of vascular compartment and later manifestation of shock.

therefore appears early in hyponatremic dehydration; for a given amount of volume loss, shock will appear sooner in hyponatremic dehydration than in isonatremic or hypernatremic dehydration because of the fluid shifts; clinical assessment of the degree of dehydration therefore tends to be overestimated in hyponatremic states. CNS symptoms may also appear on the basis of altered CNS function from hyponatremia. Fluid does move from the ECF into the cells, but the brain usually does not swell to the point of producing intracranial pressure (ICP) elevation because cell volume (brain size) was low secondary to dehydration. (In contrast, hyponatremia caused by water excess, i.e., water intoxication, intracranial hypertension and the risk of brain herniation exist because the cell/brain volume is greater than normal.)

The fluid shifts account for the differences in timing in the appearance of shock and the alteration in assessment of degree of dehydration. They also explain the CNS findings found in states of dehydration. The altered osmolality states are reviewed individually later in the chapter.

E. Hypernatremia

Hypernatremia can produce several clinically significant problems that affect the CNS: (1) CNS dysfunction caused by Na^+ abnormality alone, (2) CNS damage through vascular insults (e.g., tears and thromboses of the surface bridging vessels and parenchymal vessels).

The brain responds to hypernatremia and to serum hyperosmolality in a unique way. This response creates the major dilemma encountered in the treatment of hyperosmolar states: The hyperosmolar state, left untreated, can produce significant morbidity and death; correction of the hyperosmolar state can also cause significant morbidity and death. Consequently, special therapy and careful monitoring during therapy are imperative to prevent iatrogenic problems during correction.

The hypernatremic state can result from three well-recognized problems; each hypernatremic state requires different therapy.

1. Hypernatremic dehydration: the result of acute gastroenteritis and the most commonly encountered cause of hypernatremia. Therapy is reviewed in detail in this chapter.

2. Hypernatremia secondary to salt poisoning: occurs through excessive salt intake/administration; not commonly encountered. Therapy may include the need for dialysis to remove excess Na^+.
3. Hypernatremia secondary to diabetes insipidus: relatively common. Therapy is specialized and reviewed elsewhere in the chapter.

1. **Hypernatremic dehydration**

Hypernatremic dehydration is defined as dehydration with serum $Na^+ \geq 150$ mEq/L. It was reported to account for 20% to 25% of dehydration cases in the past, but the recent incidence is substantially lower, probably the result of the widespread use of lower osmolality solutions for gastroenteritis than were used in the past.

It was first described as a distinct clinical entity in 1954, and several peculiarities were observed in this form of dehydration: (1) the incidence of death was increased (i.e., 4 times the incidence observed in other types of dehydration), and (2) CNS morbidity in survivors in the follow-up study in Great Britain in the 1960s was increased. Explanations of these findings are reviewed.

Examination of the brains of hypernatremic animals shows less brain shrinkage than expected and greater intracellular osmolality than predicted by usual intracellular osmotically active particles. The higher than expected osmolality is the result of osmotically active particles called *idiogenic osmols*. Idiogenic osmols are discussed in the following paragraph, and the effects of idiogenic osmols on fluid distribution, especially in the cranium, are diagrammed in Figure 6–3.

Idiogenic osmols have the following properties:

1. They are produced in response to prolonged serum hyperosmolality, usually of greater than 6 hours' duration.
2. They are formed slowly, and they also break down slowly in response to changes in serum osmolality.
3. The compensated intracellular osmolality lags behind serum osmolality (i.e., is usually lower than the serum osmolality value).

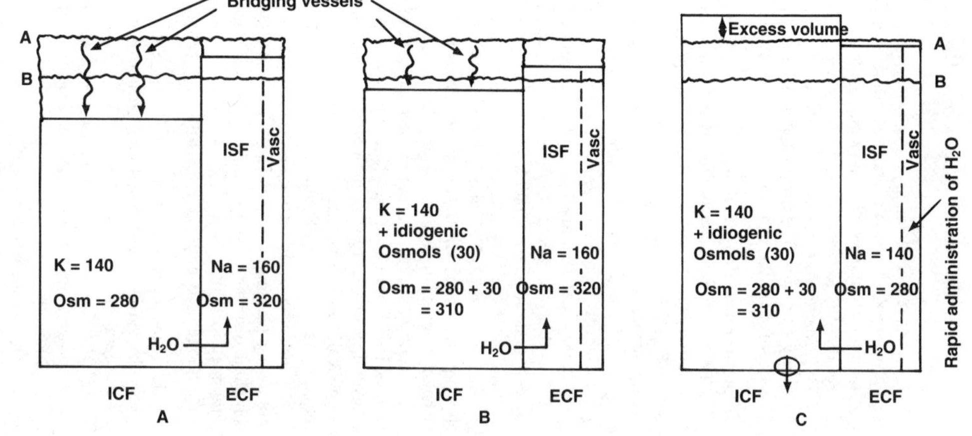
Bridging vessels
Volume
A
B
K = 140
Osm = 280
ISF
Vasc
Na = 160
Osm = 320
H_2O
ICF
ECF
A
K = 140
+ idiogenic
Osmols (30)
Osm = 280 + 30
= 310
ISF
Vasc
Na = 160
Osm = 320
H_2O
ICF
ECF
B
Excess volume
A
B
K = 140
+ idiogenic
Osmols (30)
Osm = 280 + 30
= 310
ISF
Vasc
Na = 140
Osm = 280
H_2O
Rapid administration of H_2O
ICF
ECF
C

4. Most recently, the idiogenic osmols are believed to be amino acids (e.g., taurine, aspartate, and glutamate).

The clinical consequences of idiogenic osmol formation include:

1. The presence of idiogenic osmols increases the intracellular osmolality of brain cells, decreases the osmotic gradient across the cell membrane, and results in less brain shrinkage because less water must leave the brain cells to equalize osmolalities.
2. Because idiogenic osmols break down slowly, a rapid drop of serum Na^+ (i.e., serum osmolality) can reverse the osmolality gradient: Intracellular osmolality becomes greater than extracellular osmolality, and water moves from the extracellular compartment into the cells. The result can range from cerebral edema to increased ICP and brain herniation, depending on the magnitude of fluid

---

FIG 6–3.

Ten percent hypernatremic dehydration: Effect of idiogenic osmols. KEY: ICF border represents cranium in addition to ICF volume; line AA = normal volume; line BB = 10% dehydration; FM = foramen magnum.

A, fluid shifts in absence of idiogenic osmols:

1. Brain can shrink significantly.
2. Bridging vessels stretch as brain shrinks, may tear and bleed. CNS hemorrhages and thrombosis may occur.

B, fluid shifts in presence of idiogenic osmols:

1. Formation of idiogenic osmols reduces osmolality difference and efflux of water from brain.
2. Brain shrinkage and stretching of bridging vessels are reduced. Risks of vessel tears and hemorrhage are decreased.

C, rapid rehydration and correction of serum Na:

1. Idiogenic osmols break down slowly. Rapid dehydration and correction of Na reverse osmolality gradient: ICF osmolality is greater than ECF osmolality.
2. Water moves from ECF to ICF. Brain swells. If swelling is marked, herniation through the foramen magnum occurs.

shifts. For this reason, the serum Na^+ must be lowered cautiously.

3. Glutamate and aspartate are neurotransmitters; some of the peculiar CNS irritability seen in hypernatremia may be secondary to these amino acids and not only the Na^+ values or any vascular injury.

The history of the treatment of hypernatremic dehydration is interesting. Several seemingly logical approaches used in the past led to the discovery of surprising outcomes. Rapid correction of elevated Na^+ values to normal resulted in seizures and CNS deterioration for the reasons already mentioned. Administration of solutions with Na^+ > 75 mEq/liter to avoid the previous pitfall resulted in excessive Na^+ load that resulted in persistent and worsening hypernatremia and worsening CNS status. (The results were similar to initial attempts to hydrate infants with isotonic dehydration with NS solution: Hypernatremia resulted from the administration of an excess amount of Na^+.)

Improved understanding of the pathophysiology has led to the development of a regimen proposed by Finberg that has had a high degree of therapeutic success (Finberg L: *N Engl J Med* 1973; 289:196–198.). The basic principles that form the basis of the regimen follow.

1. The replacement solution is similar in composition to the deficits incurred (see Table 6–2).
   a. The solution has a low amount of Na^+.
   b. The solution has a high amount of K^+, as tolerated, to increase the osmolality of the replacement IV solution and the intracellular compartment as the K^+ moves into the cells.
2. The Na^+ and fluid deficits are replaced *slowly* and *evenly* over 48 hours.
   a. The slow and even correction is empirically effective and avoids the sharp Na^+ and osmolality changes that produce the complications seen in therapy. 48 hours appears to be a clinically important time; attempts to repair deficits in <48 hours, especially in more severe cases, have a high incidence of complications.

The Finberg regimen of therapy is presented.

a. **Clinical and laboratory findings**
   (1) Clinical findings
      (a) Dehydration: usual clinical findings but with the following caveats:
         (i) The degree of dehydration is frequently underestimated, sometimes markedly because the vascular compartment volume is better preserved than in other types of dehydration.
         (ii) Doughy skin: classic finding of dehydration, especially over the abdomen. This is probably related to the relative preservation of the vascular volume.
      (b) CNS irritability: striking at times, frequently mistaken for meningitis. In more severe hypernatremic dehydration:
         (i) Lethargy alternating with marked hyperirritability when stimulated and awake.
         (ii) Hyperreflexia, hypertonicity, which may account for the finding of nuchal rigidity.
         (iii) High-pitched cry.
      (c) Fever: may be secondary to hypernatremia alone.
   (2) Laboratory findings
      (a) Elevated Na^+, Cl^- levels; low bicarbonate level.
      (b) Other findings indicative of dehydration
         (i) Elevated BUN and creatinine levels
         (ii) Hemoconcentration
      (c) Recognized associated abnormalities in hypernatremia
         (i) Hyperglycemia: common associated finding.
            (a) Up to 25% of infants in 1 series had glucose levels >200 mg/dL; occasionally as high as 1,200 mg/dL.
            (b) Hyperglycemia is secondary to inhibition of insulin production by beta cells caused by the hyperosmolar state.
         (ii) Hypocalcemia: not very common.

(iii) Thrombocytopenia: rare.
(a) Usually secondary to a thrombotic complication, especially CNS thrombosis.

c. **Therapy**
(1) Emergency phase
(a) Restore vascular volume if circulation is compromised.
(i) 10–20 mL/kg LR, NS, or 5% albumin solution. LR solution is preferable because it has slightly less NaCl and more base than the other solutions.
(ii) NOTE: A 10–20 mL/kg bolus of the previous volume expanders will increase serum Na^+ by an amount up to 5 mEq/L; this is not significant and does not affect further therapy or adversely affect outcome.
(2) Rehydration phase
(a) Aim to correct the water deficit and Na^+ deficit over 48 hours.
(b) Fluid volume: Calculate the volume of fluid to be administered over 48 hours.
(i) 48-hour fluid volume = Deficit volume + 48-hour maintenance fluid volume.
(a) Calculate the deficit in the usual way. Note that the degree of dehydration is likely to be underestimated on clinical grounds, that any child with significant Na^+ elevation is likely to be 10%–15% dehydrated.
(c) Fluid administration rate: The 48-hour volume is to be provided *evenly*.
(i) Hourly IV rate = 48-hour fluid volume/ 48 hours.
(ii) If the infusion falls behind schedule, do not attempt to catch up large deficits rapidly: Rapid infusion will drop serum Na^+ rapidly and may produce significant cerebral edema. Suggestion on a way to administer the catch-up fluid safely: Divide the catch-up volume by the remaining

number of hours and add this volume to the hourly IV rate.

(d) Fluid composition

(i) Na^+: 25–50 mEq/L = 0.25–0.33 NS solution.

(a) Do not use NS or LR for replacement solution.

(ii) K^+: as close to 40 mEq/L as tolerated.

(iii) Glucose

(a) 5% if glucose level is normal or slightly elevated.

(b) 2.5% if glucose level is significantly elevated.

(iv) Anions: may elect to use *lactate* or *acetate* to accompany a portion of K^+ or Na^+ if severe hyperchloremic and metabolic acidosis exist.

(a) HCO_3^- can be used in place of acetate or lactate, but it is incompatible with many medications.

(v) Rehydrating solution composition

(a) $D_{2.5}$ or D_5 ¼ or ⅓NS solution and 30–40 mEq K^+/L.

(e) Additional fluid therapy considerations

(i) Replace large ongoing gastrointestinal (GI) losses with $D_{2.5}$ or D_5 − ½NS solution + 10 mEq of K^+/L.

(ii) If circulatory compromise or hypotension develop during therapy, give 10–20 mL/kg IV push of LR or 5% albumin solution in addition to hourly IV replacement fluid.

(iii) Additional suggestion by Finberg: Add 1,000 mg calcium gluconate to each 500 mL IV fluid for possible hypocalcemia.

(a) In my experience, hypocalcemia is not seen frequently in hypernatremia; the addition of calcium gluconate does not harm the patient, but IV infiltration with calcium can produce severe tissue necrosis and slough.

(3) Laboratory monitoring during therapy

(a) Monitor electrolytes q8h in severe cases, q12h in less severe cases.

(b) Monitor glucose levels with bedside glucose strip test frequently when hyperglycemia is present to adjust IV dextrose concentrations appropriately.

(c) Follow Hgb, Hct, BUN, and creatinine levels and platelet count until rehydration is complete.

(i) Thrombocytopenia should make one suspect a CNS vascular insult, especially a thrombotic problem. Evaluate with neuroultrasound or CT scan of the head.

(4) Clinical monitoring

(a) Monitor fluid, hydration status: vital signs, inputs and outputs, weights.

(b) Monitor CNS status.

(c) Suggest using a graph (Fig 6–4) to plot results of Na^+ values and total rehydration fluid against an ideal graph. Ideal graph:

(i) Serum Na^+ values over 48 hours: hour 0 = initial Na^+ value, hour 48 = desired Na^+ value, usually 140.

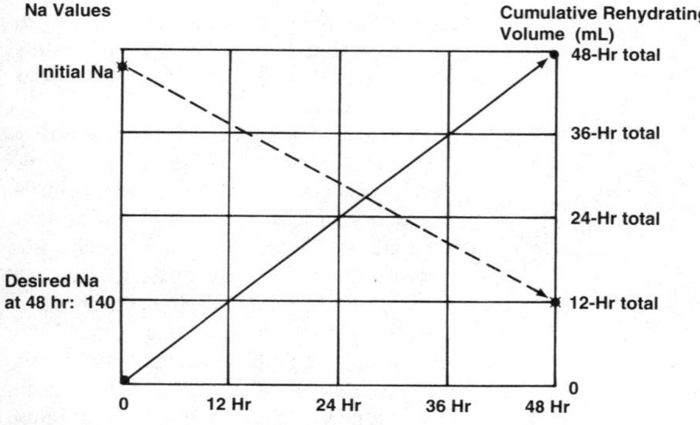

FIG 6–4.

Hypernatremic dehydration: Graph for monitoring Na correction and rehydration. KEY: x---x, ideal slope for Na fall; o—o, ideal slope for rehydration.

(ii) Cumulative fluids administered over 48 hours after the initial rehydrating fluid is given.

(iii) Plotting the actual results against ideal values on the graph indicates if and when significant deviation is occurring and warns of potential problems that may arise from therapy if they have not yet appeared.

(5) Complications seen during therapy

(a) Seizures

(i) Provide therapy.

(a) Provide usual anticonvulsant therapy to control seizure.

(b) Diazepam, 0.1–0.3 mg/kg IV, or lorazepam, 0.05–0.1 mg/kg IV, acutely to stop active seizure.

(c) Follow with a loading dose of phenobarbital or phenytoin, 20 mg/kg IV, for long-acting seizure control.

(ii) Identify the etiology of the seizure, because several problems may underlie it.

(a) Na^+: too rapid drop of serum Na^+.

(1) Make appropriate adjustment in fluid therapy dose/Na^+ concentration.

(2) Treat any associated findings of increased ICP with mannitol, 0.5–1.0 g/kg IV; if the brain stem is involved and vital signs are unstable, also provide intubation and controlled hyperventilation.

(b) Hypocalcemia: uncommon but possible cause.

(1) Calcium gluconate, 50–100 mg/kg IV over 5–10 minutes in infants, 20–50 mg/kg IV in older children, with maximum dose 2 g. Monitor heart rate and BP during Ca^{2+} infusion.

(2) Will need to provide this amount of calcium gluconate IV q6–8h to maintain normal Ca^{2+} levels.

(3) Monitor Ca^{2+} values and adjust calcium gluconate doses accordingly.

(c) Cerebrovascular insult: thrombosis, bleeds.

(1) Diagnosed by computed tomography (CT) scan.

(2) The bleed is usually not a neurosurgical problem; continue anticonvulsants for this problem.

(b) Cerebral edema and increased ICP

(i) Increased ICP will first be manifested by decreasing level of consciousness. Late findings arise from brain stem dysfunction and include abnormal pupils (decreased responsiveness and/or asymmetry), abnormal central ventilation patterns, coma, posturing. The terminal event is brain stem herniation.

(ii) Therapy

(a) Mannitol alone, 0.5–1.0 g/kg IV over 5–10 minutes, suffices for the patient with stable vital signs; place Foley catheter.

(b) Patient with unstable vital signs:

(1) Add intubation and controlled hyperventilation.

(2) Patients with these developments who are recognized and treated early can do well when the problems are caused by Na^+ value changes and cerebral edema alone (rather than by a CNS vascular insult).

(6) Final comments

(a) Once the serum Na^+ is down to the 140–150 range, if the patient is doing well clinically, significant complications are unlikely to arise.

(b) Salt poisoning: different problem from hypernatremia dehydration; dialysis may be required to remove large doses of Na^+.

(c) Oral rehydration therapy of hypernatremic dehydration is not discussed in this book.

Example: A 10 kg infant is found to have hypernatremic dehydration. Laboratory values are Na^+ 168 mEq/L, K^+ 4.3 mEq/L, Cl^- 141 mEq/L, HCO_3^- 12 mEq/L; glucose 345 mg/dL; BUN 54 mg/dL, creatinine 2.1 mg/dL. Circulation is poor in that distal pulses are weak and distal extremities are cool, although BP reading is normal. Estimated degree of dehydration: 12%.

Initial therapy: restore compromised circulation. Patient is given 200 mL LR solution (20 mg/kg), and good distal pulses return, extremities are warmer.

Course of therapy: Plan rehydration and correction of Na^+ value over 48 hours.

1. 48-hour fluid volume to be administered = Deficit volume + 48-hour maintenance volume.

$$\text{Deficit volume} = 10 \text{ kg} \times 12\% = 1{,}200 \text{ mL}$$

Because 200 mL LR solution was given, remaining deficit volume = 1,200 mL − 200 mL = 1,000 mL.

$$\text{48-hour maintenance volume} = (10 \text{ kg}) \times (100 \text{ mL/kg/24 hours}) \times (48 \text{ hours}) = 2{,}000 \text{ mL.}$$

48-hour fluid volume = 1,000 mL + 2,000 mL = 3,000 mL.

2. Hourly fluid volume for the 48 hours =

$$3{,}000 \text{ mL/48 hours} = 62 \text{ mL/hour.}$$

3. Fluid composition =

$$D_{2.5} - \tfrac{1}{4}\text{NS} + 40 \text{ mEq K-acetate/L.}$$

2.5% dextrose is used because serum glucose level = 345. K-acetate is provided for the low HCO_3^-; acetate will be converted to HCO_3^-, and acetate is compatible with most medications.

Figure 6–5 shows a graph for monitoring Na^+ correction and rehydration.

G. Hyponatremia

Like hypernatremia, hyponatremia can produce significant CNS problems: (1) CNS dysfunction, (2) cerebral swelling, and (3) ICP.

The manifestations of CNS dysfunction begin with anorexia and nausea, progress to decreasing levels of consciousness and seizures. Cerebral swelling causes irritability and headaches initially, then progressive fall in level of consciousness as edema increases, with brain stem herniation as the final event; some of the less specific early symptoms overlap those of CNS dysfunction.

There is no absolute Na^+ value at which such symptoms appear. The appearance of clinical problems is greatly af-

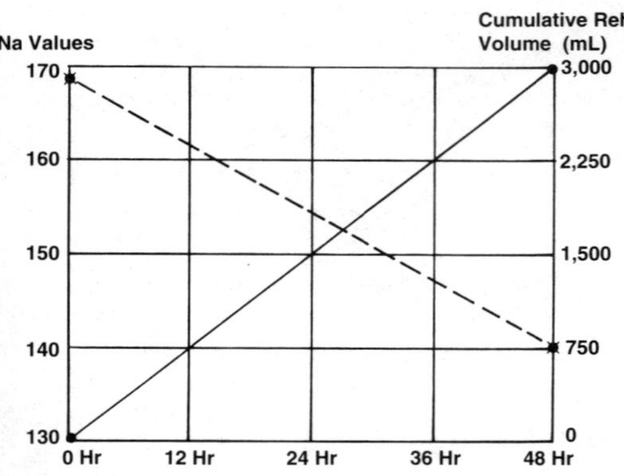

FIG 6–5.

48-Hour Na correction and rehydration.

A, Na correction:

1. Initial Na = 168.
2. Desired Na at 48 hr = 140.

B, rehydration:

3. 48-Hour rehydration volume = 3,000 mL.

fected by the rate of Na^+ fall: When Na^+ falls very slowly, symptoms may be minimal in spite of extremely low serum Na^+ values; a rapid drop in Na^+ may, however, produce major symptoms at only moderate levels of hyponatremia. ***Examples:*** The infant with salt-losing congenital adrenal hyperplasia drops Na^+ slowly. By the time the child begins to have a work-up, the Na^+ may be 110 mEq with only nonspecific findings of irritability. In contrast, the child who receives D_5W at a twice maintenance rate while having SIADH may drop the Na^+ level to 123 mEq from 140 mEq in 1 day and have status epilepticus.

Consequently, emergency intervention that raises serum Na^+ acutely is needed only for the patient with significant symptoms. More gradual correction of Na^+ is appropriate for the patient with minimal symptoms.

1. **Causes: Sodium depletion vs. dilution**

Hyponatremia is usually the end result of one of two processes: (1) *Na^+ depletion* secondary to inadequate Na^+ intake or excessive Na^+ losses (e.g., hyponatremic dehydration caused by gastroenteritis), or (2) *dilution* secondary to the presence of excess water, the result of either excess water administration and/or impaired water excretion.

It is important to note that the use of D_5W as a "maintenance" IV solution can produce significant hyponatremia in children. Feeding large volumes of water (or clear fluids with little Na^+) to young infants in place of milk can likewise produce profound hyponatremia. Both practices should be stopped.

The distinction between the two causes is important because therapy for each differs. The history will frequently enable one to identify the cause of hyponatremia. When, however, the history alone cannot identify the cause of hyponatremia, clinical findings and urine Na^+ levels are helpful in differentiating the etiologies.

The boxes in Figure 6–6 schematically illustrate hyponatremia (Na^+ = 120 mEq) resulting from two different processes and the resulting effects on the vascular compartment and intracranial volumes.

In box *A,* hyponatremia secondary to Na^+ and water losses (e.g., in dehydration from gastroenteritis), volume is decreased in all compartments. Because the serum osmolality is low, fluid moves from the extracellular com-

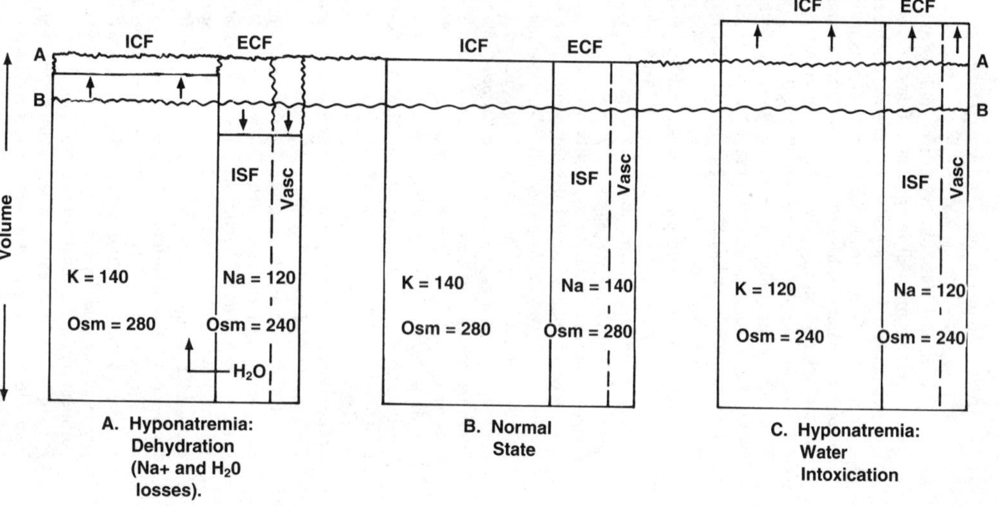
Volume
A
B
ICF
ECF
ISF
Vasc
K = 140
Osm = 280
Na = 120
Osm = 240
H_2O
A. Hyponatremia:
Dehydration
(Na+ and H_20
losses).
ICF
ECF
ISF
Vasc
K = 140
Osm = 280
Na = 140
Osm = 280
B. Normal
State
ICF
ECF
ISF
Vasc
K = 120
Osm = 240
Na = 120
Osm = 240
A
B
C. Hyponatremia:
Water
Intoxication

partment into the intracellular compartment. In addition to CNS dysfunction, additional findings that help identify water and Na^+ losses as the cause include:

1. Circulatory compromise in addition to signs of dehydration.
2. Urine characteristics: low urine volume, concentrated urine. Urine Na^+ will be low, generally <10 mEq/L, as the kidneys avidly attempt to conserve Na^+.
3. The intracranial volume is not likely to be increased; therefore, intracranial hypertension is not common, although CNS dysfunction secondary to altered Na^+ value alone may be present.

In box *C,* hyponatremia is secondary to water excess (i.e., water intoxication). Volume is increased in all compartments. In this situation, in addition to CNS dysfunction, findings that help identify water intoxication as the cause of hyponatremia include:

1. Circulation is good unless volume overload is extreme and sufficient to produce cardiac decompensation (congestive heart failure).
2. Urine characteristics vary by etiology:
   a. Urine volume and concentration
      (1) SIADH, oliguric/anuric renal failure: low volume; high concentration in SIADH, frequently isosthenuric in renal failure.

FIG 6–6.

Hyponatremia: Na depletion vs. dilution. KEY: Line AA = normal volume; line BB = 10% dehydration.

A, hyponatremia secondary to Na and H_2O losses (dehydration):

1. Total body water is decreased.
2. Vascular volume is decreased, even more so secondary to fluid shifts. Circulatory compromise is evident.
3. CNS dysfunction may be evident; brain volume is not excessive.

B, normal Na and hydration.

C, hyponatremia secondary to dilution (water intoxication):

1. Total body water is increased. Water moves into all compartments and dilutes cations.
2. Vascular volume is full, circulation is good. (When fluid overload is severe, congestive heart failure is present.)
3. CNS dysfunction may be evident, as well as increased brain volume.

(2) Excess water intake/input in the absence of the previous two conditions: high urine volume, dilute urine.

b. Urine Na^+: urine Na^+ is paradoxically high when vascular volume overexpansion exists. Urine Na^+ is generally >20–50 mEq/L, sometimes in great excess of these values (see p. 169).

3. The intracranial (intracellular) compartment is increased in size. When intracranial volume is significantly expanded, cerebral edema, intracranial hypertension, and brain herniation are possible consequences.

A smaller number of patients with Na^+ depletion are euvolemic, such as the patient with renal Na^+ wasting. These patients will usually have good circulation, normal urine output, usual urine concentrations, but low urine Na^+.

2. **Therapy**

For the child with major symptoms secondary to hyponatremia—seizures, significant depression of consciousness, respiratory arrest, brain stem herniation—the serum Na^+ must be raised acutely to improve cell function and to decrease cerebral swelling and ICP.

It is important to note that the serum Na^+ level should not be raised back to normal rapidly. Rapid full correction of serum Na^+ level is contraindicated: This could cause the brain to shrink rapidly and tear its bridging vessels; rapid Na^+ correction would contribute to potential vascular volume overload.

The hyponatremic child with major symptoms should have the serum Na^+ level acutely raised by 5–10 mEq in approximately 1 hour. This amount is usually sufficient to stop seizure activity and to reduce brain swelling by an amount that lowers ICP significantly.

Adult patients usually have their serum Na^+ levels raised more slowly because of the reported risk of central pontine myelinolysis. This complication is virtually unknown in children. It is my experience and that of many others that raising the serum Na^+ level by this value for the acutely symptomatic patient is safe and effective in children.

Sodium dose required to raise the serum Na^+ value acutely by 5–10 mEq/L: 3 mEq NaCl/kg is required to raise the serum Na^+ level by 5 mEq/L; 6 mEq NaCl/kg is required to raise the serum Na^+ level by 10 mEq/L. This amount of Na^+ should be given IV over 30–60 minutes for the acutely symptomatic child. The choices of Na^+ preparations available for administration are given in Table 6–3. Following the acute correction of symptomatic hyponatremia, the Na^+ level should more gradually be corrected to normal.

3. **Treatment plan**
   a. Assess type of hyponatremia: Na^+ depletion vs. dilutional hyponatremia.
      (1) History: frequently identifies cause.
      (2) In the absence of clarification by history, use physical and laboratory findings to help delineate etiology.
         (a) Findings associated with Na^+ depletion
            (i) Circulation: Hypovolemia is usually seen; some patients are euvolemic.
            (ii) Urine Na^+: low, usually <10 mEq/L.
         (b) Findings associated with dilutional hyponatremia
            (i) Circulation: usually excellent; occasional congestive heart failure in severe volume overload.
            (ii) Urine Na^+ level: usually paradoxically high, up to >300 mEq/L.
            (iii) May have signs of increased ICP secondary to significant brain swelling.
   b. Therapy: hyponatremia secondary to Na^+ depletion
      (1) Restore compromised circulation: 10–20 mL/kg NS or LR solution bolus IV; repeat dose as needed.

TABLE 6–3.

Sodium Preparations for Use in Hyponatremia

Na^+ Preparation	Na^+ Concentration	mL/kg Required to Raise Serum Na^+ by 10 mEq/L
0.9 NaCl solution	154 mEq/L = 0.154 mEq/mL	38
3% NaCl	500 mEq/L = 0.5 mEq/mL	12
Concentrated NaCl for IV preparation	4 mEq/mL	1.5

(2) Acute correction: Use 3% saline solution, 12 mL/kg IV over 30–60 minutes to raise serum Na^+ level by 10 mEq/L.
(3) Replace remainder of water and salt deficits as presented on p. 141.

c. Therapy: hyponatremia secondary to water intoxication
   (1) Circulation
      (a) Correct circulation that is compromised by volume overload (i.e., congestive heart failure):
         (i) Provide a diuretic if diuresis is not yet established: furosemide, 0.5–1.0 mg/kg IM, IV.
         (ii) Provide oxygen and inotropic support as needed.
      (b) Restrict fluid administration to less than maintenance rate.
   (2) Acute sodium correction:
      (a) In cases of severe volume overload, one may choose to use concentrated saline solution (4 mEq NaCl/mL), 1.5 mL/kg IV over 30–60 minutes. Provide a diuretic in conjunction with concentrated saline.
      (b) For the patient with lesser degree of volume overload and stable cardiac status, administer 3% normal saline solution, 12 mL/kg IV over 30–60 minutes.
   (3) Further correction of Na^+ value in the volume overloaded patient is dependent on:
      (a) The patient getting rid of excess fluid. This may occur through:
         (i) Spontaneous diuresis: as in the young infant who was fed copious amounts of water and is spontaneously diuresing large volumes of urine. When intake is restricted, the massive diuresis will quickly restore normal water balance.
         (ii) Administration of diuretics for the patient with impaired (inappropriately low) urine output: as in the patient with water intoxication secondary to SIADH. Fu-

rosemide, 0.5–1.0 mg/kg IV; repeat as needed.

(iii) Severe fluid restriction for the patient who is stable and unable to put out large volumes of urine: An example is the patient with oliguric renal failure. The patient may need to have fluids restricted to insensible losses or less to achieve negative water balance.

(iv) Phlebotomy: used occasionally for the patient with circulatory compromise secondary to fluid overload who is unable to diurese secondary to oliguria or anuria. Aliquots of 5 mL/kg blood may be withdrawn until circulatory stability is achieved.

(b) Providing an adequate amount of Na^+ in the IV solution: Commonly used Na^+ concentrations are ½NS or NS solution until serum Na^+ values return to the normal range.

d. **Maintenance of Na^+ correction in water intoxication: the crucial importance of eliminating excess water** (see also p. 174).

The loss of excess water alone will help raise the low serum Na^+ values in water intoxication. When, however, water excretion is impaired or interfered with (e.g., in SIADH or oliguric renal failure), awaiting water loss via urine to achieve this correction does not work with adequate rapidity to help the acutely symptomatic patient. Supplemental Na^+ must be provided to raise the serum Na^+ level acutely as reviewed. There is, however, a crucial adjunctive measure that must be provided to maintain the Na^+ correction: intervention that will reduce water overload, usually diuretic administration, occasionally measures such as phlebotomy or dialysis in the pediatric intensive care unit setting.

The physiologic explanation for this is as follows: The body protects vascular volume over osmolality. The patient with vascular volume overload is at risk of developing cardiac decompensation (Frank-Starling curve) from further volume retention. At the time that critical vascular volume overload is reached, the kidneys stop reabsorbing Na^+ at the tubular level drops as Na^+ is reabsorbed in association with water. Natriuresis follows; urine Na^+ may reach levels higher than 100 mEq of Na^+/L.

This is the explanation for the seemingly paradoxical natiuresis observed in hyponatremia secondary to water overload (i.e., the protection of vascular volume over osmolality). The clinical implications are important. The provision of supplemental Na^+ to acutely raise the serum Na^+ level will provide only transient Na^+ correction when the excess water is not eliminated. With the persistence of volume overload, natriuresis continues, and, after several hours, the serum Na^+ level drops to previous or even lower levels.

Therefore the *two* important steps that must occur to maintain Na^+ correction in hyponatremia secondary to water intoxication are:

1. Provide supplemental Na^+ to acutely raise serum Na^+ levels.
2. Eliminate excess water.
   a. For the patient with brisk diuresis, this, in conjunction with limitation of fluid intake will rapidly correct the volume overload state. ***Example:*** the child with water intoxication secondary to massive intake of water where urinary output could not keep up with massive intake.
   b. For the patient with impaired water excretion, provide a diuretic (usually furosemide or mannitol). ***Example:*** the patient with water overload secondary to SIADH.

H. Antidiuretic hormone: pathologic states

1. Physiology and pathophysiology

Antidiuretic hormone (ADH) is formed in the hypothalamus, stored in the posterior pituitary gland from where it is released as needed. It has several actions, but the one of primary interest is its effect on water balance.

ADH acts on the distal tubules and collecting ducts of the kidney to increase their permeability to water. In its presence, an increased amount of water is absorbed by the tubules into the body. The results of ADH activity are the retention of water by the body and the formation of urine that is concentrated in nature and low in volume. When released in large amounts, the urine osmolality can be raised as high as 1,400 mOsm; when absent, urine osmolality can fall as low as 50 mOsm.

There are two physiologic stimuli for ADH release. The first is increased serum osmolality; a change in serum osmolality as low as 1.2% to 2% causes a change in the amount of ADH release from the pituitary. The second physiologic stimulus is volume contraction, specifically hypovolemia. The release of ADH from the pituitary is appropriate in these circumstances because the resulting water retention will correct the problem that stimulated the ADH release.

There are other conditions in pediatrics where ADH is secreted, but in the absence of either of the two physiologic stimuli, hyperosmolality or hypovolemia. When neither physiologic stimulus exists, the secretion of ADH is physiologically excessive and inappropriate. Urine output falls, and when fluid intake is not curtailed by an amount equal to the decrease in urine volume, water retention is the net result; this can lead to hyponatremia and water intoxication, or SIADH.

The opposite pathologic condition that exists is the absence of ADH. This most frequently results from pituitary disease or damage (e.g., pituitary tumors or head trauma). In the absence of ADH, water is not absorbed by the tubules. The large amounts of water excreted by the kidney produce massive diuresis. Dehydration, shock, and metabolic abnormalities rapidly follow the development of uncompensated, nonhomeostatic, massive diuresis. This condition is diabetes insipidus (DI). Rarely, the kidney tubules cannot respond to secreted ADH; the resulting picture is clinically indistinguishable from DI but is termed nephrogenic diabetes insipidus because of the underlying pathologic condition.

Both of these pathologic conditions of ADH secretion are discussed in detail.

2. **SIADH**

As mentioned earlier, this condition is termed SIADH because ADH is secreted in the absence of the usual physiologic stimuli (i.e., hyperosmolality or hypovolemia). In SIADH, ADH is secreted reflexly in response

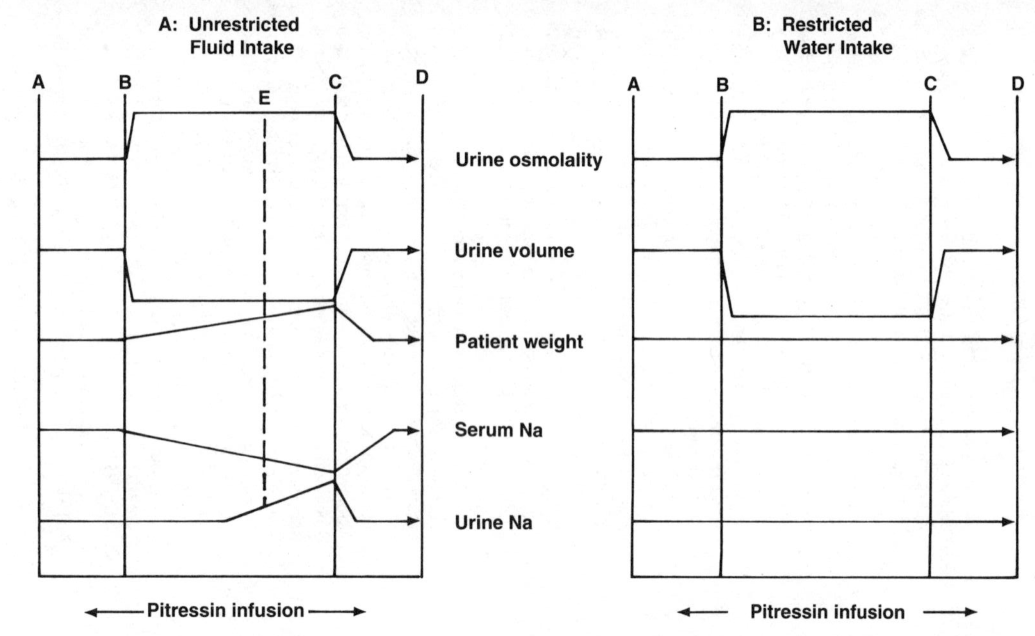
A: Unrestricted
Fluid Intake
A
B
E
C
D
Urine osmolality
Urine volume
Patient weight
Serum Na
Urine Na
Pitressin infusion
B: Restricted
Water Intake
A
B
C
D
Pitressin infusion

to certain pathologic conditions. Well-recognized conditions in which SIADH commonly occurs are:

a. CNS disorders: infection, trauma, tumors, vascular accidents, hypoxia.
b. Significant respiratory disease: usually occurs in moderate to marked respiratory disease characterized by moderate to severe retractions. The degree of respiratory difficulty produced by the disease rather than the specific respiratory disease is the factor that determines the occurrence of SIADH. SIADH may be encountered in any respiratory disease with moderate/severe dyspnea, causes that range from croup to asthma to pneumonia to hyaline membrane disease.
c. Major trauma, surgery (especially thoracotomy), or pain.
d. Certain drugs (e.g., opiates, vincristine).

The effects of SIADH can best be explained by the schematic graph in Figure 6–7. Figure 6–7 shows five parameters of patients under observation, all of which are stable (i.e., level lines) for the period a to b as they eat and drink in the usual manner.

For the period b to c, the patients have been injected with supraphysiologic amounts of vasopressin (Pitressin), which is ADH, to simulate the condition of SIADH. There are the immediate drop in urine volume and increase in urine osmolality as an increased amount of water is absorbed by the tubules. When the patient is allowed to eat and drink the same amount as during the period before the vasopressin injection (situation A), net water retention occurs. The results of water retention are increased patient weight from water and a drop in the serum Na^+ level secondary to dilution. Water intoxication is the end result of SIADH *coupled with* unrestricted water intake/administration.

FIG 6–7.
Schematic of effects of excessive pitressin infusion (SIADH). **Patient A,** no fluid restriction during SIADH. Result: water intoxication. **Patient B,** appropriate fluid restriction during SIADH; Result: no change in fluid/electrolyte status.

If in the period b to c, the patient decreases fluid intake by an amount that equals the decrease in urine output (water excretion) caused by the vasopressin injection (situation B), water balance is maintained. The patient weight and serum Na^+ level remain unchanged even with the excessive amount of vasopressin (ADH). This is the rationale for restricting fluids during SIADH: Water retention can be avoided in the face of diminished urine output by appropriate reduction of fluid intake. There is no fixed percentage by which fluid intake should be reduced that will automatically avoid water retention, because the amount of ADH secreted in these situations is variable; in each instance, the effects of fluid restriction need to be evaluated and the degree of restriction titrated accordingly.

Urine Na^+ level remains fairly stable and unremarkable until significant water retention with weight increase and hyponatremia have developed (situation A, point *E*). At that time, there is a marked surge in natriuresis.

To summarize the principle that was reviewed, once the vascular volume exceeds a critical value, the kidney decreases Na^+ reabsorption. By decreasing Na^+ reabsorption, further volume overload and cardiac decompensation are avoided because Na^+ reabsorption by the tubules is accompanied by water absorption. For this reason, when acute symptoms from hyponatremia arise, it is not sufficient to provide only concentrated Na^+ to raise the serum Na^+ level: the rise in serum sodium that follows will be transient when hypervolemia is not corrected. When critical hypervolemia fails to be corrected, profound natriuresis continues, and in hours the serum Na^+ level returns to previously low or even lower values.

For this reason, in states of water intoxication, diuresis must accompany acute Na^+ administration to *maintain* serum Na^+ corrections. If the patient has impaired diuresis (e.g., in the case of SIADH), the administration of a diuretic must accompany the administration of concentrated Na^+ for lasting correction of the acutely symptomatic patient; only then is it possible that enough excess water will be eliminated so that the patient will now be at a point to the left of point *E* on the graph, the point where volume overload is no longer critical and the point where paradoxical natriuresis does not occur.

It is critical to understand the last point. It explains the observation that administration of concentrated saline solution, even repeated doses, to patients with acute symptomatic hyponatremia from SIADH without correction of hypervolemia produces only a transient elevation of serum Na^+ levels; the serum Na^+ level falls back to previously low, or even lower values, after several hours. The concomitant administration of diuretics to these patients changes the patient response dramatically: With critical reduction of vascular volume, natriuresis halts and corrected serum Na^+ levels are maintained.

Additional comments about SIADH follow. First, SIADH, of itself, does not cause clinical problems. It is the consequence of SIADH, coupled with excessive fluid administration, that produces the undesirable clinical problems (i.e., the CNS effects resulting from hyponatremia and water intoxication).

Second, urine osmolality (and corresponding urine specific gravity) almost always will be high and urine osmolality is almost always greater than serum osmolality. This is not always the case, however. There is also no accepted urine osmolality value that clearly defines the presence of SIADH. Urine osmolality values must be interpreted physiologically. In the absence of ADH, urine osmolality is at its lowest (i.e., 50–75 mOsm). Any urine osmolality greater than 50 to 75 mOsm in the presence of excess water is inappropriately high, because ADH in this situation should not be released; urine should be maximally dilute, and a urine osmolality greater than this value suggests SIADH.

a. Findings
   (1) Conditions associated with SIADH: CNS problems, respiratory problems, trauma/pain, certain medications.
   (2) Low urine volume (which may be <50% of usual and not caused by renal disease because excessive water reabsorption is the cause of oliguria) and high urine osmolality/specific gravity in the absence of:
      (a) Hypovolemia.
      (b) Renal disease.
      (c) Adrenal disease.

(3) Laboratory and clinical findings of water overload when water retention occurs.
   (a) First findings are laboratory findings:
      (i) Hyponatremia: Serum Na^+ level falls progressively as more water is retained.
      (ii) Paradoxically high urine Na^+ level—usually in excess of 20–30 mEq Na^+/L—in the presence of hyponatremia secondary to volume overload.
      (iii) BUN and creatinine levels are in the normal range; K^+ and Cl^- levels are usually normal; HCO_3^- level is normal to slightly elevated over normal.
   (b) Clinical signs
      (i) Changes in CNS function are the primary problem.
         (a) Signs begin with anorexia, nausea; progress to headache, decreasing level of consciousness.
         (b) Severe hyponatremia: seizures, coma, brain stem herniation.
         (c) The serum Na^+ value at which signs appear is not absolute: It is dependent on the rapidity of the drop in Na^+ value.
      (ii) Vascular status: usually excellent cardiovascular status, clearly well hydrated.
         (a) Edema: uncommon; usually seen in only severe water overload.

b. Management
   (1) Know the conditions with which SIADH is commonly seen. Anticipate SIADH and restrict fluid intake from the beginning. Monitor the following to assess effectiveness of fluid management:
      (a) Measure fluid intake and output.
         (i) Urine output is expected to fall in SIADH and may fall to <50% usual amount.
            (a) This is not caused by renal disease (i.e., renal parenchymal disease or decreased blood flow to the kidneys) but by avid absorption of water from

the tubules because of large amounts of ADH present. BUN and creatinine values will support this.

(b) Urine specific gravity (occasionally osmolality) as needed.

(c) Daily patient weight.

(d) Serum electrolyte levels.

(e) Values for BUN, creatinine, Hgb, and Hct, and chest x-ray studies (for heart size, pulmonary vasculature) for further assessment if fluid status is not clear.

(2) Restrict fluid intake to avoid retention of excess water. 50% to 75% of the usual maintenance fluid volume is commonly chosen as the restricted rate with which to begin. Further adjustments in fluid administration are made according to patient monitoring.

(3) If water retention is already present (i.e., mild weight increase and hyponatremia), but the patient is clinically stable and not having significant CNS dysfunction, restrict fluid intake even more to achieve negative water balance. Fluid restriction may have to be very severe (i.e., limited to less than insensible losses).

(4) If the serum Na^+ level is low enough to cause significant CNS problems (i.e., seizures, coma, or signs of herniation), the serum Na^+ value needs to be raised by 5–10 mEq/L acutely. *Two* acute interventions are needed to raise serum Na^+ values and maintain corrected serum Na^+ level.

(a) Administer furosemide, 0.25–1.0 mg/kg IV or IM.

(i) SIADH patients are frequently very sensitive to furosemide. Frequently a low dose of furosemide, $\leq$0.5 mg/kg, will produce massive diuresis in SIADH; the dose will have to be increased if diuresis does not follow.

(ii) Both water and Na^+ are lost, but the state of vascular volume overload may be improved to the point that natriuresis stops and correction of the low serum Na^+ value can be maintained.

(b) Administer concentrated NaCl solution IV. Raise serum Na^+ level by 5–10 mEq/L in 1 hour.

(i) Concentrated NaCl (4 mEq NaCl/mL) preparation

(a) 0.75 mL/kg IV over 1 hour to increase serum Na^+ level by 5 mEq/L. Add this to 1 hour's volume of "maintenance" IV solution.

(b) 1.50 mL/kg IV over 1 hour to increase serum Na^+ level by 10 mEq/L. Add this to 1 hour's volume of "maintenance" IV solution.

(ii) 3% NaCl (500 mEq NaCl/L)

(a) 6 mL/kg IV over 1 hour to increase serum Na^+ level by 5 mEq/L.

(b) 12 mL/kg IV over 1 hour to increase serum Na^+ level by 10 mEq/L.

I. Diabetes insipidus

ADH deficiency is the usual cause of diabetes insipidus (DI). Common causes of ADH deficiency include CNS trauma, CNS surgery, CNS infection, and severe asphyxia. Very rarely, DI is caused by the inability of the kidneys to respond to ADH rather than its absence; this uncommon condition is called nephrogenic DI to distinguish it from the more common central DI. The resulting clinical picture is indistinguishable regardless of the underlying etiology. In both cases, water fails to be reabsorbed by the distal tubules and collecting ducts of the kidneys, and large amounts of water are lost in the urine.

The water loss that results from full-blown DI is massive and completely nonhomeostatic. Water balance can be maintained by older individuals who have intact thirst mechanism and the ability to obtain and drink the appropriate quantity of fluids to match the massive water losses. For the individual unable to maintain intake that keeps up with massive urinary water losses, untreated or uncompensated DI leads to the following within a few hours: (1) dehydration, followed by hypovolemic shock; (2) hemoconcentration of vascular constituents, most notably elevation of serum Na^+ levels and serum osmolality.

In the absence of ADH, the distal tubules and collecting

ducts are unable to reabsorb water and concentrate urine. The characteristics of urine formed in DI follow.

1. Massive volumes of urine with large free water excretion. Urine volumes may be increased by as much as 10 to 20 times the usual volume. The adult may maximally put out slightly more than 1 L/hour of urine compared with the usual 50 to 100 mL/hour in the normal state. Because of the magnitude of water losses, dehydration, shock, and hemoconcentration of vascular constituents quickly develop in the untreated patient.
2. Low urine osmolality, usually 50 to 100 mOsm, and low specific gravity, usually <1.005.
3. Low urine Na^+ concentration, usually ≤ 20 mEq/L. Urinary K^+ concentration is also usually low, 5 to 10 mEq/L. Neither value provided is absolute and must be checked in the individual patient for accuracy. Urine Na^+ and K^+ concentrations may be much higher in the presence of glucosuria.

Medical management of DI is tricky. IV fluid replacement therapy is especially treacherous: Extraordinary fluid volumes are needed; IV solutions needed to replace voluminous urine losses require formulations that break with rules that guide conventional IV fluid composition, and large Na^+ imbalances can result from the disparity between the Na^+ content of IV replacement solutions and the Na^+ content of urine, which can waver over time. For these reasons, important caveats in the therapy of DI are presented before proceeding with a suggested regimen for the management of DI.

1. **Therapy**
   a. *Therapy with hormone replacement: vasopressin, or desmopressin acetate (DDAVP).*

      After the administration of replacement hormone therapy, an appropriate rise in urine osmolality/specific gravity and drop in urine volume should follow shortly. For the patient without intact thirst and drinking mechanisms, fluid administration must be appropriately adjusted after administration of the hormone. If the replacement hormone dose is insufficient, excessive water loss, although in smaller amounts than previously, will still occur; when the replacement dose is in excess of physiologic needs, the excessive amount of ADH creates the situation analogous to SIADH, and fluid administration must be accordingly restricted.

b. *Fluid therapy: volume guidelines*

The patient with full-blown DI loses massive amounts of water and can rapidly develop dehydration and shock.

Example: The usual 70 kg adult who must be kept NPO usually receives 2,400 mL IV fluid/24 hours, or 100 mL/hour; urine output averages 1,200 mL/24 hours, or 50 mL/hour.

With DI, the same adult can put out 24 to 28 L of urine/24 hours, or approximately 1,000 mL of urine/hour. In 6 hours, this patient, who is unable to drink, will lose 6 L of fluid, which amounts to 8.5% weight loss, enough to place him or her in a state of advanced shock. If DI continues unabated for another 2 to 3 hours, death can be expected.

For this reason, the patient who is dependent on medical fluid administration for stability should have massive urine losses replaced on an hourly basis. A regimen that meets fluid needs is suggested.

2. **Regimen**

a. Provide the patient's insensible water losses by administering the usual maintenance IV solution at 20% to 30% of the maintenance fluid rate.

b. Replace the patient's urine output volume for volume (milliliter for milliliter) on an hourly basis. Waiting for more than 1 hour to replace the massive urine losses will increase the chance of the patient developing dehydration, shock, and greatly fluctuating metabolic values.

The milliliter for milliliter urine replacement regimen is useful, because when the urine output falls or rises dramatically, the following hour's fluid replacement is adjusted accordingly. This method minimizes the development of large fluid imbalances. Insertion of a bladder catheter may facilitate urine volume measurements and is mandatory for the obtunded or comatose patient.

c. *Hypernatremia*

Hypernatremia >150 mEq/L can develop in a few hours in full-blown DI. In this situation, idiogenic osmols do not have time to form in brain cells, so the child with hypernatremia resulting from recent onset or breakthrough of DI can usually have the serum Na^+ level corrected to normal rapidly and safely with relatively hypotonic (low Na^+ and low glucose) solutions unlike the case of more usual hypernatremic dehydration. This statement is valid as long as the hypernatremia is of less than about 6 to 8 hours' duration.

If the hypernatremia is marked and of longer duration, fluid therapy is more complex, and the serum Na^+ level will have to be dropped slowly (see p. 151). Modifications for DI follow: (1) volume expanders must be administered to restore compromised circulation; (2) urine output should be replaced milliliter for milliliter as described earlier; and (3) additional "background" fluid therapy must be provided to correct the Na^+ and water deficits, as well as to provide ongoing insensible fluid needs. The background fluid volume is the fluid deficit plus 48 hours of insensible losses; this volume is to be replaced evenly over 48 hours using the solutions described on p. 156.

d. *Sodium concentration in urine replacement IV solution*

It is imperative that the replacement solution's Na^+ concentration closely match the urine Na^+ concentration. Because the volumes of fluid lost and replaced in DI are very large, failure to closely match the Na^+ content of these solutions can produce large net Na^+ deficits or excesses. Large Na^+ imbalances in either direction significantly alter serum Na^+ values; the rapid and sometimes very large changes in serum Na^+ levels can profoundly affect CNS function.

The urine Na^+ and K^+ concentrations should therefore be checked routinely and frequently (e.g., q6–8h) in the patient who is having the massive diuresis of DI treated with IV fluid replacement. The periodic urine electrolyte concentration checks are important because urine Na^+ concentration does not remain constant during DI; the IV replacement solution's Na^+ concentration must be changed accordingly to maintain Na^+ balance.

Example: 10 kg child with DI has 200 mL of urine/hour, or 4.8 L of urine/day. Initial urine Na^+ is 10 mEq/L. The IV solution selected to replace the urine losses has 10 mEq of Na^+/L and is run at 200 mL/hour. Over the first 24 hours, the child continues to have urine replaced with this IV solution at 200 mL/hour, or 4.8 L/day.

At hour 3 into therapy, the urine Na^+ concentration rises to 20 mEq/L and stays at that value. If, over the next 24 hours, the urine Na^+ level continues to be 20 mEq/L and the IV replacement solution Na^+ level continues to be 10 mEq/L, a significant body Na^+ deficit develops.

4.8 L of urine are produced; 4.8 L of IV fluid are infused over 24 hours. Urine Na^+ losses will be 96 mEq (4.8 L × 20 mEq Na^+/L). Na^+ infused via the IV is 48 mEq (4.8 L × 10 mEq Na^+/L). The net Na^+ balance is a deficit of 48 mEq in 24 hours, or 4.8 mEq/kg. This Na^+ deficit drops the serum Na^+ level by 8 mEq/L (6 mEq Na^+/kg changes the serum Na^+ value by 10 mEq/L).

If the therapy continues unchanged for 48 hours, the Na^+ deficit will result in a drop of serum Na^+ by 16 mEq/L. The large serum Na^+ drop will produce CNS symptoms caused by hyponatremia.

The reverse situation holds true when the replacement solution contains more Na^+ than is lost via the urine: Na^+ excesses can produce significant hypernatremia.

The urine Na^+ values can be much greater than 20 mEq/L and fluctuate over an even wider range when glucosuria is present. Therefore, in the presence of glucosuria, even greater changes in serum Na^+ levels can occur.

e. *Dextrose concentration of the IV replacement solution*

The hourly IV volumes that must be administered to keep up with water losses in the urine are tremendous.

Example: The 70 kg man has maintenance fluid needs of 2,500 mL/24 hours, or about 100 mL/hour.

The same man who develops DI can produce 24 L of urine in 24 hours, or 1 L of urine/hour. The fluid replacement for urinary losses alone is 1,000 mL/hour, which amounts to 10 times the usual maintenance fluid volume. Appropriate replacement of water, Na^+, and K^+ solutions has been reviewed. The dextrose (glucose) component of IV replacement solutions, however, needs special considerations in DI; if it is not attended to, significant iatrogenic problems can follow.

If, for this patient, the dextrose concentration of the IV replacement solution is kept at 5%, the administration of a 5% dextrose solution at 10 times the maintenance rate (1,000 mL/hour) provides the same amount of glucose contained in a 50% dextrose solution running at usual maintenance rate (100 mL/hour). This exceedingly large dextrose load produces hyperglycemia, which progressively increases if the same IV solution is continued. A major effect of hyperglycemia is massive osmotic diuresis that further complicates DI. Hyperglycemia >180 mg/dL is so potent an osmotic diuretic that an osmotic diuresis will overcome the effects of ADH replacement and persist well into the state of profound hypovolemia and shock, as seen in diabetic ketoacidosis (DKA). It also complicates Na^+ balance.

To avoid this iatrogenic problem, the dextrose concentration of IV solutions used to replace urine losses in DI must be appropriately lowered, frequently to levels that are far lower than are customarily used. There is no absolute rule for dextrose concentration of urine replacement solutions. A guideline is provided.

Most unstressed individuals can tolerate a 10% dextrose-containing solution run at maintenance rate without developing osmotically significant hyperglycemia. This is the glucose load most unstressed individuals can tolerate and the amount of glucose to place in the hourly volume of urine replacement solution.

Example: A 10 kg child has an hourly maintenance fluid rate of approximately 40 mL. 40 mL/hour of a 10% dextrose solution (10 g of glucose in 100 mL of fluid) provides the patient with 4 g of glucose/hour.

The amount of glucose provided by a 10% dextrose solution run at maintenance rate in 1 hour can serve as the guide to the glucose load to provide in the urine replacement IV solution. This amount of glucose placed in the anticipated average hourly urine volume is used to determine the dextrose concentration of the replacement solution. In this instance, the child is expected to tolerate 4 g of glucose/hour. If urine output is 200 mL/hour, the replacement solution should have 4 g of glucose/200 mL solution = 2 g dextrose/100 mL = 2% dextrose solution.

The IV replacement solution is likely to be: D_2 + 10–20 mEq Na^+/L + 10 mEq K^+/L.

If the serum glucose is very high, the glucose concentration will have to be lowered further empirically, occasionally as low as 0.5%–1%. The glucose concentration needs to be increased when the serum glucose level is low. Serum glucose levels must be monitored frequently during IV replacement therapy of DI.

f. *Hypotonic composition of IV replacement fluid in DI*

The fluid composition of the replacement solution may be D_1 + 10 mEq NaCl/L + 10 mEq KCl/L. The osmolality of this solution is 90 mOsm, which is very hypotonic compared with serum osmolality and the majority of usual IV solutions. In usual circumstances, very hypotonic IV solutions are to be avoided because of the risk of producing red blood cell (RBC) lysis and hypotonicity.

In DI, because the kidneys behave as a sieve—water loss is massive and nonhomeostatic—the replacement fluid must closely resemble urine losses to maintain water and electrolyte balance. It is for this reason that these very unusual and hypotonic solutions can be used safely and in large volumes. When one is using these fluids, it is important that outputs be monitored and urine losses be replaced *on an hourly basis* rather than over longer periods of time. This way the fluctuations in water and electrolyte balance are lessened and the problems that arise from injudicious use of hypotonic solutions are minimized.

3. Management of diabetes insipidus
   a. Diagnosis
      (1) Urine characteristics
         (a) Large volume: usually 5–10 times usual volume; persistent diuresis.
         (b) Low specific gravity, osmolality
            (i) Specific gravity <1.005.
            (ii) Urine osmolality usually 50–100.
         (c) Absence of glucosuria
      (2) Blood tests: findings of hemoconcentration
         (a) Hypernatremia
         (b) Elevated Hct and Hgb values
         (c) Elevated BUN and creatinine levels
      (3) Clinical findings
         (a) Hydration: ranges from normal (early) to dehydrated to frank hypovolemic shock (late).
      (4) Obtain stat urine Na^+ and K^+ values; values will be of use in formulation of IV replacement solutions when needed.
   b. Fluid and electrolyte management

      Fluid and electrolyte management will be needed in nephrogenic DI, in the patient with central DI waiting to have the diagnosis established and when replacement hormones are not available for the patient with central DI.
      (1) Stable patient with intact thirst and drinking ability
         (a) Allow the patient to regulate oral intake.
         (b) Monitor inputs and outputs, weights, and electrolyte levels.
            (i) If they are stable, continue with patient regulation via po intake.
            (ii) If water and electrolyte balance worsen, proceed with IV therapy and/or hormone replacement therapy.
      (2) IV therapy
         (a) Shock: rapid infusion of volume expanders in usual manner.
            (i) Restore circulation.

(ii) Volume: 20 mL/kg IV push; follow with 10–20 mL/kg IV pushes until circulation is adequately restored.

(a) The severely dehydrated patient may require up to 60 mL/kg of volume expanders acutely to restore circulation.

(iii) IV solution: NS, RL, or ½NS solution.

(a) ½NS solution can be used acutely because recent urine losses are hypotonic; therefore, some of the hypernatremia, if present, is of very recent origin without the corresponding brain formation of idiogenic osmols.

(3) IV replacement of urinary losses (serum Na^+ level in 125–159 mEq/L range): 2 simultaneous IV solutions needed.

(a) Insensible fluid needs

(i) Use usual maintenance solution (e.g., D_5–⅓ NS + 20 mEq/L solution + 20 mEq/L).

(ii) IV rate: 30%–40% of maintenance rate.

(iii) Continue this fluid throughout IV therapy phase.

(b) Initial urine replacement IV solution

(i) Solution: Suggest D_2 + 20 mEq NaCl/L. (KCl can be added later as needed after electrolyte values return.)

(ii) IV rate: Adjust the hourly rate to replace the volume of the previous hour's urine output.

(4) Modifications of replacement IV solution: to be made subsequently based on urine Na^+, K^+ levels; serum Na^+, K^+, glucose levels.

(a) Na^+ and K^+

(i) Prepare solution with Na^+ and K^+ concentrations that closely match urine Na^+ and K^+ concentrations within a range of ±5 mEq/L.

(ii) Obtain stat urine Na^+ and K^+ q6h and change the IV Na^+ and K^+ concentrations accordingly.

NOTE: If glucosuria is present, urine Na^+ and K^+ values may vary to a far greater extent than in plain DI, and serum Na^+ and K^+ values are at risk of fluctuating even more than usual. In this situation, urine glucose and electrolyte levels may have to be followed more frequently than q6h and IV solutions changed correspondingly.

(b) Dextrose concentration: usually low.

(i) Suggested calculation of dextrose concentration:

(a) Calculate hourly glucose load: 10% dextrose solution (10 g of dextrose in 100 mL) at maintenance rate. Call this value "A."

(b) Select likely hourly urine volume that needs to be replaced. Call this value "B."

(c) IV solution dextrose concentration = (A/B) × (100 mL) = Dextrose %.

(ii) Dextrose concentration may be as low as 0.5%–1% ($D_{0.5}$–D_1)in the presence of massive diuresis.

(iii) The calculated dextrose concentration will have to be further modified for:

(a) Hyperglycemia: Dextrose concentration must be lowered.

(b) Hypoglycemia: Dextrose concentration must be increased.

(iv) Glucose values should be checked q2–4h and more frequently when significantly abnormal values exist.

(v) At its most extreme, a very hypotonic solution may be needed: $D_{1/2}$ + 10 mEq Na/L + 10 mEq K/L.

(5) IV replacement of urinary losses (serum Na^+ ≥160 mEq/L): 2 simultaneous IV solutions are needed.

The DI patient who has not yet been treated or has received inadequate fluids/hormone replacement will have hypernatremia on the basis of dehydration. When hypernatremia is of significant degree (serum $Na^+ \geq 160$ mEq/L) and likely to be of significant duration (>12 hours), it is wise to correct the *water deficit* and *hypernatremia* over 48 hours in a manner similar to that recommended for hypernatremic dehydration. The following are modifications in the therapy of DI associated with significant hypernatremia:

(a) Correct shock: ½NS or NS solution, 20 mL/kg IV push; repeat 10–20 mL/kg boluses as needed.

(b) Replace ongoing urine losses secondary to DI as suggested in the previous section: Use solutions and volumes as recommended.

(c) Rehydration and correction of Na^+: to be accomplished over 48 hours. (Twenty-four hours may be safe when serum Na^+ level is in the 160 mEq/L range or lower because hypernatremia develops very rapidly in full-blown DI, leaving relatively little time for brain idiogenic osmols to form.)

   (i) Rehydrating volume = *fluid deficit volume + 48-hour insensible fluid volume*.

      (a) Insensible losses for 48 hours = 48 hours maintenance fluid volume × 30%–40%.

      (b) Fluid deficit volume for mild, moderate, or severe dehydration

         (1) Infants, toddlers: 5%, 10%, and 15% of patient weight.

         (2) Preschoolers and older: 3%, 6%, and 9% of patient weight.

      (c) Administer this fluid evenly over 48 hours.

         (1) Hourly IV rate for the 48-hour rehydrating period = rehydrating volume/48 hours.

      (d) IV rehydrating solution

         (1) D_5 + ¼NS or ⅓NS + 30–40 mEq/L.

         (2) Fluid composition needs to be modified for glucose, Na^+, and

K^+ values as they are obtained in the course of therapy.

(6) Additional IV therapy considerations
   (a) Provide fluid boluses as needed to restore recurrences of compromised circulation that may occur: ½NS or NS solution in amounts of 10–20 mL/kg.
   (b) Further adjustments in glucose, Na^+, or K^+ concentrations may have to be made in the insensible and/or urine replacement IV solutions according to serum electrolyte and glucose values.

(7) Patient monitoring during IV replacement therapy
   (a) Insert Foley catheter to know hourly urine outputs.
   (b) Monitor hourly:
      (i) Measured inputs and outputs.
      (ii) Vital signs, with special attention to the circulatory status.
      (iii) Neurologic status.
   (c) Electrocardiogram (ECG) monitor: special concern for rhythm or ECG complex changes that may affect K^+ levels.
   (d) Urine evaluation
      (i) Urine glucose, specific gravity q2–4h; suggest q1h monitoring if glucosuria is present.
      (ii) Urine Na^+ and K^+ values q6h; may need more frequent evaluation when glucosuria is present.
   (e) Blood tests
      (i) Bedside glucose strip determinations
         (a) q1–2h when the patient is hyperglycemic or hypoglycemic.
         (b) q4–6h when the patient is euglycemic.
      (ii) Serum glucose and electrolyte values
         (a) q3–4h when hypernatremia and/or osmotic hyperglycemia is/are present.
         (b) q6h when laboratory values are fairly normal.

c. Hormone replacement therapy

DI, especially initial manifestation, is sometimes transient and lasts for only several hours. This phenomenon is quite commonly observed after major head trauma or major CNS infection. For this reason, a short trial of IV fluid replacement therapy may be warranted for the initial manifestation of DI until its persistence is established.

Therapy with hormone replacement is desirable after the diagnosis of DI is (fairly well) established because a prolonged course of IV fluid replacement therapy is fraught with problems difficult to control once they arise: IV access quickly becomes a problem in small children and children with poor veins; hyperglycemia is common and wreaks havoc on fluid and electrolyte control; maintenance of stable serum Na^+ values is frequently difficult to achieve, and significant Na^+ abnormalities are common.

Hormone replacement therefore offers many benefits to the patient with DI; the only exception is the patient with nephrogenic DI who, in the emergency setting, has fluid therapy as the only recourse. Two medications are available for DI.

(1) Aqueous vasopressin
  (a) Relatively short acting: 2–8 hours, but length of effect is highly variable.
  (b) Dose
    (i) 2.5–10 units IM or SC or 0.05–0.1 unit/kg IM or SC.
      (a) Dose must be titrated to the individual according to his or her response.
    (ii) Frequency: Repeat dose whenever diuresis breaks through (i.e., urine output 5–10 mL/kg/hour, urine specific gravity <1.005 or urine osmolality 50–100 mOsm, and absence of glucosuria).
  (c) Side effects: Hypertension and pallor are commonly observed in the first half hour after its administration.

(2) DDAVP
  (a) Newer drug than vasopressin.
  (b) Effects last for 8–20 hours and are again widely variable between individuals.

(c) Nasal administration: preferred route of administration.
   (i) 1–40 μg/day divided into 1 or 2 doses.
   (ii) Effects evident in about 1 hour.
   (iii) Dose to be repeated whenever breakthrough diuresis recurs (see above); subsequent doses are titrated according to patient response.

(d) Parenteral administration
   (i) Adult dose: 2–4 μg/day IV or SC divided into 2 doses.
   (ii) Effects evident in <1 hour.
   (iii) Dose to be repeated whenever breakthrough diuresis recurs; subsequent doses are titrated according to patient response.

(3) Signs of effective response to hormone administration
   (a) Urine volume and characteristics change dramatically:
      (i) Urine volume drops dramatically: Urine volumes may be in the normal range or less if excessive hormone was administered.
      (ii) Urine concentration rises: Specific gravity >1.005; urine osmolality rises dramatically >100 mOsm.
   (b) NOTE: If glucosuria is present, the effects of DDAVP or vasopressin may be overridden by the potent osmotic diuretic effects of hyperglycemia.

(4) Fluid management after response to hormone therapy
   (a) If urine output is within the normal range:
      (i) Use usual maintenance IV solution (e.g., D_5–⅓NS solution + 20 mEq KCl/L); make modifications as necessary.
      (ii) Administer fluids at maintenance rate.
   (b) If urine output drops to amounts less than normal rates (<2 mL/kg/hour in infants, <0.5–1.0 mL/kg/hour in adolescents) and urine specific gravity is very high, DDAVP or vasopressin dose was probably excessive and a state of SIADH exists.

(i) Use usual maintenance IV solution (e.g., D_5–⅓NS solution + 20 mEq KCl/L); make modifications as necessary.

(ii) Administer fluids at a restricted rate, anywhere from 50%–75% maintenance rate. Monitor patient and electrolyte values to further modify fluid administration.

4. **Summary: IV replacement therapy of DI**
   a. Treat shock: ½NS or NS solution, 20 mL/kg IV push. Follow with 10–20 mL/kg increments until circulation is restored.
   b. Follow with 2 IV solutions to maintain hydration and metabolic balance.
      (1) IV solution for insensible fluid losses.
      (2) IV solution for urine replacement.
   c. Insensible fluid losses: Use usual maintenance solution at 30%–40% of usual rate for size.
      (1) Suggest: D_5–⅓NS solution + 20 mEq KCl/L.
      (2) Rate: 30%–40% of usual maintenance rate.
   d. Initial urine replacement IV solution: Solution can be piggybacked into the same line as the insensible fluid solution.
      (1) Start empirically with D_2 solution + 20 mEq NaCl/L.
      (2) Rate: Replace the previous hour's urine volume.
   e. Subsequent modification of IV urine replacement solution.
      (1) Check urine Na^+ and K^+ values. Prepare IV replacement solution with similar Na^+ and K^+ urine concentrations:
         (a) Urine Na^+ and K^+ should be checked q6h, and IV urine replacement solution should be modified accordingly.
      (2) Modify IV dextrose concentration further according to serum and urine glucose levels: Dextrose concentration may have to be lowered even further, less commonly raised. (See text for details.)
   f. IV therapy of significant hypernatremia in DI: See text.
5. **Electrolyte problems**
   a. Hyponatremia: See p. 166.
   b. Hypernatremia: See p. 151.

c. *Hypokalemia*

Serum K^+ levels <3.0 mEq/L can produce several problems, the most critical of which are cardiac.

(1) Findings

(a) Cardiovascular system

(i) ECG changes: flattened, prolonged or inverted T waves; prominent U waves; ST segment depression; atrioventricular (AV) block

(ii) Dysrhythmias

(iii) Hypotension

(b) Neuromuscular system

(i) Weakness, hypotonia

(ii) Hyporeflexia

(iii) Paresthesias, paralysis

(c) GI system

(i) Ileus

(ii) Constipation

Not every child with a serum K^+ level <3.0 mEq/L requires acute IV correction of hypokalemia. The reasons for this are (1) children with certain medical problems will tolerate moderate hypokalemia well without any clinical problems, and (2) acute correction of hypokalemia is associated with significant risks.

(2) Guidelines for therapy

(a) Acute correction of hypokalemia should be provided in the presence of the following conditions:

(i) ECG changes of hypokalemia are present.

(ii) The child is taking digoxin: Hypokalemia significantly increases digoxin's potential to produce life-threatening dysrhythmias.

(iii) Serum K^+ level is <2.0–2.5 mEq/L, even in the absence of ECG changes.

The previously healthy child who has no cardiac involvement and is not taking digoxin can usually tolerate serum K^+ levels as low as 2.0–2.5 mEq/L without clinical problems. For these patients, one should provide extra amounts of KCl in the IV solution (up to a maximum of 60 mEq KCl/L for a peripheral IV in the emergency setting) when acute correction is not provided. The child's ECG pattern should also be closely observed on a cardiac monitor.

(3) Acute treatment
  (a) For serum K^+ value 2.0–3.0 mEq/L
    (i) Dose: 0.5 mEq KCl/kg IV over 1 hour.
      (a) KCl bolus is not to exceed 20 mEq.
    (ii) KCl concentration: not to exceed 60 mEq KCl/mL for a peripheral IV. Dilute the solution further, if possible.
    (iii) Administer the solution at an even rate over 1 hour via a pump. Rapid KCl administration can cause cardiac dysrhythmias or cardiac arrest. The child should be connected to a cardiac monitor, the ECG pattern should be closely observed, and the KCl infusion should be stopped if any signs or symptoms of hyperkalemia appear.
    (iv) Administration of the KCl bolus via a peripheral IV may produce severe pain. If this occurs, suggestions to consider are:
      (a) Dilute the KCl further.
      (b) Slow down the infusion rate for the asymptomatic patient.
      (c) For the symptomatic patient who needs the acute K^+ correction: Administer the KCl bolus through two IVs. Administer one half of the KCl bolus through each IV over the hour; a reduction of the absolute amount of KCl in a vein decreases venous irritation and pain.
  (b) For serum K^+ <2.0 mEq/L
    (i) Dose: up to 1.0 mEq KCl/kg IV over 1–2 hours.
      (a) KCl bolus is not to exceed 40 mEq.
  (c) A serum K^+ value should be obtained again 1–2 hours after the KCl bolus is administered

(not possible in the transport situation) and KCl boluses repeated if the serum K^+ level remains <3.0 mEq/L.

d. *Hyperkalemia*

Serum K^+ levels >5.5 mEq/L are abnormal but usually do not produce clinical toxicity until the serum K^+ level reaches 6.5–7.0 mEq/L. The value at which clinical signs and symptoms appear is variable, but as a guide, even in the absence of clinical findings, levels >7.0 mEq/L are medical emergencies. One must beware of factitious hyperkalemia that can result from blood sampling difficulties (i.e., capillary samples, hemolyzed blood specimens). CAVEAT: There is one instance where profound hyperkalemia can be asymptomatic—in the child with salt-losing congenital adrenal hyperplasia who develops progressive hyponatremia and hyperkalemia gradually over several weeks; this child needs extra NaCl administration, glucocorticoid, and mineralocorticoid therapy.

Several systems are adversely affected by hyperkalemia; like hypokalemia, the most pressing problems are cardiac:

(1) Cardiovascular system
   (a) ECG changes: peaked T waves, widened QRS, and depressed ST segments progressing to increasingly aberrant ECG complexes and abnormal rhythms.
   (b) Dysrhythmias: bradycardia, ventricular tachycardia, and ventricular fibrillation.
   (c) Peripheral vascular collapse and cardiac arrest.

(2) Modes of treatment: Therapeutic intervention is guided by the serum K^+ level and the clinical findings:
   (a) Discontinue K^+ administration; always take this step.
      (i) Remove K^+ from all IV fluids and diet.
      (ii) Discontinue medications that provide large sources of K^+ (e.g., penicillin G potassium).

(b) Remove K^+ from the body.
  (i) Diuresis when the kidneys are functioning (important mode when excess K^+ has been administered).
  (ii) Dialysis: not feasible during initial encounter and transport.
  (iii) Cation exchange resins: sodium polystyrene sulfonate (Kayexalate). Na^+ is exchanged for K^+: 1 g/kg should remove 1 mEq K^+.
    (a) 1 g/kg PO or NG q2–6h, or
    (b) 1 g/kg pr q2–6h as a retention enema; the enema should be retained for at least 60 minutes.

(c) Shift the K^+ from the ECF to the ICF:
  (i) $NaHCO_3$ 1–2 mEq/kg IV over 5–10 minutes.
  (ii) Glucose and insulin solution infusion.
    (a) Glucose dose: 0.5 g/kg: Use D_{25} in infants, D_{50} in older children.
    (b) Add 1 unit of regular insulin/4 g of glucose.
    (c) Infuse glucose-insulin solution IV over 15–30 minutes.
    (d) Monitor glucose levels with bedside glucose strips: Young infants are at risk of developing hypoglycemia.

(d) Protect cells against hyperkalemia:
  (i) Calcium gluconate: 0.5–1.0 mL/kg IV over 5–10 minutes.
    (a) Maximum single dose: 20 mL (2.0 g of calcium gluconate).

(3) Suggested therapy
  (a) K^+ <6.0 mEq/L; patient is asymptomatic.
    (i) Discontinue all K^+ administration.
  (b) Potassium >6.5–7.0 mEq/L; patient is asymptomatic.
    (i) Administer sodium polystyrene sulfonate.
  (c) Potassium >7.0 mEq/L; ECG changes are present but cardiac rhythm is normal.
    (i) Provide $NaHCO_3$ and glucose/insulin infusion.

(ii) Administer sodium polystyrene sulfonate.

(d) K^+ >8.0 mEq/L or cardiac dysrhythmias are present.

(i) Start with calcium gluconate infusion.

(ii) Provide $NaHCO_3$ and glucose/insulin infusion.

(iii) Administer sodium polystyrene sulfonate.

e. *Hypocalcemia*

Hypocalcemia is an especially important problem in pediatric critical care. Profound hypocalcemia produces neurologic problems. Less well recognized is the lesser degree of hypocalcemia that can profoundly depress cardiac function in the critically ill child, a condition that is easily remediable.

Defining hypocalcemia is difficult. Normal serum Ca^{2+} values are 8.5 to 10.5 mg/dL. Hypocalcemia is traditionally defined as levels <8 mg/dL in children and <7 mg/dL in neonates.

In usual states, approximately one half of the Ca^{2+} is bound to proteins (primarily albumin), and the remainder is ionized. The protein-bound Ca^{2+} is physiologically inactive, whereas the ionized Ca^{2+} affects cell membrane activity. It is the ionized fraction of Ca^{2+} that is physiologically important because it maintains normal cell membrane activity and cell function. Usual Ca^{2+} values report total Ca^{2+}, the sum of the protein-bound and ionized fractions without specifying the amount of each component.

Herein lies the difficulty in defining hypocalcemia: A low serum Ca^{2+} value, of itself, does not always signify physiologic hypocalcemia. If both fractions are low, physiologic hypocalcemia exists; when the serum albumin value is normal, the protein-bound fraction will be normal, and the decrease in Ca^{2+} value is likely to be in the ionized fraction; if the ionized fraction remains normal, as can happen in the presence of hypoalbuminemia (the protein-bound fraction, alone, is low), physiologic hypocalcemia does not exist. Ionized Ca^{2+} values, when available, are especially useful. Because they are not widely available, low total serum Ca^{2+} values must be interpreted from concomitant albumin values and via ECG patterns.

(1) Problems that arise from hypocalcemia
 (a) Neurologic
  (i) Tetany: twitching, tetany, carpopedal spasms, laryngospasm (stridor).
  (ii) Seizures.
  (iii) Weakness.
 (b) Cardiovascular
  (i) Shock secondary to decreased myocardial contractility.
   (a) Inotropic agents (e.g., dopamine) fail to correct myocardial dysfunction secondary to hypocalcemia. (IV Ca^{2+} infusion dramatically restores contractility.)
   (b) Most commonly observed in hypocalcemic patients with cardiac disease, hypoxia, or severe systemic illness.
  (ii) ECG changes
   (a) Prolonged QT interval.
   (b) AV block: uncommon.
(2) Treatment
 (a) Seizures, tetany
  (i) Calcium gluconate
   (a) Dose: 100 mg of calcium gluconate/kg, maximum dose 2,000 mg.
   (b) For peripheral IV: Dilute 1:1 with sterile water; infuse carefully (infiltration produces severe necrosis).
   (c) Administer over 10 minutes.
   (d) Place child on cardiac monitor: Monitor ECG complexes, rhythm.
 (b) Shock, hypocalcemia in child with severe systemic illness
  (i) Calcium gluconate
   (a) Neonates: 100–150 mg/kg/dose IV q8h.
   (b) Infants, toddlers: 50–100 mg/kg/dose IV q8h.

(c) Preschoolers to adolescents: 20–50 mg/kg IV q8h; maximum single dose 2,000 mg.

(ii) Calcium chloride: Consider for the child who is very ill (i.e., the child whose liver may not be able to metabolize the gluconate and liberate the ionized Ca^{2+}).

(a) Neonates: 33–50 mg/kg/dose IV q8h.

(b) Infants, toddlers: 15–33 mg/kg/dose IV q8h.

(c) Preschoolers to adolescents: 10–15 mg/kg/dose IV q8h.

(iii) Administration of Ca^{2+}

(a) Dilute 1:1 with sterile water for peripheral IV infusion; avoid infiltration.

(b) Administer dose IV over 10 minutes.

(c) Monitor ECG during Ca^{2+} infusion.

(iv) Monitor Ca^{2+} levels; adjust Ca^{2+} doses according to Ca^{2+} values. In severely ill children, hypocalcemia can be profound and subsequent Ca^{2+} doses may have to be increased beyond recommended doses to maintain values and cardiac function.

f. *Hypomagnesemia*

(1) Clinically significant problems that arise from hypomagnesemia

(a) Hypomagnesemic tetany: tetany in the presence of:

(i) Normal Ca^{2+} level and Mg^{2+} levels <1.3 mEq/L in neonates or <1.6 mEq/L in older children.

(ii) Refractory hypocalcemia.

(a) Some young infants have hypocalcemia that is refractory to Ca^{2+} supplementation alone. Provision of Mg^{2+} helps correct this disorder.

(2) Treatment

(a) Magnesium sulfate

(i) Injectable form: 50% magnesium sulfate (500 mg of magnesium sulfate/mL).

(ii) Dose
(a) Neonates: 50–100 mg/kg IV or IM q8–12h for 3–4 doses.
(b) Infants, older children: 25–50 mg/kg IV or IM q4–6h for 3–4 doses.
(iii) IV administration
(a) Dilute to <10 mg/mL concentration.
(b) Administer over 1–2 hours.
(c) Monitor BP during infusion: Hypotension may develop with rapid infusion.

II. Glucose

A. Hypoglycemia

Hypoglycemia is defined by a blood glucose measurement of less than 40 mg/dL in all infants and children (including premature and small for gestational age infants). There are many causes of hypoglycemia in a child, many related to rapid depletion of glucose stores from stress. Transient hypoglycemia is common in the newborn period. Infants and children may have hypoglycemia as a result of hepatic enzyme deficiencies (i.e., glucose-6-phosphate dehydrogenase deficiency), hepatic disease (infectious hepatitis or Reye's syndrome), endocrine deficiencies (hypopituitarism, isolated growth hormone deficiency, primary adrenocortical insufficiency), inborn errors of metabolism, or hyperinsulinism. Ketotic hypoglycemia is the most common type found in childhood. It accounts for approximately 50% of cases, usually in children 18 months to 5 years, in boys more commonly than girls. It generally has a spontaneous remission as the patient gets older, and acute episodes are treated easily with glucose. Sepsis should always be suspected and ruled out in the hypoglycemic patient. Again, hypoglycemia may be a result of any critical illness in a young child.

1. *Clinical assessment*
   a. History
   b. Symptoms of CNS glucose deficiency
      (1) Confusion
      (2) Irritability
      (3) Visual disturbances
      (4) Bizarre or psychotic behavior
      (5) Headache

(6) Seizure
(7) Coma

c. Symptoms of increased epinephrine secretion
  (1) Tremor or jitteriness
  (2) Pallor
  (3) Sweating
  (4) Tachycardia
  (5) Tingling sensations
  (6) Weakness
  (7) Anxiety
  (8) Hunger

d. Laboratory data
  (1) Serum glucose level <40 mg/dL.
  (2) Obtain a standard serum glucose measurement to back up any low rapid glucose measurement (Dextrostix, Chemstrip).

2. *Therapy*
  a. ABCs; provide 100% oxygen.
  b. Consider endotracheal intubation and mechanical ventilation for all comatose patients.
  c. Obtain IV access and administer glucose.
    (1) 2–3 mL/kg D_{10} in the young infant.
      (a) Plasma glucose level should rise by approximately 35 mg/dL.
      (b) Avoid more concentrated bolus infusions because of rapid osmotic shifts and rebound hypoglycemia secondary to stimulation of insulin secretion.
    (2) In the older child, give 0.5 g/kg of glucose as D_{25} or D_{50}.
      (a) D_{25} has 25 g of glucose/100 mL: 2 mL/kg IV.
      (b) D_{50} has 50 g of glucose/100 mL: 1 mL/kg IV.
  d. Provide continuous glucose infusion.
    (1) D_5 or D_{10}.
      (a) 7–12 mg/kg/min in neonates.
      (b) 4–8 mg/kg/min in older infants and children.
    (2) In general, maintenance volumes of D_{10} will provide these amounts.
  e. Assess serum glucose 10–15 minutes after bolus infusion.

f. Glucagon, 1 mg IM, may be effective in terminating hypoglycemia.
   (1) Glucagon will not be effective in hypoglycemia secondary to liver disease.
   (2) Glucagon should always be followed by the administration of glucose.

3. *Ongoing monitoring*
   a. Follow neurologic status closely.
   b. Check glucose level every half hour until stable.

B. Diabetic ketoacidosis

Diabetic ketoacidosis (DKA) is a very complex disease state: an underlying biochemical disorder—a complex array of metabolic derangements that arise from absent/insufficient insulin—with widespread clinical consequences. The therapy is similarly complex: management of multiple metabolic and clinical problems and the need to manage certain metabolic problems in ways that are unique to DKA. Important principles about DKA that are reviewed in this chapter are highlighted:

1. Numerous, far-reaching, and complexly interrelated problems—both metabolic and clinical—arise from uncontrolled diabetes mellitus.
2. Some of the problems that arise from insulin insufficiency (e.g., dehydration and shock) eventually become life-threatening problems and the first priority concerns in the emergency management of DKA.
3. Some of the individual metabolic problems seen in DKA require management in a manner that is unique to DKA; treatment of these problems in the usual manner would produce major complications in DKA. ***Examples:***
   a. DKA patients with low pH rarely need intubation. Correction of the metabolic acidosis with HCO_3^- can lead to multiple and major problems, including CNS deterioration, dysrhythmias from hypokalemia, tissue hypoxia, and seizures from hypocalcemia.
   b. Rapid correction of hyperglycemia can produce CNS dysfunction, brain edema, and brain herniation when the latter is severe.
4. DKA poses a dilemma. DKA, left untreated, will result in death, most commonly from hypovolemic shock. Treatment of DKA, too, can cause death, most commonly from cerebral edema and brain herniation. For the latter

reason, therapy must be meticulously administered and monitored to minimize the major complications that have come to be well recognized.

Fortunately, advances in therapy have resulted in overall excellent patient outcome and a marked decline in mortality. A regimen that has been successful in treating DKA is presented in this chapter. Understanding the pathophysiology of DKA still remains important, because unexpected problems do arise during therapy and a small number of patients still die for reasons that are not always clear. The care provider who understands the pathophysiology of DKA can knowledgeably monitor the patient during treatment and similarly provide intervention when unexpected problems arise; this allows for best patient outcome.

1. **Pathophysiology**

   Diabetes in childhood is usually type I or insulin-dependent diabetes mellitus. The cascade of events occurring secondary to absent/inadequate insulin follow.

   a. Primary problem: absent/insufficient insulin.
   b. Consequences of absent/insufficient insulin
      (1) Hyperglycemia: Hyperglycemia is increased further. As the cells fail to "see" glucose, compensatory actions are activated to increase glucose sources: gluconeogenesis and polyphagia.
      (2) Inadequate energy source for cells.
   c. Consequences of hyperglycemia
      (1) Serum hyperosmolality.
      (2) Water loss: polyuria—osmotic diuresis—develops when the glucose level exceeds the renal threshold for glucose reabsorption.
         (a) Polydipsia develops secondarily to maintain hydration.
      (3) Electrolyte losses in urine: Large quantities of Na^+, K^+, Ca^{2+}, and phosphate are lost during osmotic diuresis.
   d. Consequences of inadequate glucose (energy) source for cells: use of alternative sources of energy.
      (1) Proteinolysis.
      (2) Lipolysis: Results of lipolysis:
         (a) Lipemia.
         (b) Ketoacid production: ketones, metabolic acids.

e. Primary clinical consequences of increasing metabolic disturbances
   (1) Recurrent emesis and/or abdominal pain, which can mimic an acute condition of the abdomen. This point marks the onset of rapid deterioration.
   (2) Consequences of recurrent emesis: inability to take in fluid while brisk osmotic diuresis continues.
      (a) Rapidly progressive dehydration, shock, death.
      (b) Rapid deterioration of already abnormal metabolic status that can cause death.

   The metabolic findings at step d. in this scheme—hyperglycemia, ketonemia, metabolic acidosis, glucosuria and ketonuria—constitute DKA.

2. **Metabolic Disturbances**

   There are a large number of metabolic and laboratory disturbances in DKA, including:

   a. *Hyperglycemia:* Glucose levels are usually >200 mg/dL and may reach values >1,000 mg/dL.
   b. *Water loss:* Glucose is a very potent osmotic diuretic once the renal threshold for glucose reabsorption is exceeded. Brisk diuresis persists, even in the state of decompensated shock; oliguria and anuria occur only in far-advanced shock and are preterminal findings. For these reasons, diuresis cannot be used as a measure of the adequacy of circulation in DKA. Large amounts of electrolytes are lost in the urine in osmotic diuresis.
   c. *Hyperosmolality, idiogenic osmols:* Hyperglycemia raises serum osmolality. Elevated serum osmolality causes water to move from the cells into the ECF compartment to equalize osmolalities. Very high serum osmolalities (i.e., high glucose levels) can cause large fluid shifts that result in significant brain shrinkage with stretching and tearing of the bridging vessels. This problem, however, is rarely seen in DKA because the brain has a protective response that reduces fluid exit from the brain. In response to persistent serum hyperosmolality, the brain cells produce intracellular osmols, termed *idiogenic osmols,* that raise intracellular osmolality and reduce the exit of water from

the brain. The protective effect that idiogenic osmols provide in the hyperosmolar state do, however, pose a potentially lethal problem during therapy. Because idiogenic osmols form slowly and break down slowly, rapid correction of glucose levels, which rapidly drops serum osmolality, results in a reversal of the osmolality gradient. Intracellular osmolality will then be higher than serum osmolality, water will move from the ECF into the brain cells, and cerebral edema and brain herniation will be the clinical result when the fluid shift is large. For this reason, hyperglycemia must be corrected cautiously.

d. *Lipemia:* Lipemia is one of the results of using alternative energy sources; the blood may be grossly lipemic in DKA.

e. *Ketones:* Acetoacetate, acetone, and β-hydroxybutyrate are the ketone bodies formed in DKA. β-Hydroxybutyrate is the favored form of ketones with increasing acidosis; acetoacetate and acetone are favored with decreasing acidosis. Because only acetoacetate and acetone produce a positive reaction with ketone tablets and dipsticks, as the child improves increasing ketosis determined by these methods can be expected and is not a sign of patient deterioration. Therefore, ketone determination is not a good measure of response to therapy in DKA.

f. *Acidosis:* Acidosis in DKA is almost always metabolic in origin. Most of acids are ketoacids; lactic acid contributes to the acidosis when dehydration develops. Hyperventilation and Kussmaul's respirations are compensatory efforts to maintain normal pH. Uncompensated metabolic acidosis, however, eventually results. In advanced DKA, the pH can be as low as 6.7, the P_{CO_2} 6–10 mm Hg, the HCO_3^- <5 mEq/L. The acidotic state in DKA is, however, unique: Many patients with pH values as low as 6.8 have remarkably good mentation and cardiac function. These findings are explained by the observation that serum acidosis develops over several days rather than several minutes to hours; the CSF, especially, has time to accommodate and maintain a fairly normal pH in the face of serum acidosis. When therapy is provided—fluids to restore circulation, insulin to allow glucose utilization and cessation of lipolysis—acidosis gradually reverses; decrease in acidosis is the best measure of response to therapy.

g. *Sodium:* Initial Na^+ values are commonly low and not of clinical significance. The values are usually factitiously low because of lipemia and displacement by glucose as Na^+ is decreased by 1.6 mEq/L for every 100 mg/dL elevation of glucose. As hyperglycemia and lipemia are corrected, Na^+ values return to normal with usual rehydration therapy.
h. *Potassium:* Total body K^+ stores are invariably low, but initial serum K^+ values may range from low to high. As therapy is provided, serum K^+ levels usually fall, sometimes to dangerously low levels: K^+ moves into cells as acidosis is corrected and insulin is provided, and K^+ continues to be lost in urine through osmotic diuresis.
i. *Phosphate:* Body phosphate stores are low, and initial serum phosphate levels are variable. Phosphate levels fall during therapy in a manner similar to K^+ levels. The clinical significance of hypophosphatemia in DKA remains uncertain, but treatment of hypophosphatemia is recommended.
j. *Calcium:* Ca^{2+} is lost in the urine, but serum values are usually normal; Ca^{2+} problems are not recognized in DKA.
k. *BUN and creatinine:* The levels of both will be elevated from dehydration. The creatinine level may be spuriously elevated when measured by methods that are interfered with by ketones.
l. *Amylase:* Amylase values may be elevated. Even though abdominal pain is common in DKA, the amylase has been found to be nonpancreatic in origin and has no known clinical significance.
m. *Leukocytosis:* Elevated white blood cell (WBC) count is common with granulocytic predominance. This is most commonly a stress response and is not indicative of infection.
n. *Hemoconcentration:* Elevation of the Hgb and Hct values are found in significant dehydration.

3. **Clinical findings**

In early diabetes, few abnormalities may be detected on physical examination. History will reveal polyuria, polydipsia, and polyphagia; there may be a history of weight loss and fatigue. At this stage, laboratory abnormalities are limited to hyperglycemia, ketonemia, glucosuria and ketonuria; acidosis is absent to mild. Insulin therapy, alone, is required.

With progression to DKA, additional complaints may include malaise, weight loss, difficulty breathing; later developments are abdominal pain, nausea, and vomiting. Physical examination is remarkable for lethargy, fatigue, tachycardia, and Kussmaul's respirations; the classic odor of acetone may be present in the breath. Signs of dehydration are present to the point of early circulatory compromise. Abdominal tenderness may be pronounced at times. Laboratory findings include more pronounced hyperglycemia, metabolic acidosis, ketonemia, and ketonuria. pH value may be as low as 7.1. Emesis is a red flag because it heralds the rapid development of dehydration and shock if left untreated.

The patient with advanced DKA will have some or all of the following findings: severe dehydration with cool extremities, poor perfusion; profound Kussmaul's respirations; prostration; lethargy/obtundation. Laboratory findings include worsening of the previously mentioned laboratory test results, arterial pH <7.1, $HCO_3^- <10$ mEq/L, elevated BUN and creatinine levels, and hemoconcentration. In the prearrest state, decompensated shock, coma, or oliguria/anuria is found.

At any stage of illness, coexisting infection, which may have precipitated the decompensation, may be present.

4. **Laboratory evaluation**

The diagnosis of DKA is made on the basis of a history of known diabetes mellitus or history compatible with diabetes mellitus plus the laboratory findings of hyperglycemia, ketonemia, metabolic acidosis, glucosuria, and ketonuria. Recommended admission laboratory evaluation follows.

a. Admission laboratory tests
   (1) Glucose, electrolyte, BUN, and creatinine levels.
   (2) CBC count and differential.

(3) Arterial blood gas (ABG) values.
(4) Urinalysis.

b. Additional laboratory tests: as indicated.
(1) Phosphate, calcium values.
(2) Sepsis work-up: blood culture, other cultures, chest x-ray studies.
(3) Consider salicylate level for the patient with this picture and a history of aspirin intake.

5. **Therapy**

Therapy of DKA involves far more than insulin administration for glucose regulation. Because some of the consequences of insufficient insulin are life-threatening, they must be treated first and take priority over the administration of insulin. Some of the metabolic problems require specific management to prevent life-threatening complications. Because therapy is so complex, therapy is presented in three sections: (1) priorities and special concerns in therapy; (2) rationale for the management of the individual problems that may produce life-threatening conditions during therapy; (3) a summary of the overall management of DKA.

a. *Priorities and special concerns*
(1) *Fluid therapy:* the first priority in treating DKA.
(a) The patient with moderate to severe DKA will have moderate dehydration to decompensated shock resulting from fluid deficits. Restoration of circulation with volume expanders is the first concern in DKA. After circulation is restored, rehydration remains a major concern.
(b) The restoration of circulation with volume expanders alone will improve the metabolic and clinical status: Both the glucose level and metabolic acids are frequently reduced with initial volume expansion; neurologic status improvement and decreased work of breathing commonly follow restoration of circulation.

(2) *Insulin and glucose*
(a) Insulin is vital to restore normal metabolic pathways and normal glucose levels. It should be provided as soon as possible but follows restoration of circulation in priority.

(b) The hyperosmolar state created by hyperglycemia is of special concern: too rapid lowering of glucose levels (i.e., serum osmolality) can produce cerebral edema and brain herniation. Therefore, insulin administration and glucose level correction must be carefully regulated and monitored.

(3) *Special metabolic concerns*

Multiple derangements are present in DKA, but 3 metabolic problems need special attention and management in DKA:

(a) Metabolic acidosis
(b) K^+
(c) Phosphate

(4) Neurologic concerns: Neurologic problems may arise during therapy, some of them with clearly identifiable etiologies, others without. Neurologic problems include:

(a) Cerebral edema and herniation.
(b) Seizures.

b. *Management of specific problems*

(1) Fluid therapy

(a) Restoration of circulation: first-priority therapy

(i) Restore circulating volume *aggressively:* Patients in DKA have large fluid deficits, large ongoing losses as long as serum glucose level is >180 mg/dL (osmotic diuresis).

(a) Start with 20 mL/kg LR or NS solution IV *push*.

(b) Repeat 10–20 mL/kg pushes of LR or NS solution prn. The DKA patient in shock may need up to a total of 60 mL/kg LR or NS solution to restore circulation acutely.

(c) In the severely dehydrated patient, the end point of volume expander pushes is restoration of good central pulses. When this is accomplished, the peripheral pulses may still be weaker than central pulses, and the

extremities will still remain cool and dusky/mottled until later stages of rehydration.

(ii) Rehydration after circulation is restored

(a) Rehydration is usually accomplished in 12–24 hours by providing fluids at 2–3 times maintenance amount. Use 2 × maintenance amount for moderate DKA, 3 × maintenance amount for the patient in decompensated shock.

(b) Rehydration fluid: ½NS solution + K^+. (Discussion of K^+ and glucose addition to rehydration fluid follows.)

(c) Osmotic diuresis continues as long as serum glucose level is >180–200 mg/dL. Especially at the beginning of therapy, osmotic diuresis may be very brisk; urine volume may exceed fluid administration and cause decreased circulation. Any time signs of circulatory compromise appear during therapy, provide additional pushes of LR or NS solution, 10–20 mL/kg, to restore circulation; then resume rehydration.

(2) Insulin therapy: glucose regulation, hyperosmolality

(a) Continuous IV infusion of insulin is probably the most effective means of providing insulin reliably, correcting glucose and other metabolic derangements smoothly, thereby minimizing the occurrence of therapeutic complications.

(b) Insulin drip dose: 0.1 units/kg/hour. Infrequently a higher dose, up to 0.2 unit/kg/hour, may be required to correct hyperglycemia and ketoacidosis.

(i) Preparation of insulin drip

(a) Add 50 units of regular insulin to 250 mL bottle of NS solution.

(b) Resulting solution has 0.2 units of insulin/mL.

(c) Run solution through IV tubing to prime tubing, then attach tubing to patient IV line.

(d) IV insulin infusion can be run into the same line as the rehydrating IV solution.

(e) Dose = 0.1 unit/kg/hour = 0.5 mL/kg/hour. Regulate infusion rate with a pump.

(c) Glucose values are almost always corrected long before DKA has been corrected.

(i) When the glucose value is at the 300 mg/dL range, add D_5 to the rehydrating fluid to avoid hypoglycemia.

(ii) If after adding D_5 to the rehydrating fluid the glucose levels are low ($<150-200$ mg/dL during therapy of DKA), increase the dextrose concentration up as high as 10%.

(iii) If serum glucose values still fall to low levels on increased amounts of dextrose, proceed to decreasing the insulin dose to as low as 0.05 units/kg/hour. Remember that insulin is required to treat DKA even though hyperglycemia may have already been corrected.

(iv) Acute hypoglycemia: Give 1 mL/kg D_{50} or 1–2 mL/kg D_{25}, then raise IV dextrose concentration or decrease insulin drip dosage.

(d) Serum glucose levels and osmolality: CNS concerns

(i) Hyperglycemia produces serum hyperosmolality. The brain produces idiogenic osmols in response to serum hyperosmolality to minimize brain shrinkage. A too rapid drop of glucose (i.e., serum osmolality) will reverse the osmolality gradient because idiogenic osmols break down slowly; fluid will then move into the brain and produce cerebral edema and brain herniation if brain swelling is great. Neurologic monitoring is required during therapy of DKA.

(ii) Aim to drop serum glucose values by about 100 mg/dL/hour. This is usually accomplished with constant insulin infusion dose of 0.1 unit/kg/hour.

(iii) If serum glucose value falls by more than 100 mg/dL/hour:

(a) If the patient's neurologic status is stable, no acute intervention is needed. The insulin drip rate may have to be decreased or IV dextrose concentration may have to be increased to decrease the rate of glucose fall.

(b) If the patient develops neurologic deterioration—significant decrease in level of consciousness, seizures, focal signs (e.g., pupil inequality), brain stem dysfunction (posturing, abnormal respiratory patterns):

(1) Administer mannitol, 0.5–1.0 g/kg IV over 5–10 minutes, if cardiorespiratory system function is stable.

(2) If the patient has brain stem dysfunction and/or unstable cardiorespiratory function, intubation, hyperventilation are needed in addition to mannitol (see p. 122).

(3) Metabolic problems

(a) Acidosis: metabolic origin, ketoacids and lactic acid when dehydration is present.

(i) The patient with DKA has significant metabolic acidosis, respiratory alkalosis (Kussmaul's respirations).

(a) In moderate to severe DKA, uncompensated metabolic acidosis results in low pH values, as low as 6.7–6.8 in severe cases. These patients are unique in regard to their acidosis: DKA patients with pH values as low

as 6.8–6.9 are frequently arousable, able to converse; other patients are comatose.

(1) Explanation: The serum acidosis develops over several days, and the CSF has time to compensate and maintain a nearly normal pH value.

(ii) These patients therefore deteriorate if their pH values are acutely corrected with $NaHCO_3$:

(a) CNS deterioration: When $NaHCO_3$ is given, serum pH value increases, the drive for compensatory respiratory alkalosis decreases, and P_{CO_2} value rises. HCO_3 does not readily cross into the CSF; CO_2 rapidly crosses into the CSF, produces carbonic acid, and produces paradoxical CSF acidosis with CNS deterioration.

(b) Rapid correction of serum pH value with $NaHCO_3$ will drive K^+ into the cells and may produce profound hypokalemia and cardiac dysrhythmias.

(c) Other problems that may arise include tetany from hypocalcemia and tissue hypoxia as the oxygen-dissociation curve shifts to the left.

(iii) The DKA patient with a low pH rarely needs intubation and ventilation: Most have fairly good CNS function; most have excellent respiratory function and good respiratory muscle strength. The only DKA patient who may need intubation and ventilation is one who is in severe shock and near-arrest or the patient with profound neurologic dysfunction (e.g., Glasgow Coma Score <8–9).

(iv) Management of uncompensated metabolic acidosis

(a) If the arterial pH is >7.0 and the CNS status is good, do not give $NaHCO_3$. Metabolic acidosis and pH

will correct with rehydration and insulin.

(b) If the arterial pH is <7.0, disagreement over the best management of this state still exists.

(1) Some advocate the administration of $NaHCO_3$, 1 mEq/kg IV over 1 hour.

(2) Others advocate that $NaHCO_3$ is not needed unless signs of cardiac dysfunction are present (the concern is that the very low pH is causing cardiac dysfunction); provide 1 mEq $NaHCO_3$/kg IV over 1 hour in this case.

(3) Aside from $NaHCO_3$ pushes, the patient with pH <7.0 can have an IV solution with *acetate* anion rather than chloride. Rather than using ½NS solution as the rehydration solution (77 mEq NaCl/L), one can use 40 mEq NaCl + 35 mEq Na-Acetate/L. Acetate is converted to bicarbonate. Acetate is used because it is compatible with most medications, including insulin, whereas $NaHCO_3$ is incompatible with most medications, including insulin. Once again, many believe that if the patient is stable, acetate in the IV solution is unnecessary.

(c) Serum $NaHCO_3$ levels will rise as the patient improves, and HCO_3 values are the best laboratory indicator of patient improvement. (NOTE: When the initial HCO_3 value is very low (i.e., <10 mEq/L), HCO_3 values may fall in the first 2–3 hours before rising; then the rise in HCO_3 is very slow, frequently by 1–2 mEq/L q2–4h, until it reaches the teens when the HCO_3 rise is rapid.)

(b) K^+

(i) Body K^+ stores are depleted from urinary losses.

(ii) Initial serum K^+ values are variable (low, normal, or high) and do not reflect body K^+ stores. In the acidotic patient, H^+ moves into cells, K^+ moves into the serum; the more acidotic the patient, the more likely the serum K^+ level is falsely high.

(iii) K^+ moves into the cells as acidosis is corrected and as insulin is provided (it follows glucose into the cell). Hypokalemia can therefore become evident during therapy and reach very low values.

(iv) Management

(a) Provide K^+ in the *rehydrating solution* as soon as it is established that the patient urinates. (Do not add K^+ to the pushes of volume expanders, i.e., LR or NS solution.)

(1) Usual amount of K^+: 40 mEq K^+/L. Modify this concentration by serum K^+ values. Do not exceed 60 mEg of KCl/L in peripheral IV.

(2) K^+: Usually provide K^+ in two forms: 20 mEq KCl and 20 mEq of K-phosphate/L.

(b) For hypokalemia: K^+ <3.0 mEq/L:

(1) Give ½ mEq KCl/kg IV over 1 hour; maximum bolus dose is 20 mEq KCl. Repeat serum K^+ level; repeat this dose if K^+ value remains <3 mEq/L.

(c) Administration of large concentrations/amounts of KCl IV peripherally may produce severe pain. If this occurs, suggest:

(1) Starting a second IV. Administer half of the hourly KCl solution/bolus through each IV. A reduction of the absolute amount of

KCl in a vein decreases venous irritation and pain.

(c) Phosphate
 (i) Body phosphate stores are depleted from urine losses.
 (ii) Phosphate levels frequently fall to very low levels several hours into therapy: Phosphate moves into the cells and is used as glucose is metabolized.
 (iii) Primary concern about phosphate deficiency: tissue hypoxia.
  (a) Theoretical concern: 2,3-Diphosphoglycerate levels may fall, and the oxygen-dissociation curve will shift to the left. Hemoglobin therefore will not release oxygen to the tissues readily, thereby cause tissue hypoxia. This has been postulated as a cause of death in those DKA patients who die of unexplained causes during carefully controlled therapy. (Remarkable finding is cerebral edema; question is if this is caused by tissue hypoxia.)
  (b) Other problems associated with hypophosphatemia: Cardiac and respiratory depression are associated with chronic rather than acute hypophosphatemia.
 (iv) For the previous reason, it is recommended that one half of the K^+ be administered as K-phosphate rather than having all of it given as KCl.
  (a) NOTE: During therapy of DKA, the phosphate levels are likely to be low in the first 12–24 hours in spite of phosphate provision as recommended. This does not appear to have clinical significance as long as phosphate is being provided.

(4) Neurologic problems during therapy
  (a) Cerebral edema
    (i) Most patients being treated for DKA have some degree of cerebral edema but are asymptomatic.
    (ii) Symptomatic patients may have the usual progression of symptoms and signs: headache and irritability; decreasing level of consciousness; urinary incontinence; signs of brain stem dysfunction (pupil changes, posturing, abnormal respiratory patterns); finally, cardiopulmonary arrest. Aggressive intervention before arrest takes place can result in good patient outcome; after a cardiorespiratory arrest occurs, patient outcome is usually dismal.
    (iii) Possible causes of cerebral edema: rapid drop in glucose level, Na^+ level, osmolality; tissue hypoxia; other causes that remain yet unidentified.
  (b) Seizures
    (i) May be secondary to rapid drop in glucose level, Na^+ level, osmolality, occasional cerebral vascular complications (thrombosis, bleeds).
  (c) Management of signs of increased ICP and/or seizures
    (i) Supplemental oxygen.
    (ii) Mannitol, 0.5–1.0 g/kg IV over 5–10 minutes.
    (iii) Intubation (using ICP precautions) and hyperventilation are used in addition to mannitol if vital sign dysfunction and/or brain stem dysfunction is present (see p. 413).
    (iv) Seizure management: usual therapy. Start with benzodiazepine (diazepam or lorazepam); follow with phenobarbital or phenytoin, 20 mg/kg IV (see p. 127).
    (v) Obtain laboratory work: immediate glucose, electrolyte, and ABG values.

Summary of Treatment of DKA

a. Restore circulating volume.
   (1) 20 mL/kg LR or NS solution IV push.
   (2) Repeat 10–20 mL/kg IV pushes or LR or NS solution until circulation is restored; patient may require a total of up to 60 mL/kg.
b. Start constant infusion insulin.
   (1) Insulin drip: 50 units of regular insulin in 250 mL bottle of NS solution.
   (2) Dose: 0.1 unit of insulin/kg/hour = 0.5 mL/kg/hour.
   (3) Insulin drip may be given in the same line as the rehydrating solution.
c. Rehydration.
   (1) Solution: ½NS solution + 20 mEq KCl and 20 mEq K^+-phosphate/L.
      (a) Add K^+ after urine output is established; modify K^+ concentration by electrolyte values. Do not exceed a concentration of 60 mEq of KCl/L.
      (b) May provide some of Na^+ as acetate: e.g., 40 mEq of NaCl and 35 mEq of Na^+-acetate/L in the very acidotic patient.
   (2) IV rate: 2–3 × maintenance rate.
      (a) 2 × rate for moderate DKA; 3 × rate for DKA patient with shock.
   (3) Provide 10–20 mL/kg pushes of LR or NS solution anytime circulation is compromised. This may occur initially because urinary losses from osmotic diuresis may be very brisk.
d. Special metabolic concerns
   (1) K^+: If K^+ <3.0 mEq/L, give ½ mEq KCl/kg IV over 1 hour. Check serum K^+ value; repeat dose if K^+ level remains <3.0 mEq/L.
   (2) Add D_5 to rehydrating solution once serum glucose value reaches about 300 mg/dL.
      (a) Continue to increase dextrose concentrations up to 10% as needed and/or decrease insulin infusion rate to as low as 0.05 unit/kg/hour to avoid hypoglycemia. Do not discontinue insulin drip.
e. Treat coexisting problems (e.g., infection).

f. Other measures
   (1) Provide supplemental oxygen for the patient in shock, with altered level of consciousness.
   (2) Keep the patient npo initially.
g. Monitor the patient closely.
   (1) Vital signs: Include ECG monitoring, measured inputs and outputs.
   (2) Neurologic status: Monitor for signs of cerebral edema.
   (3) Laboratory monitoring
      (a) Hourly test-strip glucose.
      (b) Electrolyte values, glucose value q2–4h.
      (c) Repeat ABG analysis is not needed if the patient is clinically improving.
h. Neurologic complications: Treat as reviewed on p. 217.

III. Acute Adrenal Failure (Addisonian Crisis)

Acute adrenal failure results from a deficiency of endogenous glucocorticoid and mineralocorticoid, causing the signs and symptoms that follow.

NOTE: Adrenal crises may be the manifestation of chronic adrenal insufficiency.

Acute adrenal failure may represent the relative lack of adrenal glucocorticoids/mineralocorticoids. In pediatrics the most common manifestation is in the patient on a chronic corticosteroid regimen who undergoes a precipitating stress or a sudden decrease in corticosteroid therapy.

A. Clinical assessment

1. Signs and symptoms
   a. Nausea and vomiting
   b. Diarrhea, dehydration
   c. Circulatory collapse
   d. Fever or hypothermia
   e. Confusion, coma
   f. Masculinization of genitalia (in a young infant with unrecognized congenital adrenal hyperplasia)
2. Laboratory values
   a. Glucose level (hypoglycemia)
   b. Electrolyte values. (Mineralocorticoid deficiency may cause hyponatremia and hyperkalemia.)

B. Therapy

1. Before corticosteroid treatment, it is helpful to draw a red top tube to save for future cortisol determination.
2. Use 5% dextrose in ½NS solution or 5% dextrose in NS solution for treatment of tachycardia or hypotension. This is the rare case where, secondary to hypoglycemia, glucose is used in fluid boluses.
3. Hydrocortisone (Solu-Cortef).
   a. 50 mg/m^2, or 2 mg/kg as an IV bolus.
   b. Follow with 50–100 mg/m^2/day divided q4–6h, or 1.5 mg/kg q4–6h.
4. Mineralocorticoid.
   a. Not generally needed immediately.
   b. Deoxycorticosterone acetate (DOCA), 1–2 mg/day IM, or
   c. Fluorocortisone (Florinef) 0.05–0.15 mg/day po.
5. Look for cause of crises.
   a. Sepsis
   b. Trauma
   c. Other illness
   d. Withdrawal of ongoing corticosteroid therapy

C. Ongoing monitoring

1. Follow heart rate and BP.
2. Check rapid glucose test (Dextrostix) result hourly.

IV. Acute Renal Failure

Acute renal failure results from a sudden decline in the glomerular filtration rate, limiting the kidney's ability to maintain normal fluid and metabolic balance. Oliguria and acute tubular necrosis are the hallmarks of acute renal failure.

Acute renal failure may have many causes, including: hypotension/hypoxia, glomerulonephritis (i.e., poststreptococcal glomerulonephritis), hemolytic uremic syndrome, burns, transfusion reactions, toxins, and drugs (i.e., sulfonamides, bismuth, and carbon tetrachloride).

A. Clinical and laboratory assessment

1. History for etiology
2. Vital signs
   a. Hypotension or hypertension may be present.
3. Urine output
   a. Oliguria defined as <0.5 mL/kg/hour in infants and children or <500 mL/day in adults.

b. Anuria.

c. Suspect obstruction as a cause when a patient is completely anuric.

4. Laboratory values

a. Urinalysis: proteinuria, hematuria, active sediment (RBC casts, tubular cells, WBC casts, or other evidence of urinary tract infection).

b. Serum and urine electrolyte values, creatinine level, and osmolarity. If urine laboratory data are not available, save a prediuretic urine sample for later analysis. Also obtain serum calcium and serum phosphorus values. Initial abnormalities may include:

(1) Hyponatremia

(2) Acidosis, hypocalcemia

(3) Hyperkalemia, elevated BUN and creatinine levels

c. From the data in b, calculate the fractional excretion of sodium (FENa). This value is helpful in distinguishing the renal vs. prerenal state:

$$\text{FENa} = \frac{\text{urine Na}}{\text{plasma Na}} \div \frac{\text{urine creatinine}}{\text{plasma creatinine}} \times 100\%$$

Children and adults:	FENa% < 1 = prerenal
	FENa% > 2 = renal
Newborn infants:	FENa% < 2.5 = prerenal
	FENa% > 2.5 = renal

d. ECG: Look for abnormalities caused by specific electrolyte disturbances.

B. Therapy

1. Correct any nonrenal cause (i.e., volume depletion). If there is no evidence of volume overload, give 10 mL/kg of normal saline over 20–30 minutes.
2. Decrease fluid administration if patient is well hydrated but not urinating.

a. Provide replacement for insensible losses, as well as actual urine output, on an hourly basis. Use 5% or 10% dextrose in ¼NS solution.

3. Eliminate K^+ and phosphate from all IV solutions.
4. Eliminate nephrotoxins (aminoglycosides, etc.).
5. Induce diuresis using furosemide, 1–2 mg/kg IV. If there is no response in 1 hour, double the dose or give a single dose of 5 mg/kg.
6. Eliminate obstructive uropathy as a cause. Include a Foley catheter to rule out lower tract obstruction, as well as to follow urine output closely.

7. Treat hyperkalemia, hyperphosphatemia, or hypocalcemia as needed (see pp. 194, 198).

C. Ongoing monitoring

1. Cardiac monitor.
2. Strict recording of all input and output.
3. Regular glucose check: Glucose values may decrease secondary to limited fluid replacement, and, therefore, a higher concentration of glucose may be needed. Use D_{10} or $D_{12.5}$ if needed.

V. Hemolytic Uremic Syndrome

The hemolytic uremic syndrome is hallmarked by an acute hemolytic anemia, thrombocytopenia, and acute renal failure, often after a viral syndrome or GI infection. The exact cause of hemolytic uremic syndrome is as yet unknown. Many bacterial cytotoxins have been implicated in the pathogenesis of this "disease." Clinical involvement can include:

1. Renal: failure, hypertension.
2. Hematologic: anemia, thrombocytopenia.
3. GI: diarrhea (frequently bloody), colitis.
4. Cerebral: encephalopathy, seizures.

A. Clinical assessment

1. History or physical compatible with signs.
2. Laboratory data.
   a. Urinalysis: gross or microscopic hematuria with RBC casts and proteinuria.
   b. CBC count.
   c. Evaluation of peripheral smear—schistocytes.
   d. Platelet count.
   e. Electrolytes, BUN, creatinine

B. Therapy

1. As in acute renal failure, correct any volume depletion and assess degree of renal failure, fluid imbalance, and electrolyte abnormalities.
2. Treat hypertension with diuresis and antihypertensives as needed (see p. 87).
3. Transfuse with packed RBCs to keep Hct value at a minimum of 15.
4. Platelet transfusion is generally not helpful. Platelets are destroyed rapidly. Consider platelet transfusion if there is gross clinical bleeding.
5. Follow mental status closely. Look for signs and symp-

toms of increased ICP. Consider head CT scan if neurologic status is not consistent with the extent of the illness. Treat seizures with anticonvulsants (see p. 127).

C. **Ongoing monitoring**
   1. Cardiac monitor.
   2. Follow heart rate and BP.
   3. Record strict measurement of inputs and outputs.
   4. Observe for mental status and neurologic changes. Avoid sedation if possible.

REFERENCE

Freiberg L: Hypernatremic (hypertonic) dehydration in infants. *N Engl J Med* 1973; 289:196.

HEMATOLOGIC PROBLEMS 7

I. Physiologic Values

A. Blood volume: 70–80 mL/kg

1. Blood volume is closer to 80 mL/kg in small children, 70 mL/kg in larger children and adolescents.

B. Plasma volume

1. 50 mL/kg in children.
2. 40 mL/kg in adolescents, adults.

C. 1 g hemoglobin (Hgb) = hematocrit (Hct) 3%

II. Anemia

A. Routine transfusion for anemia

1. 1 mL/kg packed red blood cell (PRBC) transfusion will raise the Hct by:
   a. 1 when the patient: is euvolemic; does not have ongoing bleeding, hemolysis, or disseminated intravascular coagulation (DIC).
   b. <1 when the patient: is hypovolemic; has ongoing bleeding, hemolysis, or DIC.
2. The usual transfusion volume is 10–15 mL/kg over 2–6 hours.
   a. This can be expected to raise the Hct by 10–15 in the euvolemic patient who does not have ongoing RBC losses, by a lesser amount in patients who are hypovolemic or experiencing ongoing RBC losses.
   b. The larger transfusion volume can be given if the patient can tolerate extra volume.

B. Partial exchange transfusion: transfusion of the very anemic patient

The very anemic patient, usually one with a Hgb ≤4–5 g (Hct 12–15), is likely to be in congestive heart failure and is at great risk of developing heart failure from volume administration. Because of this danger, the usual transfusion of 10–15 mL of PRBCs/kg is almost always contraindicated. The low Hgb value must, instead, be raised very cautiously—by very slow transfusion or by partial exchange transfusion—in conjunction with measures that decrease the risk of fluid overload. A suggested approach to severe anemia is presented.

1. Provide fractional concentration of oxygen in inspired gas (Fio_2) 100%.
2. Administer furosemide, 1 mg/kg IV, IM.
3. Reduce oxygen needs: minimal patient disturbance; treat fever with acetaminophen.
4. *Slow PRBC transfusion:* may be used for the patient who is not in congestive heart failure.
   a. PRBCs: 1–2 mL/kg/hour to reach Hgb level of 6–7 g.
   b. Monitor the patient closely: heart rate, blood pressure, perfusion; urine output; pulse oximeter; clinical signs of congestive heart failure.
5. *Partial Exchange Transfusion:* A partial exchange transfusion should be performed on the patient in congestive heart failure: X mL of patient blood is withdrawn, and the same volume of PRBCs is pushed into the patient. This allows the Hgb level and Hct to be raised rapidly without giving additional fluid. (A net negative fluid balance can be achieved through the partial exchange by removing aliquots of patient blood that are larger in volume than aliquots of PRBCs infused; patient Hgb will still rise, because Hgb of PRBCs is much higher than that of patient blood).
   a. Provide supplemental oxygen, diuretic as earlier.
   b. Volume of blood to be exchanged to attain desired Hgb value:

$$\text{Volume of blood to be exchanged} = \frac{\text{Wt(kg)} \times 75\text{mL/kg} \times \text{Desired rise in Hgb value}}{22\text{g/100mL} - \text{Hgb}_M}$$

(1) 75 mL/kg = blood volume.

(2) 22 g/100 mL = Hgb value of PRBCs.

(3) Hgb_M = Mean Hgb value =

$$\frac{\text{Initial Hgb} + \text{Desired Hgb}}{2}$$

(4) Desired Hgb value is usually 6–7 g. This value is usually sufficient to get the patient out of congestive heart failure when cardiac function is good; if cardiac function is very impaired (e.g., in cardiomyopathy, cardiogenic shock), the desired Hgb value will need to be higher (e.g., 10 g).

c. Aliquots of 1 mL/kg are reasonable volumes to remove and infuse per pass. In larger children, the volume per pass is likely to be limited by the syringe size and the ease with which one can fill and empty the syringe; it is frequently impractical to use aliquot volumes >20–30 mL in large children when one is performing the exchange through regular plastic catheters. The procedure is almost always done manually.

d. Vascular line: Short lines of reasonably large caliber are preferable to long lines for exchange transfusions: Long lines only increase resistance and the difficulty of performing the exchange.

(1) For the critical situation—the patient in congestive heart failure, the patient on the brink of cardiac decompensation—*initiation* of the partial exchange transfusion is crucial: Administration of the first amounts of Hgb dramatically increase oxygen content of the blood and correspondingly reduce cardiac work and the risk of further decompensation.

Therefore, when IV access is difficult, any IV site that allows one to quickly initiate the exchange transfusion should be used; after stability and safety are attained, a more secure IV can be sought to complete the exchange.

Example: *Use of a butterfly or relatively small plastic catheter in an antecubital vein that allows one to perform 4–5 mL/kg exchange will increase the Hgb value by about 1 g, a substantial amount in the very anemic child. One can then more safely seek a better IV vein or continue to perform the exchange through this site if it is functioning effectively.*

(2) One IV line is sufficient to perform a partial exchange transfusion.

(a) Flush the line with several milliliters of NS solution if it becomes difficult to draw from or push into the line.

(b) To minimize the chance of clotting the line, remember that the patient's blood is not anticoagulated and will clot if left to sit in the line or tubing. Therefore, the amount of time the patient's blood is left to sit in the line must be minimized: After withdrawing the patient's blood, rapidly discard the patient blood, rapidly draw up PRBCs, then proceed with infusing the PRBCs at usual rate into the line.

III. Thrombocytopenia

A. Guidelines for desired platelet counts

1. Isolated thrombocytopenia: no other clinical problems. The risk of spontaneous major bleeds (e.g., a central nervous system [CNS] bleed) does not increase significantly until the platelet count falls to <10,000. Platelet transfusions are not needed for asymptomatic patients until the platelet count reaches this level.
2. Surgery, soft tissue bleeding: Keep platelet count >50,000.
3. Surgery or bleeding of CNS, major cardiac structures (heart, major blood vessels): Keep platelet count >100,000.

B. Platelet transfusion guidelines

1. 1 unit of platelets (concentrate)/7 kg of body weight will raise platelet count by 50–100,000.
   a. The platelet rise will be of lesser magnitude in the presence of platelet antibodies, ongoing platelet consumption such as DIC, and bleeding. In these instances, larger numbers of units of platelets will have to be transfused to attain the desired platelet count.

C. Platelet sources

1. Platelet concentrates: 1 unit = about 60 mL.
   a. For patients who cannot tolerate this volume, platelets may be spun down to a volume of about 30 mL. The platelet rise may be diminished slightly after spinning.
2. Pheresed platelet units: 1 unit = about 60 mL.
   a. 1 pheresed unit of platelets has a number of platelets equivalent to about 8–10 platelet concentrates.

IV. Coagulopathy

A. Coagulation factors in coagulation tests and coagulation disorders

1. Coagulation factors tested for by the following tests:
   a. Partial thromboplastin time (PTT): II, V, VIII, IX, X, XI, XII.
   b. Prothrombin time (PT): II, V, VII, X.
   c. Thrombin time (TT): I (fibrinogen).
2. Coagulation deficiencies in coagulation disorders
   a. Hemophilia A: factor VIII (prolonged PTT).
   b. Hemophilia B (von Willebrand's disease): factor IX (prolonged PTT).
   c. Liver-dependent factors:
      (1) Vitamin K–dependent factors: II, VII, IX, X; these are the liver-dependent factors that decline.

B. Therapy:

Prolonged PT/PTT (>1.5 × normal), DIC, clinical bleeding

NOTE: If in the emergency/transport situation coagulation studies cannot be obtained (inability to obtain specimens, inability to run tests) and the patient is bleeding significantly, replacement factors must be provided empirically. If the hemorrhage has been very large, PT/PTT remain prolonged or bleeding continues in spite of 20 mL/kg fresh frozen plasma (FFP), it is possible that fibrinogen levels are low. FFP, in this case, cannot provide adequate amounts of fibrinogen; cryoprecipitate contains large amounts of fibrinogen and should be given to raise fibrinogen levels to at least 100 mg/dL.

1. FFP: 10–20 mL/kg IV.
   a. 10 mL/kg suffices when patient is stable, bleeding/consumption are not ongoing.
   b. When bleeding and consumption are ongoing, the patient may need 20 mL/kg of FFP to control bleeding, and repeat doses may be needed (to be based on repeat coagulation studies and/or evidence of ongoing bleeding).
2. Cryoprecipitate: approximately 250 mg of fibrinogen/bag (1 bag = 5–10 mL).
   a. Fibrinogen level should be ≥100 mg/dL for effective hemostasis.
      (1) When fibrinogen level is <100 mg/dL in the presence of bleeding or bleeding continues after >20

mL/kg FFP and fibrinogen level is not known, cryoprecipitate should be given specifically or empirically for control of bleeding.

(2) 1 bag of cryoprecipitate/5 kg of body weight will raise the fibrinogen level by about 100 mg/dL.

3. Vitamin K:
   a. Liver synthesizes vitamin K–dependent factors. It usually takes ≥12 hours for the factors to be synthesized, so vitamin K administration is not an emergency treatment for severe coagulopathy, hemorrhage. It will also fail to be effective in the presence of liver disease.
   b. Vitamin K_1 dose: 1–2 mg IV or 2–5 mg PO.

V. Hemophilia

A. Therapy

1. Hemophilia A (factor VIII deficiency).
   a. Factor VIII activity (levels):
      (1) Normal factor VIII activity = 100%.
      (2) Desired factor activity levels for:
         (a) Soft tissue, joint bleeds: 50% activity level.
         (b) Life-threatening bleed (e.g., CNS) or surgery: 100% activity level.
   b. Factor VIII sources
      (1) Heat-treated factor VIII concentrates: the preferred source of factor VIII when available.
         (a) Heat treatment destroys human immunodeficiency virus (HIV); various hepatitis antigens can still be transmitted.
         (b) Numerous types of heat-treated factor VIII sources are available: Preparation processes and amounts/concentrations of factor VIII differ and must be looked up individually.
      (2) Cryoprecipitate: approximately 80 units of factor VIII per bag (range 60–125 units of factor VIII per bag).
         (a) Heat-treated factor VIII concentrates are greatly preferable to cryoprecipitate whenever possible.
         (b) Cryoprecipitate carries the same risk of transmitting HIV and hepatitis antigens as FFP.
   c. Treatment of bleeds
      (1) 1 unit factor VIII/kg increases factor VIII activity by 2%.

(2) Soft tissue and joint bleeds: Aim for 50% factor VIII activity level.
   (a) Transfuse 20–25 units of factor VIII/kg; use heat-treated factor VIII concentrate. (Use cryoprecipitate only when heat-treated factor VIII is not available and therapy is necessary.)
(3) Life-threatening bleeds (e.g., CNS) and surgery: Aim for 100% factor VIII activity level.
   (a) Transfuse 40–50 units of factor VIII/kg; use heat-treated factor VIII concentrate. (Use cryoprecipitate only when heat-treated factor VIII is not available.)
(4) Hemophilia A patients with inhibitors to factor VIII will require higher doses of factor VIII than just listed to achieve adequate hemostasis.

2. Hemophilia B.
   a. Factor IX activity (levels).
      (1) Normal factor IX activity: 100%.
      (2) Desired factor IX activity for:
         (a) Soft tissue, joint bleeds: 50%.
         (b) Life-threatening bleeds (e.g., CNS) and surgery: 100%.
   b. Factor IX sources
      (1) Heat-treated concentrates: Konyne, Profilnine.
         (a) 500-unit vials and 1,000-unit vials are available.
         (b) Heat treatment eliminates risk of HIV transmission; hepatitis can still be transmitted.
   c. Treatment of bleeds
      (1) 1 unit factor IX/kg raises factor IX activity by 1%.
         (a) Higher dose of factor IX is required than for factor VIII because factor IX has a larger volume of distribution.
      (2) Soft tissue and joint bleeds: Aim for factor IX activity level of 50%.
         (a) Administer 40–50 units of factor IX/kg. Use heat-treated factor if available.
      (3) Life-threatening bleed (e.g., CNS) or surgery:
         (a) Administer 80–100 units of factor IX/kg. Use heat-treated factor if available.

INFECTIOUS DISEASE

8

I. Sepsis and Meningitis

Sepsis is a bacterial infection of the bloodstream accompanied by signs of systemic toxicity. In meningitis, pathogens invade the central nervous system. Discussion in this chapter is limited to recognition and specific treatment for sepsis and meningitis. Discussion of accompanying conditions such as shock and respiratory failure are discussed separately in this manual.

A. Clinical assessment

1. Sepsis.
   a. Fever in the older child; fever or hypothermia in the neonate.
   b. Poor perfusion.
   c. Shock.
   d. Evidence of coagulopathy in the form of a petechial or purpuric eruption.
2. Meningitis.
   a. Fever.
   b. Nuchal rigidity (often not present if <1 year old).
   c. Headache.
   d. Altered mental status, including coma of unknown etiology.
   e. Sepsis.
3. Laboratory data.
   a. Complete blood cell count.
   b. Blood and urine cultures.
   c. Lumbar puncture if patient is clinically stable.
   d. Electrolyte and glucose levels.
   e. Arterial blood gas.

B. Therapy

1. Administer 100% oxygen. Assure airway patency; ventilate for evidence of respiratory failure or severe shock.

2. Obtain vascular access (peripheral intravenous line, intraosseous line, central line, cutdown).
3. Evaluate for signs of shock (poor perfusion, altered mental status, decreased urine output, hypotension, tachycardia).
   a. Give 20 mL/kg of normal saline solution for shock. Reassess and repeat as needed.
   b. Consider inotropes when fluid therapy has diminishing results. Start dopamine therapy at 10 μg/kg/min.
4. Administer antibiotics.
   a. Sepsis.
      (1) Neonate: ampicillin, 100 mg/kg, and gentamicin, 2.5 mg/kg.
      (2) Child: Ceftriaxone, 50 mg/kg.
      (3) See Table 8–1 for alternate selections.
   b. Meningitis.
      (1) Neonate or older child: ampicillin, 100 mg/kg, and cefotaxime, 50 mg/kg.
      (2) See medication table for alternate selections.
5. If venous access has not yet been obtained, give ceftriaxone, 100 mg/kg IM (child), or ampicillin, 100 mg/kg IM with gentamicin, 2.5 mg/kg IM (neonate).
6. Treat the unstable child with suspected meningitis with antibiotics without performing a lumbar puncture.
7. Be prepared to treat hypoglycemia with 0.25 g of 25% glucose/kg.
8. Treat evidence of disseminated intravascular coagulation with 10 mL of fresh frozen plasma/kg.

C. Ongoing monitoring

1. Use pulse oximeter and cardiac monitor.
2. Follow vital signs closely along with clinical examination for evidence of shock.
3. Watch closely for signs of respiratory compromise.
4. Repeat glucose checks q1–2h.
5. Use other monitoring as indicated for shock or respiratory failure.

TABLE 8–1.
Antibiotic Therapy for Infectious Disease Emergencies*

Clinical Diagnosis	Therapy
Bacterial meningitis	
Neonates	Ampicillin 200 mg/kg/day q12h for 0–7 days, q6–8h for > 7 days *and* Gentamicin 5 mg/kg/day q12h for 0–7 days; 7.5 mg/kg/day q8h for > 7 days **or** Cefotaxime 150–200 mg/kg/day q12h for <7 days, q8h for > 7 days *and* Ampicillin 200 mg/kg/day q6h
Children 1–3 mo	Ampicillin 300 mg/kg/day q6h *and* Cefotaxime 200 mg/kg/day q6h
Children >3 mo	Cefotaxime 200 mg/kg/day q6h **or** Ceftriaxone 100 mg/kg/day q12h
Bacterial sepsis	
Neonates	Ampicillin 200 mg/kg/day q12h for 0-7 days, q6–8h for > 7 days *and* Gentamicin 5 mg/kg/day q12h for 0–7 days, 7.5 mg/kg/day q8h for > 7 days **or** Cefotaxime 150–200 mg/kg/day q12h for <7 days, q8h for >7 days *and* Ampicillin 200 mg/kg/day q6h
Children	Cefotaxime 100 mg/kg/day q6–8h **or** Ceftriaxone 50–75 mg/kg/day q12h **or** Cefuroxime 100–150 mg/kg/day q8h
Endocarditis, acute staphylococcal	Nafcillin or oxacillin 200 mg/kg/day q4–6h *and* Gentamicin 5 mg/kg/day q6h **or** Vancomycin 40 mg/kg/day q6h alone or in combination with gentamicin
Encephalitis due to herpes simplex	Acyclovir 30 mg/kg/day q8h for 10–14 days

(continued)

TABLE 8–1 (cont.).

Clinical Diagnosis	Therapy
Epiglottis and bacterial tracheitis	Cefuroxime 100–150 mg/kg/day q8h **or** Cefotaxime 100 mg/kg/day q6–8h **or** Ceftriaxone 50–75 mg/kg/day q12h
Necrotizing fasciitis originating from umbilical stump	Cefotaxime 100–150 mg/kg/day q6h *and* Clindamycin 40 mg/kg/day q6h NOTE: This combination is not adequate coverage against *Pseudomonas* spp.
Orbital cellulitis	Cefotaxime 200 mg/kg/day q6h *and* Clindamycin 40 mg/kg/day q6h or Metronidazole 30 mg/kg/day q12h **or** Nafcillin 150 mg/kg/day q6h *and* Chloramphenicol 100 mg/kg/day q6h
Pertussis	Erythromycin 40 mg/kg/day PO q6h
Pneumonia and empyema	Cefuroxime 100–150 mg/kg/day q8h **or** Cefotoxime 100–150 mg/kg/day q6–8h **or** Ceftriaxone 50–75 mg/kg/day q12h
Purulent pericarditis	Cefuroxime 100–150 mg/kg/day q8h **or** Cefotaxime 100–150 mg/kg/day q6–8h **or** Ceftriaxone 50–75 mg/kg/day q12h
Retropharyngeal or lateral pharyngeal abscess/cellulitis	Clindamycin 30–40 mg/kg/day q6h
Toxic shock syndrome	Nafcillin **or** oxacillin 150–200 mg/kg/day q6h

*Recommended dosage is for empiric treatment before specific organism is cultured. Once the specific organism is known, substitute the most narrow spectrum and specific antibiotic.

MISCELLANEOUS DISORDERS 9

I. Near-Drowning and Asphyxia

A. Patient classification

Near-drowning is a leading cause of morbidity and mortality in children. *Asphyxia,* following respiratory failure/arrest, produces problems very similar to near-drowning; the review of problems and management of near-drowning is therefore applicable to the asphyxiated patient.

The primary problem posed by submersion is the inability to breathe. The following sequence of events is observed in submerged animals: an initial struggle to breathe; laryngospasm, possibly brought about by initial aspiration of water during the struggle to breathe; swallowing of large amounts of water, sometimes associated with emesis; relaxation of the larynx as muscle tone is lost with progressive hypoxia; influx of water/vomitus into the larynx and lung; the final event, cessation of cardiac activity.

When submersion is prolonged, the resulting problems are secondary to inability to breathe and the problems that arise out of the struggle to breathe. Pathophysiologically, the problems commonly seen after submersion are:

1. Hypoxia.
2. Hypothermia, except when submersion occurs in water greater than body temperature (e.g., in hot tubs).
3. Aspiration, which can impair pulmonary function and thereby aggravate existing hypoxia after breathing is restored.

Hypoxia is the primary problem. The clinical manifestations of hypoxia are related to both the severity of hypoxia and the differing abilities of individual organs to tolerate hypoxia. The brain cortex is the first to sustain irreversible damage, the lower brain next; the lungs and heart can tolerate up to 20 to 30 minutes of hypoxia and survive when provided with appropriate postrescue support. This observation explains the different outcomes of submersion victims: intact survival in those who are retrieved before any organ has sustained irreversible damage; survival with anoxic-ischemic encephalopathy in those who are retrieved after irreversible cortical brain damage has occurred but before the brain stem and other organs have sustained irreversible injury; inability to survive or be resuscitated when irreversible damage has affected all vital organs. The clinical picture of the submersion victim is therefore variable, and treatment must accordingly be tailored. The classification system provides guides to treatment.

Hypothermia is common and is reviewed in the following section. Aspiration is likewise common and seen in the majority of patients who seek medical attention. Aspiration is likely to interfere with lung function, especially oxygenation, and produce further hypoxic damage if not appropriately managed after retrieval. Experience also indicates that saltwater and freshwater aspiration do not produce clinically significant differences in near-drowning victims and do not merit special attention. Corticosteroids are not indicated. Antibiotics will be useful in cases of aspiration of grossly contaminated water; they may be provided in the initial period or later if there is evidence of developing pneumonia.

Conn and Barker devised a classification of submersion victims based on neurologic function. The classification is to be made shortly after the victim is retrieved from water. The classification is useful for 3 reasons: (1) it allows one to estimate the magnitude of the hypoxic insult; (2) it guides one in the selection of appropriate therapy; and (3) it is highly predictive of outcome. Although Conn and Barker recommend classifying the patient within the first hour of retrieval, I believe that classification is most useful for the purposes of selecting therapy and predicting outcome when the classification is made on the basis of patient findings in the first 15 to 30 minutes after retrieval.

The classification of submersion victims developed by Conn and Barker is as follows:

Category A: *Awake*. Alert, fully conscious; minimal injury.

Category B: *Blunted*. Obtunded to stuporous; normal central respiratory drive; purposeful responses to pain.

Category C: *Comatose*. Unarousable; abnormal central respiratory pattern; abnormal motor responses to painful stimuli; may have seizures. Overt respiratory failure present. Category C is further divided into subcategories based on worsening CNS function.

C1: Decorticate; Cheyne-Stoke respirations.

C2: Decerebrate; central hyperventilation.

C3: Flaccid; apneustic or cluster breathing.

C4: Deceased? Flaccid; apneic; no detectable circulation. (Manifestations of multiorgan dysfunction/failure appear at this stage.)

Patients in categories A and B almost uniformly do well with medical supportive therapy alone; intact survival is the rule. A few category B patients develop respiratory failure severe enough to require mechanical ventilatory support, usually from massive aspiration or aspiration of irritants (e.g., pool cleaning agents); some of these patients may succumb to respiratory failure.

Patients in category C are in respiratory failure and require invasive therapy and monitoring. Patient outcomes in this category vary. With appropriate cardiopulmonary resuscitation (CPR) and pediatric intensive care, the following outcomes are observed. A very high percentage of C1 and C2 patients presently survive and have normal outcome. At stage C3, a significant percentage of victims still survive intact, but a substantial increase in the incidence of death or survival with anoxic-ischemic encephalopathy is observed, even with aggressive therapy. Category C4 patients do poorly: The majority die or survive with profound anoxic ischemic encephalopthy; a small percentage of victims appear to have intact survival.

Prediction of submersion victim outcome can be reduced to the following observation: The submersion victim who has not had a cardiac arrest stands a good chance of surviving intact when appropriate resuscitation and medical care are provided. (NOTE: Many patients in categories A through C3 will be apneic when retrieved from the water but not have sustained a cardiac arrest; when the latter is true, moving the patient, chest compressions and/or assisted ventilation rapidly stimulate(s) resumption of respiratory efforts and movements.) Therefore, the patient who has a heartbeat when retrieved or immediately after basic stimulation is provided—even if the patient is seizing, posturing, hypotonic—has hypoxic changes that are reversible, and the patient can be expected to do well. Because the moving patient has cardiac activity, any patient who is moving when retrieved from the water or moves very shortly after retrieval and basic stimulation has the chance to do well. Other values—initial pH, length of submersion—are of secondary importance to this finding.

A word of caution about prediction is needed. One can predict with quite good accuracy the likely outcome of the submersion victim (i.e., the chances of intact survival, survival with anoxic-ischemic encephalopathy, or death). Predictions are more difficult to make for asphyxiated patients. The air/oxygen supply of submersion victims is interrupted abruptly and completely, and most victims are well just before the submersion occurs; resulting hypoxic changes follow well-established patterns. Asphyxia patients usually experience a gradual decline in air/oxygen supply of varying duration and degree, and many have associated systemic illness; cumulative hypoxemia and hypoxia in the already ill patient may thus inflict significant damage before cardiac arrest ever takes place. Therefore, one cannot apply submersion outcome predictors with equal validity in asphyxiated patients.

B. Immersion hypothermia

Immersion hypothermia is the phenomenon that explains the remarkably good outcome of a small number of victims who have been submerged in icy waters for up to about 45 minutes. Immersion hypothermia is observed when the temperature of the water is icy cold. The explanation for this phenomenon is as follows.

Water is an excellent conductor of heat. Small children have large surface areas and therefore lose heat rapidly in water that is cooler than their body temperatures. Movement (struggling) also increases heat loss and contributes to the rapidity of temperature drops. When submerged in icy cold water, the body temperature may plunge rapidly to the point where body activity and metabolism come to a virtual standstill on the basis of hypothermia. If this standstill develops before available oxygen is completely used, the hypothermia confers a protective effect: Because metabolism is very slow, the remaining oxygen is used slowly and the body can survive submersion for a longer period of time before anoxia develops. If the patient is retrieved and resuscitated before anoxia develops, the child may do well after prolonged submersion.

Icy cold water is key here. In these instances, resuscitation efforts must be continued until body temperature reaches 30° C before one decides cardiac activity can or cannot be restored.

In most other instances of submersion (i.e., non–cold water drowning), the patient will be cold on admission. When water temperature is lower than body temperature, the victim's temperature will drop for reasons just reviewed. The rate of temperature drop will, however, be much less than in cold water and will almost always be too slow to confer any protective effect. In fact, very low temperatures in victims of non–cold water drowning submersions are usually a poor sign rather than a good sign: They are usually indications of lengthy submersion and, therefore, severe hypoxia/anoxia. Warming the patient whose temperature is less than 30° C should still be done to confirm the presence or absence of cardiac activity.

C. **Therapy of near-drowning by patient classification**

1. **Category A patient.**

   This patient has had a fairly short submersion and quickly regains good neurologic function. Many patients are blue, apneic when retrieved, but quickly regain respiratory function with stimulation. After retrieval, neurologic function steadily and quickly returns; the child may be sleepy and lethargic but cries appropriately, answers questions if old enough to speak. The child may be mildly hypothermic. Aspiration is quite common on chest x-ray film, and some may have clinical respiratory symptoms—tachypnea, wheezes, even rales, mild retractions. Initial blood gas values may show pH values as low as 7.1 with a metabolic acidosis and moderate base deficit. If, however, neurologic function is good, restoration of oxygenation is sufficient to restore normalcy.

   a. Evaluation.

      (1) Consider arterial blood gas (ABG) values, complete blood cell (CBC) count, electrolyte values, and chest x-ray film.

(2) Look for associated problems: head, neck, other injuries; ingestions; seizures.

b. Therapy: symptomatic.

(1) Supplemental oxygen as needed.

(2) Aerosols for wheezing; diuretics, bicarbonate are not usually needed.

(3) Warming measures.

(4) $NaHCO_3$: not usually needed; patient does not require intubation for low pH value if he is waking up or awake.

(5) May observe overnight or discharge if submersion was minimal and family is reliable.

(a) Child may develop inflammatory response to aspiration over the following 24–48 hours. Respiratory problems may appear at that time and need evaluation, therapy.

2. **Category B patient.**

This patient has more severe hypoxic changes than the category A patient. The key finding is decreased level of consciousness—obtunded to stuporous, but with normal brain stem function; neurologic function returns gradually as oxygenation is restored. Blood gas values will be more abnormal, and the pH will be as low as 6.9–7.0; hypoxemia is common without supplemental oxygen. Respiratory abnormalities are likewise common: tachypnea, retractions; wheezing, rhonchi and/or rales; the chest radiograph usually shows aspiration. Much water may have been swallowed, and gastric distention may be evident. Those submerged in fresh water frequently have slightly low Na values secondary to absorption of water from the stomach. These children need medical respiratory support, intravenous (IV) fluids, close monitoring. If they deteriorate neurologically, this is almost always secondary to respiratory difficulties and hypoxia; intubation is indicated for respiratory failure and/or neurologic deterioration. The length of hospitalization is generally several days and is determined largely by the pulmonary status.

a. Evaluation.

(1) Consider ABG values; electrolyte and glucose levels, CBC count; chest radiograph.

(2) Look for associated problems: head, neck, other injuries; ingestions; seizures.

b. Therapy.
  (1) Respiratory system:
    (a) Provide supplemental oxygen. Provide mechanical ventilation for child in respiratory failure.
    (b) Provide aerosol bronchodilator therapy as needed.
    (c) Furosemide, 0.5–1.0 mg/kg IV, may be considered for marked pulmonary edema.
    (d) $NaHCO_3$, 1 mEq/kg, may be given for severe metabolic acidosis; if moderate, HCO_3 usually corrects as hypoxemia and temperature are corrected.
  (2) Warm the patient.
  (3) Start IV line; administer usual fluids at maintenance or slightly restricted rate.
  (4) Consider antibiotics for aspiration of contaminated water.
    (a) Leukocytosis is a common stress response and is not indicative of infection.
  (5) Monitor patient closely: vital signs, pulse oximeter, neurologic status; blood gas values and chest x-ray studies as indicated.
    (a) If neurologic status deteriorates, especially if patient becomes comatose or develops seizures, prepare for intubation and ventilation: Neurologic deterioration is usually caused by hypoxia, inadequate respiratory function.
    (b) Intubate, ventilate for respiratory failure due to deteriorating respiratory function: aspiration changes and deterioration in function may take several hours or days to peak.

3. **Category C patient.**

All patients are comatose and in significant respiratory failure. Hypoxemia in room air is present, pH values are generally ≤ 7.0. Brain stem dysfunction is apparent: Respiratory patterns are abnormal secondary to brain stem dysfunction; muscle tone and motor responses are clearly pathologic.

All patients require intubation and ventilation; C4 patients additionally require CPR. Virtually all have abnormal chest radiographs with changes of aspiration. Those in category C4 may have sustained enough systemic hypoxia to show evidence of multisystem organ damage ranging from laboratory abnormalities alone to overt multisystem failure.

Patients who require aggressive resuscitation—chest compressions, multiple doses of resuscitation medications—may have some significant laboratory abnormalities that are a function of the severe hypoxia and, in most cases, require nothing more than noting them. They include hyperkalemia up to 8's in patients with very low initial pH values (<6.8) and will correct when the pH is corrected; leukopenia with a white blood cell (WBC) count as low as 1,000 cells/mm^3 and neutropenia (corrects over next 1–2 days); hyperglycemia secondary to stress, which may produce massive diuresis and circulatory compromise that need correction with volume expanders; hypokalemia down to 2.0 after the pH is in the normal range—this can be treated with a potassium bolus.

a. Resucitation phase (advanced cardiac life support).
   (1) Respiratory system:
      (a) Airway: Clear mouth (vomiting is common); good suction is highly desirable.
      (b) Use bag-valve-mask ventilation.
      (c) Use fractional concentration of oxygen in inspired gas (FiO_2) 100% throughout resuscitation and stabilization.
      (d) Intubate, ventilate as soon as possible.
         (i) Patient may require high inflating pressures to move the chest (aspiration, atelectasis, bronchospasm).
         (ii) Use high ventilation rate, 1.5–2 × usual resting rate for age (see p. 27).
         (iii) Suction endotracheal tube (ETT): There may be large amounts of secretions, aspirated material.
      (e) Place nasogastric (NG) tube as soon as it is feasible to empty stomach of air, swallowed water, and food contents.

(2) Cardiovascular system.
   (a) Administer external compressions to the patient with cardiac arrest until acceptable spontaneous pulses return.
   (b) Start IV line. Any site is acceptable; consider intraosseous line.
   (c) Check electrocardiogram (ECG) pattern:
      (i) Sinus tachycardia is the expected rhythm. Normal or low heart rate is insufficient unless the child is very cold (the heart rate decreases during hypothermia).
      (ii) Ventricular dysrhythmia: Ventricular tachycardia or fibrillation.
         (a) The result of profound hypoxia and acidosis; hyperkalemia secondary to profound acidosis may be a contributory factor.
         (b) Defibrillation for ventricular fibrillation: 2 J/kg.
         (c) Lidocaine, 1 mg/kg for ventricular tachycardia; may also consider synchronized cardioversion, 0.5–1.0 J/kg.
         (d) Correct hypoxia and acidosis (increase ventilation).
   (d) Administer lactated Ringer's (LR) or normal saline (NS) solution, 10–20 mL/kg IV push for decreased circulation; repeat as needed.

(3) Laboratory work: Obtain when possible.
   (a) ABG values.
   (b) Electrolyte values:
      (i) Sodium: Hyponatremia is common after freshwater submersion (usually not <125–129); probably secondary to absorption of water from the stomach; is not usually of clinical significance. Mild hypernatremia after saltwater immersion usually is not clinically significant. Empty the stomach of water.

(ii) Potassium:

(a) Hyperkalemia: not uncommon in the severely hypoxic patient with pH usually ≤6.8. H^+ enters cells, K^+ leaves cells when pH is low. K^+ rapidly normalizes as the serum pH is corrected.

(b) Hypokalemia: frequently seen after resuscitation, especially in the patient who required vigorous CPR. If K^+ <2.5–3.0 mEq/L, give ½ mEq KCl/kg IV over 1 hour. Check serum K^+ level 1–2 hours after infusion is done; repeat dose prn.

(c) Glucose: Hyperglycemia is the commonly observed initial response to stress; requires no treatment.

(d) WBC count: Leukopenia, neutropenia are common in the child who had a full arrest and vigorous CPR. WBC count may be as low as 1,000; both correct in 1–2 days.

(e) Chest x-ray studies:

(i) Check ETT placement.

(ii) Look for lung pathologic conditions: infiltrates, pulmonary edema, atelectasis, pneumothorax.

(iii) Check NG tube placement.

(f) Other tests for associated problems, e.g., suspected ingestion (toxicology studies), known seizure disorder (anticonvulsant levels), cervical spine for suspected neck injury.

b. Therapy: Stabilization phase.

(1) Respiratory system.

(a) Aim to achieve the following values on blood gases:

(i) Partial pressure of oxygen (Po_2) >90–100 mm Hg if possible. Do not be concerned about extremely high

Po_2 values during this phase. Continue to use Fio_2 100%.

(a) Low Po_2 value may indicate the need for larger tidal volume (if chest movement is not adequate); higher positive end-expiratory pressure (PEEP), especially if there are significant atelectasis, edema, or infiltrates; or suctioning of ETT.

(ii) pH ≥7.35. pH values up to 7.59 are well tolerated by children.

(iii) Partial pressure of carbon dioxide (Pco_2) in the 20 to low 30 mm Hg range.

(b) Tidal volume/inflating pressure:

(i) Anticipate the need for high peak inflating pressures to move the chest initially.

(ii) If a ventilator is used, use a volume ventilator with delivered tidal volume 10–15 mL/kg.

(c) Bronchospasm:

(i) Fairly common response to aspiration, intubation, irritation from suctioning.

(a) Indications: wheezing, rhonchi, marked airway resistance (persistently high inflating pressures).

(ii) Administer aerosolized albuterol, terbutaline, or metaproterenol.

(d) *Control* the patient's ventilation (i.e., do all of the breathing for the patient with the ventilator [or manual ventilation] even if the patient is making respiratory efforts).

(i) Reasons: Assure good ventilation, oxygenation because the patient may not be able to do this on his or her own; decrease the work of breathing and oxygen demands.

(ii) Use sedation, neuromuscular relaxants to achieve control if the patient is fighting ventilator efforts, posturing (see p. 29).

(2) Cardiovascular system.

(a) Heart rate and rhythm: Refer to p. 83.

(b) Blood pressure (BP), perfusion: for impaired circulation:

(i) Begin with plasma volume expanders, NS or LR solution, 10–20 mL/kg, repeat prn to restore circulation. Volume may be effective because of fluid loss from capillary leaks.

(a) Fluid leaks may continue over next 1–2 days; volume expander pushes may have to be given repeatedly.

(ii) If volume expanders do not quickly restore BP, perfusion initially, quickly proceed to inotrope infusions. Inotrope drips are usually required only for patients in category C4 where profound hypoxia has damaged the myocardium.

(a) Dopamine or dobutamine is used for hypotension with tachycardia. Start at 5–10 μg/kg/min, titrate up to 20–30 μg/kg/min (see pp. 428, 429).

(b) Isoproterenol is used for hypotension with normal heart rate/bradycardia. Start at 0.05–0.1 μg/kg/min, titrate dose (see p. 430).

(c) Proceed to second, third inotrope as needed if first inotrope is insufficient to restore circulation.

(3) Central nervous system.

Of central concern in the resuscitation is the central nervous system (CNS). Restoration and maintenance of oxygen delivery to the brain is key to preventing further CNS damage and to beginning repair of those cells that remain viable. Steps that facilitate this goal follow.

(a) Seizures: Treat in usual manner (see p. 127).
   (i) Diazepam, 0.1–0.4 mg/kg, or lorazepam, 0.05–0.1 mg/kg IV, to stop the seizure.
   (ii) Follow with phenobarbital or phenytoin, 20 mg/kg IV.

(b) Control of struggling: important for control of ventilation/oxygenation, to reduce oxygen demands.
   (i) Sedation for the struggling, fighting patient:
      (a) Narcotic: morphine sulfate, 0.1 mg/kg IV q1–2h, or fentanyl, 1–5 μg/kg IV qh and/or
      (b) Diazepam, 0.1–0.2 mg/kg IV q1–2h; lorazepam, 0.05–0.1 mg/kg IV q6h; or midazolam, 0.1 mg/kg IV qh.
   (ii) Neuromuscular relaxant: for the patient who fails to be adequately controlled with the previously listed sedation, for the patient who is posturing.
      (a) Pancuronium or vecuronium, 0.1 mg/kg IV prn movement.
      (b) Always use sedation in conjunction with neuromuscular relaxant.

(4) IV fluids:
   (a) Usual maintenance fluid (e.g., 5% dextrose in ⅓NS solution + KCl).
   (b) Rate: Limit volume: two thirds maintenance to maintenance *after* circulation is restored.

(5) Renal function:
   (a) Most patients, except those in category C4 with profound anoxia, will be urinating well, especially if stress hyperglycemia is present (osmotic diuresis).

(b) If urine output is low or absent *after* circulation is established, consider a trial of furosemide, 1 mg/kg IV, or mannitol, 0.5–1.0 g/kg IV, to restore urine output.
   (i) If a large diuresis follows diuretic and compromises circulation, restore circulation with 20 mL/kg of LR or NS solution.

(6) Metabolic status:
   (a) Electrolyte values: See pp. 245–246.
   (b) Glucose levels: Refer to p. 201.
      (i) Monitor test-strip glucose qh initially because hypoglycemia may develop.
   (c) Calcium: not likely to present a problem in initial phase. Significant hypocalcemia may develop later in postresuscitation phase (see p. 198).

(7) Temperature.
   (a) Aim for euthermia.
      (i) Hypothermia: Provide external warming sources.
         (a) If patient temperature is <30° C, see p. 265.
      (ii) Hyperthermia: Fever commonly develops after 6–12 hours. It may be caused by infection but is most commonly a postasphyxial inflammatory response. Provide acetaminophen, 10–15 mg/kg q4h prn.

(8) Antibiotics: Consider use for aspiration of contaminated water (e.g., from a dirty lake).

(9) Corticosteroids: not indicated.

(10) Computed tomography scan of head: not indicated for routine submersion because there is no useful information provided. Consider it for associated head injury.

(11) Intracranial pressure (ICP) monitoring, barbiturate coma: not indicated in drowning, asphyxia.

(12) Treat other associated problems (e.g., injuries, ingestion).

c. Postresuscitation care.
   (1) See discussion of postresuscitation care on p. 95.
   (2) Monitor patient closely: vital signs, neurologic status, laboratory values as per postresuscitation section.

II. Carbon Monoxide Toxicity

A. Interference with oxygen-hemoglobin binding Pathophysiology and caveats regarding blood gas determinations and pulse oximetry values.

Under usual circumstances, one can correctly assume that the patient who has both an adequate Po_2 and adequate *hemoglobin (Hgb) value* has adequate *oxygen content of the blood*. The basic assumption is that a certain (known) amount of oxygen is bound to Hgb for a given Po_2 value (see Chapter 1).

There are times, however, when this assumption is not valid. They occur when there are substances that interfere with Hgb's ability to bind oxygen: Substances may bind to Hgb and occupy the sites normally taken up by oxygen; or substances may alter the configuration of Hgb and reduce the amount of oxygen it can carry. In both ways, oxygen-binding sites are diminished, the amount of oxygen carried by Hgb is decreased, and the oxygen content of blood is decreased. With a significant drop in oxygen content, tissue hypoxia and anaerobic metabolism follow; the end results are lactic acid production (metabolic acidosis) and cell damage. Two situations where this occurs are *carbon monoxide toxicity* (oxygen displacement from Hgb, as well as change in hemoglobin configuration) and *methemoglobinemia* (change in hemoglobin configuration).

Carbon monoxide and methemoglobin do not affect lung function. In the absence of lung pathologic conditions, oxygen tension of the blood (the amount of oxygen dissolved in plasma, i.e., Po_2) is unaffected. Therefore, when either carbon monoxide or methemoglobin is present in the presence of normal lung function: (1) the Po_2 value will be normal; (2) oxygen saturation value will be reduced because the amount of oxygen that Hgb carries is reduced; (3) the oxygen content of the blood will be reduced; and (4) metabolic acidosis (lactic acid) will be present when the reduction in oxygen content is significant. *The presence of an interfering substance should be readily detected by the discrepancy between the* Po_2 *and oxygen saturation values (i.e., a low oxygen saturation value for a given* Po_2 *value).*

Unfortunately, the ready detection of the presence of substances that interfere with Hgb's ability to bind oxygen is not possible with usual blood gas determinations. Of the parameters of interest, routine blood gas determinations directly measure only the oxygen tension (i.e., Po_2). The HCO_3^- and base excess/deficit values are calculated from the measured pH and Pco_2 values. The oxygen saturation value is not measured but is derived from the O_2-Hgb dissociation curve using measured Po_2 and pH values; the calculation assumes that there are no substances that interfere with the ability of Hgb to bind oxygen. Therefore, when carbon monoxide or methemoglobin is present, the reduction in oxygen saturation will not be reported by usual blood gas determinations. The caveat:

Usual blood gas determination cannot be relied on to detect the presence of substances that interfere with Hgb's ability to bind oxygen: The reduced oxygen saturation and the discrepancy between Po_2 *and oxygen saturation values will not be reported by routine blood gas determinations. Therefore, the presence of a normal* Po_2 *value and normal oxygen saturation on a routinely run blood gas sample does not rule out the presence of carbon monoxide toxicity or methemoglobinemia.*

Confirmation of the presence of carbon monoxide or methemoglobin and accurate oxygen saturation measurements require requesting and performing *direct oxygen saturation measurements of blood* on a blood gas machine. Direct measurements of Po_2, oxyhemoglobin (oxygen saturation), carboxyhemoglobin, and methemoglobin are made. A heparinized blood specimen is required, usually larger in volume than that used for routine blood gases. Either an arterial or venous specimen can be used to determine the amount of abnormal Hgb present; only an arterial specimen can be used for accurate determination of oxyhemoglobin (oxygen saturation).

The presence of an abnormal hemoglobin level may be suspected from the history (e.g., a fire for carbon monoxide, certain ingestions for methemoglobin), dark or brown blood in the presence of high Po_2 values (methemoglobin), marked metabolic acidosis that is otherwise unexplained.

Pulse oximeters, similarly, have been found to be inaccurate in measuring oxygen saturations in the presence of abnormal Hgb values. The pulse oximeter tends to give falsely elevated oxygen saturation readings in this setting and cannot be relied on to provide valid or useful information. Blood gas measurements must be used to monitor oxygen values when carbon monoxide or methemoglobin are present.

B. Sources of carbon monoxide

1. Fires: incomplete burning of carbon-containing materials.
2. Motor vehicle exhaust.
3. Gas leaks.

C. Carbon monoxide and carboxyhemoglobin

1. Carbon monoxide properties: nonvisible, odorless, tasteless, nonirritating.
2. Avidly binds to Hgb: CO + Hgb = CO-Hgb (carboxyhemoglobin).
   a. Carbon monoxide binds to Hgb 240 times more avidly than does oxygen; it therefore preferentially binds to Hgb and displaces oxygen.
3. Carboxyhemoglobin half-life.
   a. In room air: 4 hours.
   b. In Fio_2 100%: 40 minutes.
   c. In hyperbaric oxygen at 3 atm: 23 minutes.
4. Carbon monoxide shifts the oxygen dissociation curve to the left (i.e., decreases oxygen release to the tissues).
5. Carboxyhemoglobin classically produces a cherry red skin color; this finding is not common, and is unreliable.
6. Tachypnea is not seen in spite of the low oxygen content because the Po_2 is not affected: The carotid body responds to the Po_2 value.

D. Clinical picture of carbon monoxide toxicity

1. Carbon monoxide poisoning is present when carboxyhemoglobin levels are elevated to the point of causing symptoms.

2. A fairly good correlation exists between the carboxyhemoglobin level and the clinical picture. See Table 9–1 for clinical manifestations.
   a. Mild toxicity: corresponds with CO-Hgb levels <20%.
   b. Moderate toxicity: corresponds with CO-Hgb levels of 20%–40%.
   c. Severe toxicity corresponds with CO-Hgb levels of 40%–60%.
   d. Fatalities are associated with CO-Hgb levels >60%.

E. Therapy

1. Remove patient from contaminated environment.
2. Provide Fio_2 100% immediately (see p. 14 for methods of delivering high Fio_2 in the awake patient.) Use of Fio_2 100% is critical for the following reasons:
   a. It corrects hypoxemia that may be present.
   b. It raises oxygen content of the blood moderately by increasing the dissolved Po_2 level.
   c. It greatly decreases the half-life of carboxyhemoglobin and thereby increases the oxygen content of the blood significantly.
3. Provide bag-valve-mask ventilation, followed by intubation and ventilation if the patient is comatose and/or if respiratory efforts are poor.
4. Maintain, restore cardiovascular stability.
5. Treat neurologic problems (e.g., seizures).
6. Assess the patient for related injuries from a fire, jumping from a burning building, etc.
7. Laboratory evaluation.
   a. Obtain a heparinized blood specimen for *direct measurement* of Po_2, oxyhemoglobin (oxygen saturation), carboxyhemoglobin (CO-Hgb), in addition to other blood gas values.
      (1) If a routine blood gas test has been performed, be aware that the Po_2 and oxygen saturation values may be normal and, thereby, misleading (see p. 252).
         (a) In this case, until a direct oxygen saturation or carboxyhemoglobin level is determined, the presence of metabolic acidosis on the routinely run blood gas specimen,

in conjunction with depressed level of consciousness, suggests cell hypoxia and significant CO-Hgb levels.

b. Obtain CBC count, other laboratory values as needed.

8. Consider transporting patient to a hyperbaric oxygen chamber if the patient has severe symptoms.
   a. NOTE: Any given carboxyhemoglobin level may produce different manifestations in different people.
9. Continue Fi_{O_2} 100% until the carboxyhemoglobin level is down to 5%–10% (Table 9–1).

III. Methemoglobinemia

Methemoglobinemia is uncommon but can manifest dramatically and present a very confusing picture when its presence is not obvious. It can also be just as dramatically reversed with relatively simple therapy. The presence of dark blood, classically brown, in the presence of high P_{O_2} values should make one suspect methemoglobinemia. It is important to note that methemoglobinemia is seen in neonates and young infants in association with diarrhea and dehydration.

A. Methemoglobin (MetHgb)

1. Altered form of Hgb: iron is in the ferric rather than ferrous form.

TABLE 9–1.
Carboxyhemoglobin Levels and Clinical Findings

CO-Hgb Level (%)	Clinical Findings
1–2	Normal nonsmoker.
5–10	Smoker, truck driver, or anyone regularly exposed to high levels.
	In nonsmokers, this level may result in impairment of judgment and fine motor skills.
20	Headache, mild dyspnea, visual changes, confusion.
20–40	Drowsiness, weakness, nausea/vomiting, dulled sensation, decreased awareness of danger.
40–60	Poor coordination, recent memory loss.
>60	Coma, convulsions, cardiovascular and neurologic collapse, death.

2. MetHgb cannot bind oxygen.
3. Normal MetHgb level: ≤2%.
4. Regulation of MetHgb level:
   a. MetHgb reductase: usual regulator.
      (1) MetHgb reductase activity is low in cord blood; adult values are reached between 2 and 6 months of age.
      (2) Reduced nicotinamide adenine dinucleotide phosphate MetHgb reductase: Alternate regulator when MetHgb reductase level is deficient.

B. Cause

1. Inherited etiologies: baseline cyanosis; may be exacerbated by exposure to oxidant drugs.
   a. MetHgb reductase deficiency.
   b. Hgb M disorders
      (1) Increased spontaneous oxidation of Hgb to MetHgb.
      (2) Benign disorder; needs no therapy, does not respond to antioxidants.
2. Toxic etiologies: predominant etiology.
   a. Drug, chemical exposures:
      (1) Numerous drugs, including benzocaine, aniline dyes, nitrates, nitrites, nitroglycerin, sulfonamides, naphthalene.
      (2) Newborns are more susceptible to drugs than older children and adults.
   b. Diarrhea and acidosis in neonates, young infants.
      (1) No specific toxin, etiology identified.

C. Clinical picture, laboratory findings

1. Clinical picture:
   a. Cyanosis, slate gray color
      (1) Cyanosis appears when MetHgb level reaches 10%–15%. (Cyanotic heart disease is frequently suspected.)
   b. Fatigue, dyspnea, depressed neurologic function.
      (1) MetHgb level approaches 50%.
   c. Fatalities:
      (1) Seen when MetHgb levels are >70%.
2. Laboratory findings:
   a. Blood color:
      (1) Brown (sometimes dark, not brown).
      (2) Does not turn red when aerated.

b. Blood gas findings:
   (1) Po_2 value may be very high (≥100 mm Hg), but the child remains cyanotic. (This finding is not cyanotic heart disease.)
   (2) Metabolic acidosis: suggests tissue hypoxia and high MetHgb level.
   (3) Elevated MetHgb level when direct blood gas measurements are performed.
   (4) Directly measured oxyghemoglobin level (oxygen saturation) is low.

D. Therapy

1. Remove offending agent.
2. Methylene blue: for rapid conversion of MetHgb to Hgb.
   a. Indication: MetHgb level ≥30%.
   b. Dose: 1% methylene blue solution for infusion.
      (1) 1–2 mg/kg IV over 5–10 minutes; color improves within the hour after its administration.
      (2) May repeat dose in 1–2 hours if cyanosis persists.
   c. CAUTION: Patient with glucose-6-phosphate dehydrogenase deficiency (primarily males):
      (1) Methylene blue can cause a hemolytic anemia.
      (2) Methylene blue will not correct methemoglobinemia.
   d. Alternatives to methylene blue:
      (1) Ascorbic acid: slow action; therefore, not useful in the emergency situation.
      (2) Exchange transfusion.
3. Exchange transfusion:
   a. Indication: MetHgb level ≥50%.
      (1) Use in addition to methylene blue.
      (2) Use in place of methylene blue.

E. Diagnostic work-up for methemoglobinemia.

1. To be done, as indicated, in ward or pediatric intensive care unit setting.
   a. Enzyme studies.
   b. Hgb electrophoresis.

IV. Acute Life-Threatening Event (Near-Miss Sudden Infant Death Syndrome)

An acute life-threatening event (ALTE) is any unexplained, sudden, near death of a young child, usually age 1 to 6 months. This section presents a brief overview of assessment and therapy. See the appropriate section for therapy of known underlying cause.

A. **Clinical assessment**

1. Vital signs.
   a. May be normal.
   b. Shock of different etiologies may be present.
2. Clinical appearance: anywhere on a continuum from normal to clinically dead.
3. Signs of increased ICP may be present.
4. Laboratory data.
   a. Arterial blood gas values.
   b. Blood, urine, and possibly cerebrospinal fluid (CSF) cultures.
   c. Electrolyte, glucose, calcium, magnesium, and phosphorus levels.
   d. CBC count with differential.
   e. Save blood, if possible, for endocrine studies.
   f. ECG.
   g. Chest x-ray film.

B. **Therapy**

1. ABCs and CPR, if needed (see Appendix II–6).
2. Correct hypothermia (see p. 265).
3. Correct hypoglycemia (see p. 201).
4. Correct acidosis:
   a. Provide adequate ventilation.
   b. When ventilation is established, give $NaHCO_3$, 1–2 mEq/kg.
5. Tracheal intubation is indicated for any infant with poor respiratory effort, hypoxemia or hypercapnia.
6. Seek etiology.
   a. Hypothermia.
   b. Sepsis.
   c. Trauma/abuse.
   d. Adrenal insufficiency.
   e. Overwhelming pneumonitis (respiratory syncytial virus [RSV]).
   f. Seizure.
   g. Aspiration.
   h. Toxin ingestion.
7. Give glucose and naloxone.

8. Administer ampicillin, 100 mg/kg IV, and cefotaxime, 50 mg/kg.
9. Consider Solu-Cortef, 4 mg/kg IV.
10. Obtain detailed history.

C. Ongoing monitoring

1. Pulse oximeter and cardiac monitor.
2. Monitor BP and vital signs continuously.
3. Keep patient warm.

V. Reye's Syndrome

Reye's syndrome is a postinfectious disorder marked by an acute metabolic encephalopathy and fatty degeneration of the viscera, most notably the liver. Its incidence peaked in the late 1970s and early 1980s, dwindled in the mid- and late 1980s; it may be reappearing again at this time. Its etiology remains unidentified. It ranges in severity from mild to lethal, it may progress rapidly, and its course is unpredictable during the early stages. It typically affects children ranging from several months to 16 years of age.

A. Clinical picture

A biphasic clinical history is classically found. The first phase of illness is typically a viral illness. The infection is most commonly an upper respiratory tract infection, less often varicella or acute gastroenteritis. The most commonly identified organisms are influenza B and varicella.

As the child appears to be recovering from the viral illness, the second phase begins. It is marked by recurrent and intractable vomiting; medical attention is usually sought for this distressing problem. Altered CNS function may become apparent at this stage; it begins with lethargy, then can progress to agitation, delerium, coma, and, finally, death. Gastrointestinal (GI) and CNS problems dominate the clinical picture, but extensive multisystem involvement is common.

Lovejoy classified Reye's syndrome into 5 progressive stages based on CNS involvement; a list of them follows. It is important to note that (1) patients do not always go through all stages of the disease; the disease process can halt at any stage; and that (2) the disease may progress from stage 1 through stage 5 at variable rates ranging from several hours to 48 hours.

1. *Lethargy:* Sleepy, vomiting. Liver function test results (LFT) are abnormal.
2. *Disorientation:* Delerious, combative; hyperventilating, hyperactive reflexes. Appropriate responses to noxious stimuli. LFT results are abnormal.
3. *Coma.* Comatose, decorticate rigidity; hyperventilating. Preserved pupillary and oculovestibular reflexes. LFT results are abnormal.
4. *Decerebrate rigidity.* Deepening coma, decerebrate rigidity. Large, fixed pupils, loss of oculocephalic reflexes. LFT results are minimally abnormal.
5. *Respiratory arrest:* Flaccid, loss of deep tendon reflexes, respiratory arrest. LFT results are often normal.

Seizures may occur at several stages, typically stages 3 through 5.

Infantile Reye's syndrome: Infants occasionally have Reye's syndrome. Their clinical picture is very different from that of older children. Their preceding illness is frequently an acute gastroenteritis rather than an upper respiratory tract infection. They may have vomiting, but it may not be pernicious or easily distinguishable from the preceding illness. Seizures are common and may be the presenting sign; seizures and encephalopathy may be severe. In most instances, Reye's syndrome is not suspected and is diagnosed only incidentally when the child is found to be hypoglycemic. In this situation, evaluation of hypoglycemia leads to the discovery of liver function abnormalities characteristic of Reye's syndrome. Laboratory abnormalities are the same as in older children, but hypoglycemia is prominent. In infants, a liver biopsy may be required for confirmation of this disease.

B. Pathology

Mitochondrial damage appears to be the basis of the extensive changes seen in Reye's syndrome. At the electron microscopic level, the mitochondria are structurally damaged. Metabolically, mitochondrial disruption alters metabolism and results in the widespread accumulation of metabolic byproducts, notably metabolic acids. Metabolic acidosis is prominent.

At the organ level, brain and liver pathologic conditions dominate the picture, but widespread organ involvement is present.

Fatty deposition is the prominent finding in involved viscera. The liver is swollen and yellow because of fatty infiltration; little evidence of inflammation or necrosis is present. Fatty degeneration of the kidneys, heart, and pancreas may also be present.

The brain is edematous and may show evidence of herniation in fatal cases. Cells are swollen or damaged; the changes are noninflammatory in nature. CSF values are normal. Fatty deposits in brain blood vessels are seen.

C. Laboratory findings

1. *Elevated aspartate aminotransferase (AST) and alanine aminotransferase (ALT) levels.*
2. *Elevated ammonia level.*
3. *Prolonged PT.*
4. *Hypoglycemia (most common in children <4 years old).*
5. Bilirubin level: usually normal.
6. CSF: normal (if a lumbar puncture is done).
7. Metabolic acidosis.
8. Elevated WBC count.
9. Elevated blood urea nitrogen (BUN) and creatinine levels.
10. Elevated amylase level.
11. Elevated creatine phosphokinase (CPK) and lactic dehydrogenase levels.
12. Cerebral edema on computed axial tomography (CAT) scan of head.

D. Diagnosis

The diagnosis is made on the basis of the clinical picture and laboratory values.

1. Clinical picture:
   The biphasic picture is important, and a preceding illness can usually be identified. Pernicious vomiting is a cardinal feature of the disease. Changes in the sensorium generally follow the stages outlined.
2. Laboratory values:
   The laboratory abnormalities in italics are required to confirm the diagnosis. AST, ALT, and ammonia

should be at least 2.5–3 times higher than normal. Hypoglycemia is common in young children but may not be seen in older children. Initial laboratory studies should include glucose, AST, ALT, and ammonia levels, PT/PTT, electrolyte levels, and CBC count; additional laboratory tests may include ABG values, BUN level, creatinine clearance, and CAT scan of head.

Diagnoses that must be ruled out include viral encephalitis, varicella hepatitis, metabolic disorders, salicylism, plumbism, acetaminophen poisoning, other drug ingestions, and other liver diseases.

E. Therapy

Therapy is supportive. Therapy is guided by the clinical stage of the disease. Those with stages 1 and 2 disease need supportive medical care and noninvasive monitoring. Those in stages 3 to 5 require invasive support and monitoring in addition to general supportive medical measures. Close monitoring of vital signs, neurologic status, and laboratory values is vital because deterioration may rapidly develop.

Correction of metabolic and hematologic abnormalities is important. Control of cerebral swelling and ICP in stages 3 to 5 has proved to be crucial in improving outcome. Initial therapy of Reye's syndrome follows.

1. Stage 1 and 2 therapy.
   a. Respiratory: Provide oxygen as needed.
   b. Cardiovascular: Restore circulation. Provide crystalloid boluses to replenish volume deficits incurred by emesis.
   c. Glucose: Treat hypoglycemia with 50% dextrose, 1 mL/kg.
      (1) Provide 10% dextrose concentration in IV solution.
      (2) Monitor test-strip glucoses qh; treat hypoglycemia, increase IV dextrose concentration further as needed.
   d. Coagulopathy:
      (1) Fresh frozen plasma (FFP), 10 mL/kg IV (immediately effective) or
      (2) Vitamin K_1, 1–2 mg IV (which takes at least 12 hours to be effective; it may not be effective with hepatic disease).

e. Hyperammonemia: Neomycin, 20 mg/kg NG.
f. Anticerebral edema measures:
  (1) Elevate patient's head 30 degrees.
  (2) Restrict fluids to two-thirds to three-fourths maintenance rate.
  (3) Mannitol, 0.25–1.0 g/kg IV, can be considered, primarily for the child whose condition is deteriorating; must place Foley catheter when mannitol is given.
  (4) Dexamethasone: not indicated.

2. Stage 3 through 5 therapy.
  a. Use previously listed measures. Additional measures follow.
  b. Intubation: Perform facilitated intubation (see p. 413).
  c. Ventilation:
    (1) Controlled hyperventilation:
      (a) Keep P_{CO_2} 20–30 mm Hg.
      (b) Keep pH >7.4 (up to 7.59).
      (c) Keep P_{O_2} >100 mm Hg.
    (2) Sedation, neuromuscular paralysis.
      (a) A neuromuscular relaxant is usually required to provide controlled hyperventilation and to minimize intracranial hypertension in the nonflaccid (stage 3, 4) patient.
        (i) Vecuronium, 0.1 mg/kg IV prn movement; preferable over pancuronium because the latter may increase ICP if pushed rapidly.
      (b) Sedation is needed to blunt sensation of noxious stimuli that can increase ICP.
        (i) Morphine sulfate, 0.1 mg/kg IV q1–2h prn and/or
        (ii) Benzodiazepine (e.g., midazolam), 0.1 mg/kg IV qh.
  d. Seizures:
    (1) Diazepam, 0.1–0.4 mg/kg IV acutely.
    (2) Follow with phenobarbital, 20 mg/kg IV.
      (a) Phenobarbital has some ICP-lowering effects.

e. Mannitol, 0.25–1.0 gm/kg IV, may be helpful because the likelihood of ICP elevation is significant in these patients.
   (1) Place Foley catheter.
   (2) Give 20 mL/kg LR or NS solution bolus if large diuresis and signs of circulatory compromise follow administration of mannitol. Cerebral perfusion pressure must be maintained.

f. Maintain euthermia.
   (1) Fever: Avoid use of antipyretics, especially aspirin, to reduce fever; use external cooling measures instead.

g. Antacids, especially with bloody NG drainage.
   (1) Cimetidine: Use lower doses (e.g., 20 mg/kg/day in 4 divided doses) because renal function may be impaired, or
   (2) Such agents as aluminum hydroxide and/or magnesium hydroxide, 0.5–1.0 mL/kg NG, maximum dose 30 mL, q2–4h.

VI. Hypothermia

Hypothermia, defined as core body temperature <35.5° C, can be secondary to exposure to low environmental temperature, immersion, sepsis, malnutrition, CNS dysfunction (including head trauma), or metabolic derangements (including hypoglycemia, hypothyroidism, addisonian crisis).

A. Clinical assessment

1. History of incident.
2. Vital signs.
   a. Measure rectal temperature 3–5 cm into rectum.
   b. Bradycardia may be present.
3. Physical examination.
   a. Note mental status changes, including disorientation, agitation, obtundation and coma.
   b. Pupils may be dilated and sluggishly reactive to light.
   c. Deep tendon reflexes may be decreased or absent.
   d. Pulses may be decreased.
   e. Patients are pale, sometimes cyanotic.
4. Laboratory data.
   a. ABG values may show a mixed metabolic and respiratory acidosis.

b. Electrolyte values (hypokalemia may be present).
c. CBC count and coagulation studies (disseminated intravascular coagulation [DIC] may be present).
d. ECG.
   (1) Pathognomonic J wave—camel hump immediately after the QRS complex.
   (2) Ventricular fibrillation is the most common dysrhythmia.

B. Therapy

1. General: Careful handling of hypothermic patients is necessary to avoid precipitation of dysrhythmias in an irritable myocardium.
2. Assess ABCs.
3. Immobilize cervical spine if appropriate from history.
4. Tracheal intubation is usually necessary only for severe hypothermia with respiratory depression, hypoxemia, and hypercapnia.
   a. Intermittent mandatory ventilation is delivered at one-half the usual rate. Adjust upward with ABG values as patient is rewarmed.
5. Continue external cardiac massage for sinus bradycardia, ventricular fibrillation, or asystole until the core body temperature is ≥30° C.
6. Fluids.
   a. NS or LR solution warmed through a blood-warming coil (45° C).
   b. 10–20 mL/kg increments.
   c. FFP is used in the presence of bleeding abnormalities.
7. Assess for hypoglycemia, especially in the small child.
8. Attempt to maintain pH ≥7.25 with careful use of $NaHCO_3$ (1–2 mEq/kg).
9. Rewarming.
   a. Most hypothermic patients can be successfully externally warmed.
      (1) Hot water bottle.
      (2) Overhead warmers.
      (3) Thermal blankets/mattresses.
   b. Too vigorous warming may cause "after drop" of core temperature; some suggest warming head and trunk only.

c. Core rewarming for patients with body temperature <32° C:
   (1) Warm humidified oxygen (42° C–48° C) inhalation, or
   (2) Warm aqueous NS aerosol administration.
   (3) Gastric irrigation is contraindicated because of the risk of inducing dysrythmias.
   (4) Colonic and bladder irrigation with warmed NS solution is described in most texts.
   (5) Peritoneal dialysis with warmed dialysate or NS solution (43° C–45° C) is very effective.
d. Most patients can be managed with external warming and warm inhalation therapy.
e. Consider glucose and naloxone in the obtunded, comatose patient.
f. Transport the patient when temperature is >32° C and cardiac rhythm is normal.

C. Ongoing monitoring

1. Pulse oximetry and cardiac monitors.
2. Frequently assessed perfusion and BP. Vasodilatation may require additional fluid resuscitation.
3. Maintain the patient in a warm environment.

VII. Heat Excess Syndromes

Classic heat stroke is defined as impaired heat dissipation secondary to high ambient temperature and high humidity. Exertional heat stroke adds excessive heat production in the context of high ambient temperature along with extreme activity in a poorly conditioned person. Heat exhaustion often precedes heat stroke.

A. Clinical assessment

1. History of exposure and patient's past conditioning.
2. Vital signs.
   a. Hyperthermia rarely exceeds 39° C in heat exhaustion.
   b. Hyperthermia usually >41° C for heat stroke.
3. Physical examination.
   a. Heat exhaustion.
      (1) Patient complains of weakness, lethargy, thirst, headache, nausea, and vomiting.
      (2) Tachycardia and hypotension may be present.

(3) Mental status changes include agitation, incoordination, and psychosis.

b. Heat stroke.

(1) Tachycardia with thready, rapid pulse.
(2) Hypotension and circulatory collapse.
(3) Usually hot, dry skin.
(4) CNS dysfunction: headache, dizziness, confusion, agitation, seizures, and coma.

4. Laboratory data.

a. Electrolyte values, glucose levels (hypernatremia, hyperchloremia, hyperglycemia).
b. CBC count and coagulation studies (hemoconcentration, DIC).
c. CPK level (rhabdomyolysis).
d. Urinalysis (myoglobinuria).

B. Therapy

1. Assess ABCs. Provide 100% oxygen.
2. Cardiovascular support.

a. Volume expansion with 10–20 mL/kg IV bolus of LR, NS, or 5% albumin solution.
b. Isoproterenol is the optimum inotrope.

(1) Increases cardiac output.
(2) Maintains peripheral vasodilatation.
(3) Dose: 0.1–0.5 μg/kg/min.

c. Dopamine as drug of second choice.
d. α-Agonists are contraindicated.

3. The treatment for hyperthermia is rapid cooling.

a. Ice bath or ice massage, especially to large pulse points; consider chlorpromazine (Thorazine) to prevent shivering.
b. Keep skin moist.
c. Use fans to increase evaporative heat loss.
d. Continuously monitor core body temperature; discontinue cooling when temperature has been lowered to 38.5° C.

4. Renal function.

a. Maintain urine output >1 mL/kg/hour via fluid therapy.
b. Diuresis with furosemide, 1 mg/kg IV, or mannitol 0.5–1 g/kg IV, may be necessary for myoglobinuria or acute tubular necrosis.

5. Consider glucose and naloxone in the obtunded or comatose patient.
6. Transport the patient when cooling has been initiated and cardiovascular status is stable.

C. **Ongoing monitoring**

1. Use pulse oximetry and cardiac monitor.
2. Cool the ambient temperature of the room and transport vehicle.

VIII. Acute GI Bleeding

Loss of blood from the GI tract is identified by the presence of hematemesis or hematochezia. It usually is classified as either upper or lower, depending on location of blood loss. GI bleeding can be secondary to anatomic lesions (ulcer, intussusception, tumor), toxic exposures (aspirin, iron), coagulopathy (decreased platelets, elevated PT or PTT), or failure of other organ systems (liver failure with bleeding varices or secondary coagulopathy; multiple system failure with poor GI tract perfusion and secondary sloughing).

A. **Clinical assessment**

1. History of prior GI bleed or of underlying cause.
2. Physical examination.
   a. Obvious passage of gross blood or coffee ground material orally or rectally. Note appearance of blood (i.e., bright red, dark, clotted).
   b. Signs and symptoms of illnesses associated with GI bleeding.
   c. Associated signs of volume loss: pallor, tachycardia, tachypnea, hypotension, weak pulses, poor capillary refill, depressed mental status.
3. Laboratory data.
   a. Hematocrit.
   b. Platelet count, PT, PTT.
   c. Liver function tests.
   d. Toxicology screen, if appropriate.

B. **Therapy**

NOTE: Although diagnostic methods and specific therapies may vary for upper vs. lower GI bleeding, the principles of initial management are the same. Therapy here is limited to symptomatic treatment of the GI bleed. Refer to the appropriate section for the treatment of any known underlying cause.

1. Respiratory. Provide 100% oxygen, because patient's Hgb concentration may be low.
2. Circulation.
   a. Estimate volume loss and evaluate perfusion status by vital signs and initial physical examination.
   b. Establish IV access with 2 large-bore lines.
   c. Administer volume until perfusion has stabilized.
      (1) 20 mL/kg of NS or LR solution. Reassess and repeat as needed.
      (2) 5% albumin, FFP, and packed red blood cells (PRBCs) may be substituted when available.
      (3) For catastrophic blood loss, type O negative fresh whole blood is best before type and cross.
      (4) For every 70–100 mL/kg of blood replaced, transfuse 1 unit of platelets to avoid secondary dilutional effects.
      (5) Remember that shock from GI bleeding is secondary to intravascular volume depletion. Pressors will *not* be effective without appropriate volume replacement.
3. Nasogastric lavage.
   a. If bleeding site is unclear, place NG tube to assess for upper GI bleeding.
   b. If ongoing bleeding is present, perform gastric lavage.
      (1) Use room temperature NS solution.
      (2) Infuse and evacuate 50–100 mL at a time.
      (3) Lavage until clear.
      (4) Leave NG tube in place to easily assess if bleeding restarts.
4. Medications.
   a. For upper GI bleeding: H_2 blockers.
      (1) Cimetidine, 10 mg/kg/dose (maximum 300 mg) q6h IV.
      (2) Ranitidine, 0.5 mg/kg/dose (maximum 50 mg) q6h IV.
   b. Antacids may be considered, but may interfere with anticipated endoscopy.

c. Sucralfate.
5. Serial hematocrit values.
   a. Initial hematocrit may not represent equilibrated state if blood loss was recent.
   b. Hematocrit may appear to fall further, secondary to dilutional effects from initial nonblood fluid resuscitation.
6. Treat underlying cause of GI bleeding as appropriate.

C. Ongoing monitoring

1. Cardiac monitor.
2. Frequent assessment of vital signs and perfusion.
3. Attempt to stop bleeding (if reasonable) before transport.

IX. Small Infant

This section is devoted to the small infant because of the very different signs these infants sometimes manifest in response to significant illness. The signs of major problems may be very subtle (i.e., nonspecific in nature and not the usual ones that are associated with illness in older patients). For this reason, the absence of clear-cut signs of illness is commonly misinterpreted to mean that the small infant is not significantly ill; the patient is sent home only to return moribund.

Because small infants have very limited reserve, immature responses to stress, and limited abilities to combat infection—far greater limitations than the general infant population—they are highly susceptible to developing devastating decompensation when illnesses go unchecked. Because increasing numbers of infants are discharged from hospitals at low weights, it is important to be alert to the findings that serve as warning signs of potentially significant illness; follow-through with appropriate evaluation, careful monitoring, and early intervention may avert later major disasters.

Low weight is the feature that characterizes the group of infants that responds uniquely to significant illness. There are other features, which, in association with low weight, greatly increase the likelihood of the infant responding in this manner to illness. Characteristics that should alert the care provider of this possibility include:

1. Low weight: Small infants include those up to about 4.0 kg, occasionally larger. Those infants $\leq$2.5 kg

are highly prone to responding to illness in the manner described in this section.

2. Prematurity: Low weight is not always equated with prematurity. Those who are preterm (<38 weeks corrected gestational age) are especially likely to respond to illness in the manner described in this chapter. Infants up through the neonatal period (equivalent to 44 weeks' gestation) can manifest these unique responses to illness, more so if the infant is a former premature infant.
3. Little to absent subcutaneous (SC) tissue: The small infant with little SC tissue is far more likely to respond to illness in this unique manner than an infant of equal weight with good SC tissue and muscle. Older infants of low weight secondary to failure to thrive may manifest these unique responses to illness, especially if they are developmentally delayed and/or less active than usual.
4. Severe neurologic disability: The young infant with severe neurologic incapacitation is at great risk of responding to illness and stress like the very small or premature infant.
5. Specific infections: Many infections may produce the clinical response described in this section. Two specific infections, however, have especially been recognized to produce hypotonia, hypoventilation, and hypothermia in a significant number of its young victims: pertussis and RSV pneumonia. Although the usual clinical picture is the rule for this age/size patient, a significant number of small and young infants respond uniquely to these infections.

A. Signs of illness in the small (premature) infant

1. Poor feeding: This alone can produce illness: dehydration, hypoglycemia.
2. Decreased tone.
3. Decreased activity, responsiveness: includes decreased feeding, decreased movement, decreased cry (both strength and amount of crying), decreased wakefulness, decreased response to stimulation.
4. Tachypnea or decreased respirations (depth and rate): Tachypnea is the expected response to illness in older children; it is seen in small infants. However, a significant number of small/premature infants develop hy-

poventilation, periodic breathing, even apnea in response to illness. This can occur in either the absence or presence of pulmonary disease.

5. Temperature instability: Fever may occur with infection. However, hypothermia may occur in many small infants and can be an ominous sign. The absence of fever in a small infant does not rule out infection.

B. Concerns and management

1. Infection: Either a viral or bacterial infection can produce this picture.
   a. Consider sepsis work-up: blood culture; urinalysis and urine culture; lumbar puncture; chest x-ray film; CBC count, differential and platelet count.
   b. Provide parenteral antibiotics for suspected infection (see Table 8–1).
2. Glucose level: Hypoglycemia is a nonspecific response to illness, stress, as well as poor feeding, and develops rapidly in small infants.
   a. Perform test-strip glucose test and laboratory glucose test.
   b. Treatment of hypoglycemia: 1–2 mL/kg D_{10} IV; follow with IV solution containing D_{10} + electrolytes. Continue to monitor test-strip glucoses q30–60min until stable; provide glucose boluses as needed.
3. Hypoventilation, respiratory failure: common response to illness and stress; may be a primary or secondary problem.
   a. Obtain blood gas values; obtain pulse oximeter reading.
   b. Provide oxygen: Hypoventilation, apnea may be the result of hypoxemia; in some cases, restoring normal Po_2 values may improve ventilation.
   c. Intubate and ventilate if a patient is in respiratory failure or continues to have recurrent apnea.
4. Hydration: The patient who has not fed well may be dehydrated.
   a. Restore circulating volume in volume-depleted patient: 10–20 mL/kg LR or NS solution; repeat as needed.
   b. Replace remaining fluid deficit (see p. 141).

5. Electrolyte values: most common abnormalities.
   a. Hypernatremia is fairly common when po intake has been very low. Rehydrate as per p. 151.
   b. Hyponatremia: not very common but may be seen in association with pneumonia, meningitis secondary to syndrome of inappropriate secretion of antidiuretic hormone. Hyponatremia may cause hypoventilation in addition to seizures.
      (1) When hyponatremia is the result of water intoxication, give furosemide. If infant is clinically stable, avoid NaCl bolus and use NS solution + K^+ and glucose IV solution to correct serum Na^+ gradually (see p. 167).
   c. Metabolic acidosis: evidence of illness. Generally does not require $NaHCO_3$ correction but requires correction of underlying problem (e.g., dehydration, infection, hypoglycemia).
6. Hematologic system:
   a. Anemia: commonly found in infection/sepsis.
      (1) Anemia, by itself, can cause hypoventilation, apnea, decreased activity.
      (2) Transfuse the symptomatic patient with PRBCs.
7. Temperature: Small infant may respond to infection or stress with fever or hypothermia.
   a. Hypothermia: may be a sign of significant infection or significant problem (e.g., CNS bleed).
   b. Temperature variation is also frequently environmental in origin. Temperature variation—fever or hypothermia—can adversely affect the infant's behavior and clinical picture. In these instances, correction of environmental temperature or removal/addition of extra covering may correct the temperature and improve the infant's clinical condition.
8. Seizures: Infant's seizures can be very subtle, ranging from staring, rhythmic mouth/tongue movements, hypotonia/hypertonia, or hypoventilation/apnea to generalized tonic/clonic seizures. Clinical diagnosis of seizures is a judgment based on observation and clinical suspicion; treat with phenobarbital (see p. 127).

9. Trauma: must be in the differential diagnosis; examine skin, note bones and bone/joint tenderness; examine fundi. Perform diagnostic imaging studies as indicated.
10. If, after an unrevealing evaluation, the infant still remains quiet, does not feed well, and/or still has trouble maintaining body temperature, it is prudent to continue to closely observe the patient in the emergency department or in the inpatient ward rather than to send the patient home.

REFERENCES

Conn AW, Barker GA: Fresh water drowning and near-drowning: An update. *Can Anaesth Soc J* 1984; 31:538.

Lovejoy F: Clinical staging in Reye syndrome. *Am J Dis Child* 1974; 128:36.

TRAUMA 10

I. Major Trauma

Trauma continues to be the leading cause of death in children, and it is also responsible for a great deal of morbidity. The care given in the stabilization period may have a major impact on long-term outcome.

There are several differences between the pediatric and adult trauma patient that should be kept in mind during evaluation. The young child often cannot communicate except to cry, making assessment of injuries more difficult. Blunt trauma accounts for about 80% of pediatric trauma, with penetrating injuries being relatively rare. The airways of a child have a smaller diameter and are therefore more likely to be compromised by a given amount of edema (e.g., in an inhalation injury or blunt tracheal trauma). The head of the child has a greater mass relative to the rest of the body. As a result, a child who falls or is thrown (in a motor vehicle accident [MVA] or off of a bicycle) will frequently land on his or her head and sustain head trauma. Head trauma accounts for 50% of pediatric trauma.

The thorax and abdomen of a child are more susceptible to major injury despite relatively minor external signs. Because the ribs are more cartilaginous (and therefore flexible) and there is less muscle and SC tissue, forces applied to the chest wall are easily transmitted to underlying structures. The liver and spleen are relatively lower in the abdomen and are more anterior than in adults. Therefore, those organs are more susceptible to injury.

A. Priorities in stabilization

1. Evaluate for immediate life-threatening conditions.
   a. Assure a patent airway, maintaining cervical spine control if appropriate.
   b. Assess respiratory effort and assist if needed.
   c. Assure adequate circulation and perfusion.

   d. Assess neurologic status for treatable signs of increased intracranial pressure (ICP) (see p. 420).
2. Determine if immediate surgical intervention is likely to be required. If so:
   a. If the appropriate surgical capabilities exist at the referring hospital, proceed accordingly.
   b. If not, select a mode of transport designed to get the patient to a tertiary care center as quickly as possible, even if the transport personnel are not highly experienced in pediatrics (they *must,* however, be able to control the patient's airway and circulation).

   This is one of the few cases where waiting for a pediatric team might not be beneficial to the child.
3. Perform a "secondary survey" for non-life-threatening injuries.
   a. Include a complete head to toe examination of every organ system.
   b. Stabilize as appropriate for transport (minor bleeding, wounds requiring cleaning, fractures).
   c. Remove all of patient's clothing to avoid missing injuries.

B. Assessment and management

1. Airway.
   a. Use 100% oxygen for all patients.
   b. Apply pulse oximetry and cardiac monitors.
   c. Keep the airway open and clear via head positioning, jaw thrust manuvers, and suctioning.
   d. Use bag and mask ventilation if respiratory effort is inadequate.
   e. Endotracheal intubation may be necessary for airway control or for increased ICP (see p. 413 for intubation criteria, and p. 122, medications).
      (1) Secure tube well for transport.
      (2) Remember to remove some air from the pilot balloon on cuffed tubes (before transport) if the transport involves high-altitude flight.
      (3) If there is significant facial trauma and the cervical spine cannot be cleared, a cricothyrotomy is the safest way to secure an airway. The need for open cricothyrotomy is rare, and it should be performed only in children >12 years of age; under this age, a needle-catheter cricothyrotomy is pre-

ferred (see p. 345) with subsequent surgical tracheostomy within 30 minutes.

2. Circulation.
   a. Control ongoing hemorrhage.
   b. Establish 2 routes of large-bore intravenous (IV) assess, preferably in the upper extremities.
      (1) Peripheral IV line.
      (2) Central venous line (see p. 351).
      (3) Intraosseous line (see p. 349).
      (4) Saphenous vein cutdown (see p. 353).
   c. Monitor perfusion (see also the discussion of hypovolemic shock on p. 61):
      (1) Capillary refill should be <3 seconds unless the patient is cold.
      (2) Heart rate above normal value for age, especially in the nonagitated patient, may represent attempted compensation for hypovolemia.
      (3) Altered mental status out of proportion to known injuries may signal decreased cerebral perfusion.
      (4) Hypotension is a late sign of shock in the pediatric patient.
      (5) Decreased urine output: <0.5–1.0 mL/kg/hour.
   d. Therapy (see also p. 66).
      (1) If perfusion is good, use lactated Ringer's (LR) solution initially at the patient's maintenance rate. Switch to 5% dextrose in ¼ NS solution after stabilization.
      (2) For signs of poor perfusion and shock:
         (a) LR or NS solution, 20 mL/kg; reassess and repeat as needed.
         (b) Add packed red blood cells (PRBCs) when available.
         (c) For known massive hemorrhage, use type O negative blood until crossmatch is available.
         (d) Remember that shock from hemorrhage is secondary to intravascular volume depletion and pressors will *not* be effective without appropriate volume replacement.
            (i) Pressors are indicated for the patient whose shock was severe enough to cause poor myocardial perfusion with secondary myocardial dysfunction.

(ii) Adequate volume replacement is still required before use of pressors in this situation.

(iii) Consider use of dopamine or dobutamine (see pp. 428, 429).

(3) Spinal shock is rare and is a diagnosis of exclusion.

(4) Use of military antishock trousers (MAST) is not of proven benefit in children but may be considered in severe cases of shock.

(5) "Unnoticed" sites of significant blood loss in children:

(a) Blood lost at scene of accident (especially from large lacerations to the face and head).

(b) Bleeding into the chest, abdomen, or retroperitoneum.

(c) Soft tissue bleeding around a femur fracture.

(d) Intracranial bleeding in the young infant (<6 months).

3. Cervical spine.
   a. The cervical spine deserves special attention in stabilization and transport of trauma patients.
   b. The only safe assumption is that the cervical spine is injured.
   c. A lateral cervical spine x-ray film of all seven cervical vertebrae should be cleared at the referring institution as part of the initial trauma survey.
   d. Regardless of result of this film, the neck should be immobilized completely for the transport.
   e. A small percentage of cervical spine injuries will be missed by a lateral radiograph; only a full cervical spine series, including anteroposterior plus oblique and open-mouth views, can exclude a cervical spine injury. Therefore, the safest option is cervical spine immobilization for the transport.
4. Secondary survey.
   a. Examine the head, neck, chest, abdomen, pelvis, rectum, extremities, back, skin, and neurologic system for any evidence of injury.
   b. Obtain a past history for allergies, medications, illnesses, last meal, and events preceding the injury.

c. Laboratory data:
   (1) Hematocrit or hemoglobin value.
   (2) Urinalysis.
   (3) Amylase, cardiac, and liver enzymes.
   (4) X-ray studies as appropriate for injuries (usually a minimum of chest and cervical spine films).

5. Foley catheter.
   a. 8 F for infants.
   b. 10 F for school-aged children.
   c. 12–14 F for teenagers.
   d. If there is any suspicion of urethral injury in male patients, a retrograde urethrogram should be obtained before Foley insertion. If the urethra is injured, urinary drainage is obtained by a suprapubic catheter, not by a urethral catheter.
6. The stomach should be decompressed with a nasogastric or orogastric tube to prevent vomiting. This is doubly important in the patient with an unintubated airway. Avoid using a nasogastric tube in the patient with massive facial or nasal trauma.
7. Keep the patient warm throughout stabilization and transport.
   a. Children have a higher surface area/mass ratio; this means that pediatric patients are much more prone to cooling.
   b. Fatal coagulopathy can result from:
      (1) Dilution from IV fluids.
      (2) Extensive cooling from exposure.
8. Potential complications of chest and abdominal trauma.
   a. Pneumothorax.
      (1) Suspect pneumothorax in the presence of any chest trauma, rib fractures, or sudden worsening of respiratory status in the traumatized or intubated patient.
      (2) Any pneumothorax visible on chest radiograph requires placement of a chest tube before transport, especially for air transport.
         (a) Changes in barometric pressure on ascension will cause trapped air to expand.
         (b) Placement of a chest tube in a patient while in a moving vehicle is more difficult than when the patient is in the stable emergency department environment.

(3) *Tension* pneumothorax.
   (a) Suspect in case of sudden hemodynamic instability.
   (b) Trachea deviates *away* from the pneumothorax.
   (c) Evacuate by placing a large-bore needle in the chest (see p. 346) before placement of a chest tube.

b. Flail chest.
   (1) Treat with intubation and positive pressure ventilation to avoid sudden respiratory failure from fatigue.

c. Internal hemorrhage.
   (1) Suspect when hypovolemia, anemia, or shock are out of proportion to obvious blood loss.
   (2) Bleeding may be into the chest (pulmonary contusion or hemorrhage), abdomen (hepatic, splenic, or inferior vena cava laceration), or retroperitoneum.

d. Pericardial tamponade.
   (1) Secondary to either blunt or penetrating trauma.
   (2) Hallmark is Beck's triad:
      (a) Hypotension.
      (b) Distended neck veins.
      (c) Distant heart sounds.
   (3) Volume and pressors may be helpful.
   (4) Fluid restriction or diuresis is *contraindicated.*
   (5) Pericardiocentesis may be needed as a life-saving measure (see p. 348).

9. Fractures.
   a. Spinal cord: Thoroughly immobilize with cervical collar, sand bags, tape, and backboard.
   b. Long bones.
      (1) Assess distal perfusion.
      (2) Splint and elevate if possible.
      (3) Open fractures.
         (a) Dress in sterile manner.
         (b) Splint.
         (c) Transport for definitive care quickly, because the risk of osteomyelitis increases significantly in untreated open fractures after 6 hours.

   c. Pelvic and femur fractures can be causes of significant occult blood loss. Placing these patients in MAST may help to splint the fractures and may minimize blood loss.
10. Open wounds should be dressed and bleeding stopped with pressure dressings or suturing.
11. Amputated body parts.
   a. Wrap in moist sterile gauze.
   b. Place inside a plastic bag in an iced saline bath. Do not place in ice alone because the body part may freeze.
   c. Transport with the patient for possible reimplantation.

II. Head Trauma

Central nervous system injury is frequent and can occur alone or in association with other injuries in the pediatric trauma victim. Therefore, it is extremely important for the patient to have an initial thorough neurologic examination, followed by frequent serial examinations during stabilization and transport.

A. Assessment and management

1. ABCs: Assure that hypoxia and shock are not contributing to the diminishing sensorium. Maintain in-line cervical spine stabilization for any patient requiring intubation.
2. Immobilize cervical spine in all head trauma.
3. Assess sensorium via the Glasgow Coma Scale (GCS) (see p. 437).
   a. Increasing ICP leads to decreasing GCS.
   b. Intubation and ventilation are required for patients who have or are developing a GCS of ≤ 8. See the section on increased ICP if needed (p. 122).
4. External signs of significant head injury.
   a. Battle's sign.
   b. Hemotympanum.
   c. Orbital ecchymoses.
   d. Cerebral spinal fluid otorrhea or rhinorrhea.
5. Seizures.
   a. Will increase the metabolic demands of brain tissue.
   b. Will often interfere with the ability to ventilate effectively.

c. Treatment.
   (1) Administer 100% oxygen.
   (2) If the airway is not intubated, use phenytoin, 20 mg/kg IV, at a maximum rate of 1 mg/kg/min.
   (3) If the airway is intubated, use phenobarbitol, 20 mg/kg IV. If seizures continue, give an additional 10 mg/kg dose 1 or 2 more times.
   (4) For second medication use phenytoin or phenobarbitol as just listed.
   (5) If patient continues having seizures, give lorazepam, 0.1 mg/kg IV, or diazepam, 0.1 mg/kg. Watch for hypotension when combining phenobarbitol and a benzodiazepine.
   (6) In major head trauma, consider using prophylactic phenytoin.

6. Corticosteroids:
   a. Not indicated for head trauma.
   b. For spinal cord trauma: Administer methylprednisolone 30 mg/kg loading dose, followed by 5.4 mg/kg/hr for 24 hours.

III. Burns

Approximately 2,500 children die every year as a result of burns; a greater number suffer permanent damage. Because of their thinner skin, children sustain greater injury than adults from a similar burn incident. The outcome from burns is often quite dependent on the early management of the patient; appropriate initial stabilization plays a significant role.

A. Clinical assessment

1. ABCs.
2. History of event.
   a. A patient burned in a closed space will be predisposed to inhalation injury.
   b. The patient may have other injuries if burned in an MVA, in an explosion, or before a jump from a burning building.
   c. Management at scene of burn.
3. Assess extent of burn.
   a. Degree.
      (1) First degree: Superficial, involving only the epidermis (most sunburns).
      (2) Second degree: Involves epidermis and part of dermis; skin is red, blistered, and painful.

(3) Third degree: Full-thickness burn destroying both skin layers; has a whitish or charred appearance with tough, leathery feel. Sensory nerves are destroyed so there is no pain.

(4) Fourth degree: Involves muscle or bone.

b. Initially it may be impossible to tell a deep second-degree burn from a third-degree burn.

c. Percent body surface area burn (for purposes of treatment) refers to second-degree burns or worse.

d. See Tables 10–1 and 10–2 for calculation of percent of burn and guidelines for hospitalization or transfer.

e. For patchy or small burns, the area of the patient's palm represents approximately 1% of the body surface area.

B. Treatment

1. Administer 100% oxygen. Assure airway patency and adequate respiratory effort.
2. Maintenance/placement of an airway is of special concern in the victim of a burn. Inhalation injury can cause airway edema, which may progress rapidly (in minutes) to obstruction. This can preclude intubation. It is absolutely crucial to establish an artificial airway immediately.

a. Absolute criteria for intubation.

(1) Erythema or swelling of the oropharynx or nasopharynx.

(2) Soot in the pharynx.

(3) Mechanism suggesting possible inhalation injury (e.g., a burn in a closed space).

(4) Hoarseness, stridor, or brassy cough.

(5) Wheezes or rales.

(6) Agitation, tachypnea, stupor, cyanosis.

(7) Grunting, flaring or retracting.

(8) Oxygen saturation <90%.

b. Relative criteria for intubation (not needed only if the burn mechanism was localized).

(1) Singed eyebrows or nasal hair.

(2) Facial burns.

c. Nasotracheal intubation is preferred; however, time should not be wasted attempting this route if the practitioner is not experienced.

TABLE 10–1.
Lung-Browder Chart

	% Body Surface Area Burn							
Area	0–1 yr	1–4 yr	4–9 yr	10–15 yr	Adult	2nd Degree	3rd Degree	Total
Head	19	17	13	10	8			
Neck	2	2	2	2	2			
Trunk (front/back)	13	13	13	13	13			
Buttock (R/L)	2.5	2.5	2.5	2.5	2.5			
Genitalia	1	1	1	1	1			
Arm (R/L)	4	4	4	4	4			
Forearm (R/L)	3	3	3	3	3			
Hand (R/L)	2.5	2.5	2.5	2.5	2.5			
Thigh (R/L)	5.5	6.5	8.5	8.5	9.5			
Leg (R/L)	5	5	5	6	7			
Foot (R/L)	3.5	3.5	3.5	3.5	3.5			
					TOTAL			

TABLE 10–2.
Guidelines for Hospitalization/Transfer of Burn Patients

Classifications	
Major burn injury	>25% BSA* (children: < 10 yr, > 20% BSA). Full thickness ≥ 10%. All significant burns of face, eyes, ears, hands, feet, perineum or joints, likely to result in functional or cosmetic impairment. All significant high-voltage electrical burns. All burns complicated by inhalation injury or major trauma or associated illness. **Refer patients to burn center after initial stabilization.**
Moderate uncomplicated burn injury	15%–20% BSA (children: < 10 yr, 10%–20% BSA). Full-thickness 3%–10% BSA. All significant burns of face, eyes, ears, hands, feet, perineum or joints that do not threaten significant functional or cosmetic impairment. **Can be managed on an outpatient basis at a general hospital, if staff is comfortable.**
Minor burn injury	< 15% BSA (children: < 10 yr, 10%) Full thickness < 2%. Very minor burns of face, eyes, ears, hands, feet, perineum or joints that do not threaten significant functional or cosmetic impairment. **Can be managed on an outpatient basis.**

*BSA = body surface area.

3. Stop the burning process. Remove smoldering clothing or debris to prevent increasing the depth of the burn.
4. For patients with an inhalation injury, obtain a blood carboxyhemoglobin level. If it is elevated, maintain the patient on 100% oxygen via endotracheal tube or nonrebreathing mask. See p. 254 for treatment of carbon monoxide poisoning. Note that pulse oximetry measurements may be falsely reassuring in the patient with carbon monoxide poisoning. Oximetry measures the percent of binding of hemoglobin *available* for oxygen binding. So a patient with 40% carboxyhemoglobin may show an O_2 saturation of 100%, but that means only that 100% of his

or her normal hemoglobin is oxygen bound (i.e., O_2 delivery to the tissues is only 60% of the oximetry reading).

5. Vascular access in order of preference.
   a. Peripheral IV access through nonburned tissue.
   b. Peripheral IV access through burned tissue.
   c. Central venous access.
   d. Intraosseous infusion.
   NOTE: The order of c. and d. depends on the experience of the practitioner.
6. Fluid resuscitation.
   a. 4 mL/kg/% burn in the first 24 hours.
      (1) Administer this amount *in addition* to daily maintenance requirements in the young child.
      (2) Administer one half of this solution in the first 8 hours *from the time of the burn.*
      (3) Resuscitation fluid should be crystalloid solution (LR or NS), not colloid.
   b. The most frequent mistake is underresuscitation of the burn victim, with resultant renal failure, and a considerably higher mortality.
   c. ***Example:*** a 10 kg patient who has sustained a 50% total body surface area burn requires 2,000 mL in the first 24 hours, one half of which is given in the first 8 hours (i.e., during the time of stabilization and transport). Therefore, the IV should be run at 125 mL/hour from the time of the injury and deficits should be made up. Remember, this is in addition to the patient's maintenance fluids.
7. Assessment of adequacy of fluid resuscitation.
   a. Insert a Foley catheter.
   b. *Maintain 1.0 mL/kg/hour of urine.*
   c. Other means of assessing fluid status do not always apply in the burn patient.
      (1) Peripheral perfusion (capillary refill) may be diminished secondary to proximal edema of burned tissue.
      (2) Blood pressure may be difficult to obtain because of proximal edema and because of difficulty in using a cuff and stethoscope on burned skin.
      (3) Mental status may be altered because of hypoxic injury or pain medication.

(4) Tachycardia may be present secondary to pain and anxiety.

d. If urine output is <1 mL/kg/hour, *assume the patient needs more volume* and increase the infusion rate.

e. Red or pink pigment in the urine indicates myoglobinuria from myonecrosis and should be treated with IV mannitol (0.5–1 g/kg) and IV sodium bicarbonate to keep urine pH ≥ 7 (see p. 289).

8. Treatment of burned skin.
   a. Personnel should wear sterile gloves, as well as gowns and masks, when caring for a burned patient.
   b. During the ABCs of resuscitation, the only treatment for the burn should be covering with a clean sheet.
   c. Later, the burns themselves should be wrapped in sterile gauze moistened with saline solution over which is wrapped some type of barrier to evaporation (e.g., plastic wrap).
9. Check a rapid glucose test (Dextrostix, Chemstrip) on every child with a burn.
   a. Young children are predisposed to hypoglycemia when stressed.
   b. If glucose level is low, give 0.5 g of glucose/kg as 25% dextrose.
10. Check tetanus immunization status and administer tetanus toxoid if needed.
11. Systemic antibiotics are not indicated in the initial treatment of a burned patient unless other injuries (open fracture, etc.) warrant their use.
12. Pain control.
    a. Morphine: 0.05–0.1 mg/kg IV q1h prn.
    b. Meperidine: 1–2 mg/kg IM q1h prn.
    c. Observe closely for signs of respiratory depression.
13. Escharotomy may be required for signs of ventilatory (circumferential chest burns) or circulatory (circumferential extremity burns) compromise.
14. Laboratory data.
    a. Complete blood cell count.
    b. Arterial blood gas value with carboxyhemoglobin.
    c. Electrolyte values.
    d. Urinalysis.
    e. Chest x-ray film.

C. Chemical burns.

1. Chemical reactions with the skin or exposed areas leading to tissue destruction.
2. ABCs and fluids as for thermal burns.
3. Cardinal rule: *Stop the burning process.*
   a. Remove chemical-soaked clothing.
   b. Most acids and lyes can be treated with copious water lavage.
   c. Neutralize according to specific instructions on container or from poison control center.
   d. Exceptions to water lavage rule.
      (1) Oxalic acid and hydrofluoric acid should be neutralized by injection of 10% calcium gluconate solution into the involved areas.
      (2) Phenol should be covered with oil.
      (3) Sulfuric acid should be neutralized with soda lime.
      (4) Chlorox should be neutralized with milk, egg-white, or starch paste.
      (5) The unfortunate patient exposed to sodium metal should have this immediately excised.
      (6) Tar should first be cooled and later removed with lard.
4. Chemical burns to eyes:
   a. Flush continuously with saline solution for 20 minutes.
   b. Alkali burns to eyes will require 8 hours of continuous irrigation.

D. Electrical burns.

1. ABCs as for thermal burns.
2. Usually the extent of injury is much greater than is visible from the surface burns.
   a. Deep body structures in between entrance and exit wounds can be severely damaged.
      (1) Muscle.
      (2) Nerve.
      (3) Internal organs.
   b. Often there are other associated injuries (e.g., electrocuted patients often fall from heights).
3. Hydration is crucial.
   a. Insert a Foley catheter.
   b. Provide liberal fluids IV.
      (1) Urine output should be 1–2 mL/kg/hour.

(2) If any pink or red urine appears:
   (a) Administer mannitol (0.5–1.0 gm/kg); urine output should be maintained consistently at ≥2 mL/kg/hr.
   (b) Institute urine alkalinization; keep urine pH ≥7. Give $NaHCO_3$, 1–2 mEq/kg IV followed by IV solution with 40 mEq $NaHCO_3$/L at one to two times maintenance rate.

4. Locate entrance and exit wounds.
   a. Provide local care.
   b. Elevate affected extremities.
5. Obtain initial electrocardiogram and provide continuous cardiac monitoring, because myocardial damage may be present.

BIBLIOGRAPHY

Friedman AH, Wilkins RH: *Neurosurgical Management for the House Officer*. Baltimore, Williams & Wilkins Co, 1984.

Kim S, Lund D: Pediatric surgical emergencies, in Wilkins EW (ed): *Emergency Medicine: Scientific Foundations and Current Practice*, ed 3. Baltimore, Williams & Wilkins Co, 1989, pp 568–582.

Lee G: Transport of the critically ill trauma patient. *Nurs Clin North Am* 21:741–749.

TOXIC AND UNKNOWN INGESTIONS

11

Stabilization and transport of the child with a toxic ingestion can present several management difficulties. The history of the ingestion may be unclear with regard to timing, amount ingested, or identification of the substance or substances ingested.

Most children with a history of an ingestion appear clinically well. However, many substances can cause sudden life-threatening complications, such as cardiac arrest, respiratory arrest, cardiac arrhythmias, and seizures. For this reason, certain well-appearing children may need intensive monitoring and sophisticated interhospital transport.

This chapter presents a general discussion of decontamination procedures, followed by sections on identification (by clinical signs) of unknown ingestions and treatment of common known ingestions. *It is assumed that therapy in all cases will include consultation with the hospital's regional poison control center.*

I. Decontamination Procedures

A. ABCs

1. Establish and stabilize airway.
2. Cardiac monitor.
3. Obtain intravenous (IV) access.
4. Fluid bolus with normal saline (NS) solution if indicated.

B. First things first

1. Naloxone (Narcan): for unknown ingestion, especially if opioid is suspected or in patient with respiratory depression.
   a. 0.1 mg/kg IV push.
   b. If unsuccessful, may be repeated after 5 minutes.

2. Glucose.
    a. 2–4 mL/kg 25% aqueous dextrose solution ($D_{25}W$) IV if > 1 month old.
    b. 1–2 mL/kg $D_{10}W$ IV for neonates.
3. Consider multiple ingestion.
    a. Obtain good history.
    b. Consider toxic syndromes.

C. Gastric decontamination

1. Ipecac.
    a. Dose.
        (1) 6–12 months: 10 mL with 15 mL/kg clear fluid.
        (2) 1–12 years: 15–30 mL with 240 mL clear fluid.
        (3) >12 years: 30–60 mL with 240–480 mL clear fluid.
    b. Technique.
        (1) Give appropriate amount po, preferably within 1 hour of ingestion.
        (2) Keep patient in upright position.
        (3) Supervise children after administration of ipecac.
        (4) If no emesis after 20 minutes, repeat once and give more fluids.
    c. Contraindications.
        (1) Age < 6 months.
        (2) Caustic ingestion (strong acid or alkali).
        (3) Patient comatose and/or central nervous system (CNS) depression (no gag reflex).
        (4) Seizures.
        (5) High risk for coma and/or seizures.
        (6) Hemorrhagic diathesis.
        (7) Foreign body ingestion.
        (8) Significant vomiting before ipecac administration.
        (9) Camphor/strychnine.
        (10) Hydrocarbons.
        (11) Late-stage pregnancy.
        (12) Uncontrolled hypertension.
2. Gastric lavage.
    a. Nasogastric/orogastric (NG/OG) placement.
        (1) *Protect airway* (intubate if necessary).
        (2) Keep patient in left lateral decubitus position with head slightly lower than feet.
        (3) Use large-bore OG/NG tube (16–26 F in children).

(4) Measure/check placement of tube. After insertion, aspirate all stomach contents.

b. Technique.
   (1) Lavage with NS (0.9%) solution.
   (2) Use 15 mL/kg/cycle aliquots to maximum 400 mL/cycle. Continue gastric lavage until clear.
   (3) Initial pass may be sent to toxicology for identification.

c. Indications.
   (1) Ipecac unsuccessful.
   (2) CNS depression.
   (3) Unprotected airway (intubate before perfoming lavage).
   (4) Seizures.
   (5) Urgent removal (tricyclics, camphor, cyanide, strychnine).
   (6) Concretion formation (meprobamate, ferrous sulfate).

d. Complications.
   (1) Nasal trauma.
   (2) Esophageal perforation.
   (3) Tracheal intubation.
   (4) Aspiration.
   (5) Electrolyte imbalance.
   (6) Hypothermia.

3. Activated charcoal.
   a. Dose.
      (1) 1 g/kg body weight *or* 5–10 g/g drug ingested NG or po.
      (2) Mix with cathartic or water in 1:4 solution.
   b. Administration.
      (1) May be given NG or po.
      (2) If ipecac has been given, do not give charcoal before emesis.
   c. Contraindications: *Do not give if:*
      (1) Poorly absorbed substance (alkalis, acids, lithium, DDT, iron, cyanide, alcohols).
      (2) Endoscopy to be performed.
   d. Multiple-dose activated charcoal.
      (1) Indicated for severe ingestion of theophylline, tricyclics, phenobarbital, digoxin, carbamazepine (Tegretol).

(2) Give 0.5 g/kg q4h.
(3) End point:
(a) Nontoxic blood level or
(b) No signs/symptoms of toxicity
(4) Complications.
(a) Adynamic ileus.
(b) Hypernatremia.

4. Cathartics.
a. Dose.
(1) Sodium sulfate: 250 mg/kg, maximum 30 g.
(2) Magnesium sulfate: 250 mg/kg, maximum 30 g.
(3) Magnesium citrate: 4 mL/kg, maximum 200 mL.
(4) Sorbitol:
(a) 70% solution with appropriate dose of activated charcoal or
(b) 10–20 mL for children, 50 mL for adult.
b. Administration: Give NG/OG/po with appropriate dose of activated charcoal.
c. Contraindications.
(1) Adynamic ileus, intestinal obstruction, recent gastrointestinal surgery, or abdominal trauma.
(2) Congestive heart failure (sodium sulfate).
(3) Renal failure (magnesium sulfate or magnesium citrate).
(4) Severe diarrhea.
(5) Caustic ingestion.

D. Other detoxification procedures

1. Forced diuresis; may be indicated for ingestions of salicylate or phenobarbital.
2. Alkalinization.
a. Indicated for tricyclics, salicylates.
b. 2 mEq/kg sodium bicarbonate in D_5W over 1 hour.
c. Goal: serum pH 7.45–7.50.
d. Potassium replacement may be needed.
3. Hemodialysis: may be necessary in severe ingestions of (partial list of common ingestions) amphetamines, long-acting barbiturates, boric acid, ethylene glycol, fluorides, isoniazid, methanol, paraldehyde, potassium, salicylates, strychnine.
4. Hemoperfusion: may be necessary in severe ingestions of theophylline, salicylates, phenytoin, chloramphenicol, short-acting barbiturates.

E. Chemical burns

1. *Stop the burning process!*
   a. Remove exposure (e.g., clothing).
   b. Flush exposed area for 15 minutes with copious amounts of water or 0.9% NS solution at body temperature.
   c. After irrigation, neutralization usually not helpful (sometimes harmful), except for:
      (1) Hydrofluoric acid (HF) burn: Rinse exposed area off with lime water (CaOH solution), calcium chloride, magnesium sulfate, or calcium gluconate solution. If HF penetrated skin, infiltrate area involved with 10% calcium gluconate SC (0.5 mL/m^2).
      (2) Phenol exposure (phenol, lysol, creosote): Remove substance with polyethylene glycol or propylene glycol (diluted 1:1).
2. *Call the poison control center!*

F. Laboratory data

1. Toxicology screen.
   a. May send urine, gastric sample, serum for identification.
   b. Discuss with laboratory what substances will be screened for (which ones immediately).
2. Serum drug levels: Helpful in certain ingestions: acetaminophen, ethanol, methanol, ethylene glycol, carbon monoxide, digoxin, iron, salicylates, theophylline, thyroxine.

APPENDIX 11–1.

Evaluation of the Patient With an Unknown Ingestion*

Vital Signs†	
T	↑ 'd→ASA, phenothiazines, cocaine, PCP, TCAs, MAO inhibitors, lithium, NMS.
	↓ 'd→Narcotics, barbiturates, TCAs, phenothiazines, hypoglycemia.
BP	↑ 'd→Cocaine, amphetamines, PCP, TCAs, MAO inhibitors.
	↓ 'd→Alcohol, barbiturates, phenothiazines, meprobamate, antihistamines.
RR	↑ 'd→CO, CN, ASA, hydrocarbons,
	↓ 'd→Alcohol, barbiturates, opiates.
HR	↑ 'd→Cocaine, amphetamines, xanthines, MAO inhibitors, belladona, alkaloids.
	↓ 'd→Barbiturates, Ca channel blockers, chloral hydrate, arrhythmias→digitalis, TCAs, quinidine.
Eyes	
Pupils	Miosis→Narcotics, phenothiazines, barbiturates, organophosphates, opiates, clonidine, nicotine, pontine hemorrhage.
	Mydriasis→Cocaine, amphetamines, LSD, TCA, atropine, antihistamines.
EOMs	Strabismus→botulism.
	Nystagmus→phenytoin (Dilantin), alcohol, PCP, lithium, sedative hypnotics.
GI	Vomiting/pain/diarrhea→Alcohol, caustics, digoxin, ASA, xanthines, metals, insecticides, mushrooms, arsenic.
Skin	Dry→Anticholinergics, antihistamines, narcotics.
	Diaphoretic→Organophosphates, cholinergics, ASA, sympathomimetics, arsenic.
	Cyanotic→Hypoxia, nitrates, nitrites, benzocaine, methemoglobinemia.
	Erythematous→Anticholinergics, CO, CN.
Neurologic system	Fasciculations→Lithium, organophosphates.
	↑ 'd Tone→PCP, strychnine, haloperidol, NMS.
	Paralysis→Botulism, organophosphates, carbamates, poison hemlock.
	Dystonia→Phenothiazines, haloperidol, PCP, TCA, heavy metals.
	Seizures→Cocaine, TCAs, Pb, PCP, INH, propoxyphene, lithium, lindane, antihistamines, hypernatremia, hyponatremic, hypoglycemia.

*TCA = tricyclics; MAO = monoamine oxidase; NMS = neuroleptic malignant syndrome; CN = cyanide; ASA = acetylsalicylic acid.

†T = temperature; BP = blood pressure; RR = respiratory rate; HR = heart rate; EOMs = extraocular movements; GI = gastrointestinal.

APPENDIX 11–2.

Toxic Syndromes and Management Guidelines

Substance	Symptoms or Complaints	Potential Early Adverse Events	Initial Laboratory Values or Studies	Pretransport and Transport Management	Comments
Acetaminophen	Can be asymp. N/V Lethargy	Vomiting		Mucomyst if known toxic level or if level will not be back by 10 hr after ingestion.	IV metoclopramide (Reglan) or droperidol for vomiting.
Anticholinergics	Dry skin/mouth Hyperthermia Dilated pupils Tachycardia	Delirium Respiratory failure Seizures Tachyarrhythmias		Supportive therapy. Consider physostigmine (to be used with extreme caution).	
Antihistamines	Drowsiness N/V/D Flushing Tachycardia	Hallucinations Seizures Respiratory/circulatory collapse		Supportive therapy. Consider physostigmine (to be used with extreme caution). Seizures⟶ diazepam/ phenytoin.	*Avoid:* phenothiazines, quinidine, disopyramide, CNS depressants (i.e., phenobarbital).

(Continued.)

APPENDIX 11–2.—cont'd

Substance	Symptoms or Complaints	Potential Early Adverse Events	Initial Laboratory Values or Studies	Pretransport and Transport Management	Comments
Aspirin	Agitation Disorientation Tinnitus N/V Kussmaul's respirations Hyperthermia	Hallucinations, seizures, coma 2° to cerebral edema Pulmonary edema Dysrhythmias 2° to acidosis or hypo-K^+ or -Ca^+	ABG Serum K^+ Serum Na^+ Serum HCO_3^- Glucose/Dextrostick Urine pH	Charcoal q4h. Alkalinize urine (see HCO_3^-). Goal: urine pH 8. Consider adding KCl to IV fluids (especially during alkalinization). Run total IV fluids at maintenance or 1.5–2.0 × maintenance.	Watch for hypernatremia from HCO_3^- administration. Must have K^+ in normal range to achieve an alkaline urine.
Barbiturates	Lethargy Ataxia Nystagmus Miosis Hypothermia	Respiratory/circulatory collapse Hypoglycemia	ECG Glucose/Dextrostick	Charcoal q4h. Alkalinize urine (see HCO_3^-). Goal: urine pH 7.5 Consider adding KCl to IV fluids (especially during alkalinization). Run total IV fluids at 1.5–2.0 × maintenance.	Watch for hypernatremia from HCO_3^- administration. Must have K^+ in normal range to achieve an alkaline urine.

β-Blockers	Bradycardia Decreased SA or AV conduction Apnea Seizures Hypoglycemia	Hypotension Ventricular dysrhythmias (especially with Isotolol) Asystole Bronchospasm	ECG/BP Glucose/Dextrostick Serum K^+	Bradycardia/heart block⟶ *Atropine*/ *isoproterenol*/pace. Hypotension⟶fluids/ *glucagon*/and/or *epinephrine*. Seizures⟶*diazepam*. (Check glucose.) Bronchospasm⟶ aminophylline/ nebulizers.	Use lidocaine cautiously because membrane stability effects may be synergistic with β-blockers. Watch for hyperglycemia, hypo-Ca^+ and -K^+ with glucagon administration.

APPENDIX 11–2A.

Toxic Syndromes and Management Guidelines

Substance	Symptoms or complaints	Potential Early Adverse Effects	Initail Laboratory Values or Studies	Pretransport and Transport Management	Comments
Ca channel blockers	Flushing Headache Palpitations Syncope	Hypotension Conduction abnormalities Bradycardia	ECG/BP Serum Ca^+ Serum K^+	Bradycardia/heart block ⟶ atropine/isoproterenol/pacer. Hypotension → Ca gluconate.	*Avoid:* digoxin, class I drugs, β-blockers, and other Ca channel blockers.
Carbon monoxide	Headache Nausea Dizziness Palpitations	Hypotension Dysrhythmias Pulmonary edema/ARDS	ABG COHgb ECG CXR Pulse oximeter: spuriously high saturation	100% O_2. Symptomatic therapy. ICP precautions ⟶ consider: hyperventilation, mannitol, 30° head elevation.	PO_2 usually normal or slightly decreased. O_2 saturation (measured) decreased. Avoid overcorrection of acidosis because alkalosis shifts O_2 curve left.
Clonidine	Sedation Dry mouth Miosis Mydriasis Hypothermia	Bradycardia Hypotension Hypertension AV block Apnea Seizures Coma	ECG/BP	Bradycardia ⟶ atropine. Hypotension ⟶ fluids/dopamine. Hypertension ⟶ furosemide/diazoxide/nitroprusside. Naloxone (Narcan): for apnea, cardiovascular toxicity, and coma.	Watch for hyperglycemia with diazoxide use. Hypertension seen with high serum levels of clonidine.

Cocaine	Agitation Mydriasis Tremor Hyperthermia Hyperreflexia	Seizures Hypertension Hypotension Dysrhythmias Pneumothrax Pneumomediastinum	ECG/BP CXR?	Seizures⟶*diazepam/ phenytoin (Dilantin)/ phenobarbital/? pancuronium.* Hypertension⟶ *nitroprusside/ labetalol.* Hypotension⟶ *fluids/dopamine/ norepinephrine.* Dysrhythmias⟶Use ACLS/APLS guidelines.	Intractible seizures in the presence of hyperthermia are an indication for neuromuscular paralysis. Propranolol may cause an increase in BP secondary to unopposed α stimulus. Lidocaine is a common adulterant of cocaine, so use it cautiously.
Digitalis	Fatigue N/V Confusion Delirium Hyperkalemia	Bradycardia Heart block Tachydysrhythmias Ventricular dysrhythmias	Serum K^+ ECG/BP	Charcoal q4h. Digoxin-specific antibodies. (See dosage information for indications.) Bradycardia⟶ atropine/ pacemaker. Ventricular irritability⟶ phenytoin/lidocaine.	If KCl administration is necessary, give slowly and in NS solution because glucose increases movement of K^+ intracellularly.

APPENDIX 11–2B.

Toxic Syndromes and Management

Substance	Presenting Symptoms or Complaints	Potential Early Adverse Effects	Initial Laboratory Values or Studies	Pretransport and Transport Management	Comments
Ethanol	Drowsiness Ataxia Flushing Mydriasis Hypothermia	Respiratory depression Hypotension Atrial fibrillation Hypoglycemia, seizures	Glucose/Dextrostick	Supportive therapy. Watch respiratory/CV status. Watch Dextrosticks. Seizures→ anticonvulsants, glucose	
Ethylene glycol	N/V Nystagmus Myoclonic jerks Acidosis Inebriation	Seizures Coma Cerebral edema	ABG ECG	Supportive therapy. Ethanol drip. (See dosage information for indications.) HCO_3^- for acidosis. Ca^{2+} for prolonged Q-T interval and/or tetany.	Hypocalcemia has been reported. Metabolites cause toxicity. ETOH blocks the metabolism of ethylene glycol.
Iron	V/D Melena Tachycardia	Hypotension Lethargy Coma	KUB Hct	Hypotension⟶ *fluids*/dopamine. Serum Fe > 350, or TIBC > serum Fe⟶desferoxamine. KUB + for pills/	Watch for blood loss. IV deferoxamine (Desferol) itself can cause hypotension, however; would treat hypotension with fluids and

				bezoars⟶lavage with HCO_3^- solution. (Add 50 mEq HCO_3^- to 1 L D_5-½NS.)	dopamine instead of decreasing deferoxamine.
Isoniazid	N/V Dizziness Slurred speech Dilated pupils Nystagmus	Hypotension Respiratory collapse Seizures	ABG	*Pyridoxine* (even if asymptomatic). Supportive therapy. Seizures⟶diazepam/pyridoxine. Metabolic acidosis⟶HCO_3^- if acidosis is not responsive to pyridoxine.	Clinical triad of isoniazid overdose is seizures, metabolic acidosis, coma.
Lithium	Tremor V/D Drowsiness	Myoclonus Dysrhythmias Seizures Hypotension	ECG	NS solution IV at 1.5 × maintenance. Supportive therapy for seizures and hypotension.	Sodium Na^+ blocks the renal reabsorption of lithium and thereby enhances excretion.
Methanol	Headache Vertigo Blurred vision N/V	Seizures Coma	ABG Glucose/Dextrostick	Supportive therapy. Ethanol drip. (See dosage information indications.) HCO_3^- for pH < 7.2.	Watch for hypoglycemia. Metabolites cause toxicity. ETOH blocks the metabolism of methanol.

APPENDIX 11–2C.

Toxic Syndromes and Management

Substance	Presenting Symptoms or Complaints	Potential Early Adverse Effects	Initial Laboratory Values or Studies	Pretransport Transport Management	Comments
Monoamine oxidase inhibitors	Agitation Dilated pupils Hyperthermia Hyperreflexia Tachycardia	Seizures Hypotension Hypertension Cardiac arrest	ECG	Hypertension⟶ nitroprusside/ phentolamine. Hypotension⟶ norepinephrine/ high-dose dopamine. V-tachyarrhythmias⟶ lidocaine/ procainamide/ phenytoin. Malignant hyperthermia⟶ dantrolene. Muscle rigidity⟶diazepam/ phenytoin.	*Avoid* bretylium, meperidine, sympathomimetics, and sedative hypnotics.
Opiates	Pinpoint pupils Hypothermia	Bradycardia Respiratory depression Hypotension Seizures Coma		Supportive therapy. Naloxone.	

Organophosphates	Bronchorrhea Wheezing N/V/D Miosis Salivation Muscle weakness	Fasciculations Tachycardia Hypertension Bradycardia Respiratory depression		If significantly symptomatic⟶ atropine and pralidoxime. (See dosage information for indications for pralidoxime.)	*Avoid* physostigmine, succinylcholine, CNS depressants, antihistamines and phenothiazines.
Phenothiazines	Sedation Dystonia Ataxia Delirium	Seizures Hypotension Dysrhythmias Neuroleptic malignant syndrome	ECG	Charcoal q4h. Hypotension⟶ norepinephrine. Dysrhythmias⟶ lidocaine. Seizures⟶diazepam/ phenytoin.	*Avoid* quinidine, procainamide, disopyramide, isoproterenol. Epinephrine and dopamine may worsen hypotension. Asystole has been seen w/physostigmine.
Theophylline	N/V Agitation	Seizures APCs/VPCs/SVT	ECG Serum K^+	Charcoal q4h. Seizures⟶diazepam/ phenytoin. Tachyarrhythmias⟶ propranolol/verapamil. Hypotension⟶fluids/ norepinephrine.	Watch for hypokalemia.

APPENDIX 11–2D.

Toxic Syndromes and Management

Substance	Symptoms or Complaints	Potential Early Adverse Effects	Initial Laboratory Values or Studies	Pretransport and Transport Management	Comments
Tricyclic antidepressants (TCAs)	Agitation Mydriasis Dry mouth Tachycardia	Hypotension Dysrhythmias Seizures Delirium	ECG/BP	Hypotension⟶ fluids/norepinephrine. Keep serum pH 7.45–7.50 with HCO_3^-. Charcoal q4h.	QRS > 0.16 is associated with high risk of ventricular dysrhythmia. Serum alkalinization reduces the amount of active unbound TCA. Hypotension in TCA overdoses tends to be more responsive to norepinephrine than dopamine.

*N/V = nausea and vomiting; IV = intravenous; N/V/D = nausea, vomiting, and diarrhea; CNS = central nervous system; ABG = arterial blood gas; ECG = electrocardiogram; SA = sinoatrial; AV = atrioventricular; BP = blood pressure; COHgb = carboxyhemoglobin; CXR = chest x-ray film; ARDS = adult respiratory distress syndrome; ICP = intracranial pressure; PO_2 = partial pressure of oxygen; ACLS = advanced cardiac life support; APLS = Advanced Pediatric Life Support; NS = normal saline; CV = cardiovascular; ETOH = alcohol; KUB = kidney, ureter, and bladder x-ray film; Hct = hematocrit; TIBC = total iron-binding capacity; D_5–½NS = 0.5% dextrose in 0.5% normal saline solution; APCs = atrial premature contractions; VPCs = ventricular premature contractions; SVT = supraventricular tachycardia.

NEONATAL EMERGENCIES 12

I. Care of the Premature Infant

An infant is considered to be premature if he or she is less that 38 weeks' gestational age. A low birth weight infant weighs less than 2,500 g. A *very* low birth weight infant weighs less than 1,500 g, and a *very very* low birth weight infant weighs less than 1,000 g. It is important that an accurate birth weight and gestational age be obtained. Infants who are small or large for gestational age are at risk for hypoglycemia, hypocalcemia, and polycythemia.

A. Clinical assessment

1. Obtain a prenatal history.
   a. Gestational age.
   b. Maternal medical problems during pregnancy.
   c. Medications during pregnancy.
   d. Complications of labor and delivery.
   e. Infection potential (premature rupture of membranes, maternal fever).
2. Obtain a complete set of vital signs, including temperature, heart rate, blood pressure (BP), and respiratory rate.
   a. Premature infants are at high risk of hypothermia because of relative lack of SC tissue and inability to promote themogenesis.
3. Physical examination.
   a. Emphasize cardiorespiratory status.
      (1) Grunting, flaring, retractions.
      (2) Peripheral perfusion, murmurs.
      (3) General activity level and neurologic assessment.
4. Laboratory data.
   a. Rapid glucose determination.
   b. Arterial blood gas (ABG) determinations if indicated.

c. Complete blood cell (CBC) count and blood cultures if indicated.
d. X-ray studies, especially of the chest.
e. Electrolyte values.

B. Treatment

1. Respiratory system.
   a. Ideal range for partial pressure of oxygen (Po_2) is 60–80 mm Hg.
   b. Avoid hypoxia or hyperoxia.
   c. Treat respiratory acidosis with positive pressure ventilation.
   d. Treat metabolic acidosis with an isotonic fluid bolus (10 mL/kg) and/or a dose of sodium bicarbonate (1–2 mEq/kg).
   e. Hypoventilation and/or apnea lead to hypoxia. Hypoxia leads to bradycardia. *Most neonatal bradycardia is related to respiratory failure,* not primary cardiac failure.
2. Cardiovascular system.
   a. Assess perfusion by capillary refill, heart rate, and BP.
   b. Treat signs of hypovolemia with 10 mL of normal saline (NS) solution/kg. Repeat if needed (see p. 66).
3. Maintenance fluids.
   a. Low to very low birth weight infants require 80–100 mL/kg/day.
   b. Very low to very very low birth weight infants require more fluid, generally 120–140 mL/kg/day (secondary to increased insensible losses).
   c. For first 24 hours after delivery, use 10% or 5% aqueous dextrose solution ($D_{10}W$ or D_5W) for maintenance fluids.
4. Glucose: Avoid hypoglycemia (<40 mg/dL) and hyperglycemia (>150 mg/dL).
   a. Most premature infants require 5–8 mg/kg/min, which is provided by an IV infusion of $D_{10}W$ at 80–100 mL/kg/day.
5. Temperature: Prevention of hypothermia is crucial.
   a. Dry the infant well after delivery and place in heated environment.
   b. Cover the infant's head with a stocking cap.

c. Cover very low birth weight infants with plastic wrap.
d. Use prewarmed blankets.
e. Work through isolette port holes as much as possible.
f. Use warm humidified oxygen.
g. During transport, maintain a warm environment in the ambulance or aircraft.

C. Ongoing monitoring

1. Assess vital signs frequently. Remember to follow temperature carefully.
2. Monitor patients on oxygen with transcutaneous oxygen monitors or pulse oximetry.
3. Cardiac monitor.
4. Use clinical assessment of patient's status, especially during transport, rather than relying completely on mechanical devices.

II. Resuscitation of the Newborn

The general principles of neonatal resuscitation are essentially the same as those for pediatric and adult patients. The gold standard acronym for airway breathing circulation and drugs, ABCD, has served this process well for many years. The major point to remember in neonatal resuscitation is **almost all episodes of bradycardia are related to hypoxia.** Therefore, if an adequate airway is obtained and successful ventilation is established, most bradycardic episodes can be treated without the use of pharmacologic agents. The emphasis on obtaining an adequate airway must be paramount (Table 12–1). Thus, establish an airway, ventilation, and circulation. Administer drugs only if the patient does not respond.

A. Indications for resuscitation

1. Bradycardia.
   a. Heart rate <70 beats/min in a term infant.
   b. Heart rate <100 beats/min for a premature infant.
2. Inadequate or ineffective respirations that result in bradycardia, hypoxia, or acidosis.
3. Hypovolemia resulting in decreased BP and a severe metabolic acidosis. Examples include hemorrhage and severe enteric losses.

B. Management

1. Airway.
   a. Place infant in supine position and extend the neck.
   b. Do not hyperextend the neck.

TABLE 12–1.
Resuscitation of the Newborn

Drug	Dose*	Comments
Atropine	0.1–0.2 mg/kg/IV/ET	Use only for *vagal* bradycardia. Minimum dose should be 0.1 mg to avoid further bradycardia.
Sodium bicarbonate	1–2 mEq/kg IV	Give as 1:1 dilution to decrease osmolarity. Repeat dose prn if ventilation adequate.
Calcium	10 mg/kg elemental Ca (0.3 mL/kg CaCl or 1.0 mL/kg Ca gluconate)	Infuse *slowly* to avoid bradycardia and do not mix with $NaHCO_3$.
Epinephrine (1:10,000)	0.1 mL/kg IV/ET	Less effective when severe acidosis present.
Naxolone (Narcan)	0.01 mg/kg IV/IM	*Never* use in suspected cases of maternal drug abuse, because it may precipitate seizures.
Defibrillation	2 J/kg	May double the energy prn each time to treat ventricular fibrillation or ventricular tachycardia.

*IV = intravenously; ET = via endotracheal tube; IM = intramuscularly.

   c. Clear the airway of secretion or vomitus by the use of liberal suctioning.
2. Breathing.
   a. Bag and mask ventilation should be attempted first. This may be accomplished more easily by thrusting the lower jaw forward.
   b. Always listen to the chest to make sure that the ventilation is effective.
   c. If the patient does not respond quickly, endotracheal intubation should be performed.
3. Circulation.
   a. Check BP and capillary refill (normal is <3 seconds).
   b. Bradycardia unresponsive to oxygenation and ventilation requires closed chest cardiac massage.
      (1) Compress at a rate of 100–120/min.
      (2) Use respiratory rate of 40–60 breaths/min.

4. Drugs.
   a. Access via umbilical vein catheter is usually fastest.
   b. Atropine and epinephrine can be given down the endotracheal tube.

III. Neonatal Shock

As in the older child, shock in the neonate manifests as peripheral vascular collapse secondary to a loss of circulating volume or derangement of circulatory control. Common causes in the neonate include hemorrhage, sepsis, perinatal asphyxia, and congenital heart disease.

A. Clinical picture

1. Perinatal history.
   a. Hypovolemia can be secondary to perinatal hemorrhage, fetal maternal transfusion, twin/twin transfusion.
   b. Significant perinatal asphyxia may predispose the patient to loss of circulatory control mechanisms.
2. Physical examination.
   a. Check vital signs, pulses, and capillary refill. Remember that BP can be normal in a shock state.
   b. Evaluate respiratory effort.

B. Treatment

1. Consider endotracheal intubation and mechanical ventilation.
2. After the airway is secure, use volume resuscitation.
   a. 10 mL/kg NS solution every 5–10 minutes until BP has stabilized.
   b. Alternatives to NS solution include whole blood, packed red blood cells, 5% albumin solution, fresh frozen plasma, and lactated Ringer's solution.
   c. If condition is not improved after 30–40 mL/kg of volume or if primary circulatory etiology of shock is present, administer:
      (1) Dobutamine, 20–30 μg/kg/min (see p. 429) or
      (2) Dopamine, 10–15 μg/kg/min (see p. 428).
   d. Review laboratory data for other correctable etiologies.
   e. Obtain blood cultures and begin broad-spectrum antibiotic coverage with ampicillin, 100 mg/kg, and gentamicin, 2.5 mg/kg.

C. Ongoing monitoring

1. Use cardiac monitor and pulse oximeter or transcutaneous oxygen monitor.
2. Frequently reassess vital signs and perfusion.
3. Prepare volume expanders in advance, especially for transport.

IV. Neonatal Sepsis.

Sepsis is a generalized bacterial or viral infection spread throughout the body via the bloodstream. Meningitis is commonly associated with this condition. Sepsis should be considered in any infant born with the following risk factors: prematurity, prolonged rupture of membranes, maternal fever, meconium aspiration, or other perinatal problems. Common neonatal pathogens include group B *Streptococcus* and *Escherichia coli*.

A. Clinical assessment

1. Obtain history for possible causes of perinatal infection, including the presence of premature rupture of membranes or maternal fever. Also ask about sources for congenital viral infections, such as cytomegalovirus, toxoplasmosis, and rubella, as well as herpes, group B *Streptococcus,* or gonorrhea infections.
2. Physical examination.
   a. Vital signs, pulses, and capillary refill.
   b. Tachypnea, grunting, flaring, retracting, or apnea.
   c. History of lethargy or poor feeding.
   d. Temperature instability.
   e. Petechae.
   f. Signs of septic shock (pallor and/or cyanosis, hypoxia, hypercarbia, acidosis, hypotension).
3. Laboratory data.
   a. White blood cell count $<5{,}000/mm^3$ or $>30{,}000/mm^3$ with elevated band count.
   b. Glucose instability.
   c. Thrombocytopenia with increased prothrombin time and partial thromboplastin time. Decreased fibrinogen level and elevated level of fibrin split products may suggest disseminated intravascular coagulation.
   d. ABG values.

B. Treatment

1. Evaluate airway breathing and circulation.
2. Consider mechanical ventillation.

3. Support perfusion with volume (see p. 311).
4. If necessary, begin a pressor infusion (see p. 311).
5. Administer broad-spectrum antibiotics (i.e., ampicillin, 100 mg/kg IV, and gentamicin, 2.5 mg/kg IV or IM).

C. Ongoing monitoring

1. Cardiac monitor and pulse oximeter.
2. Follow vital signs and peripheral perfusion regularly, because the septic neonate may become unstable quickly.

V. Neonatal Respiratory Distress Syndrome: Hyaline Membrane Disease

Neonatal respiratory distress syndrome (RDS) is seen in premature infants and infants of diabetic mothers. It is caused by a lack of surfactant in the aveoli of the lungs and results in alveolar collapse and decreased lung compliance. Therefore, the infant has to work harder to breath because the surface area for gaseous exchange progressively decreases. The occurrence of RDS may be predicted by the prenatal use of the amniotic L/S ratio or the presence/absence of saturated phosphatidyl glycerol.

A. Clinical picture

1. History of prematurity or maternal diabetes.
2. Physical examination.
   a. Hallmarks of RDS: grunting, flaring, and retracting.
   b. Cyanosis.
   c. Coarse breath sounds with poor air entry.
3. Laboratory data.
   a. ABG values, CBC count, blood cultures, electrolyte values, glucose level.
   b. Chest x-ray film.
      (1) The chest x-ray film in classic RDS shows a diffuse fine reticulogranular pattern with the presence of air bronchograms and low lung volumes.
4. Evaluate the infant's overall respiratory status by combining the perinatal history, physical examination, and laboratory data to make this clinical diagnosis.

B. Treatment

1. Consider continuous positive airway pressure or endotracheal intubation and mechanical ventilation for respiratory support.
2. RDS in the premature infant is a progressive process. Consider intubation for transport even if absolute intubation criteria have not yet been met.

3. Deliver sufficient oxygen to keep the arterial oxygen level between 60 and 80 mm Hg and/or the oxygen saturation >90%. If the infant requires >60% oxygen or has a partial pressure of carbon dioxide (Pco_2) >60 mm Hg, mechanical ventilation should be provided.
4. Treat metabolic acidosis with a volume bolus (10 mL/kg) of NS solution and/or 1–2 mEq/kg of $NaHCO_3$.
5. Begin broad-spectrum antibiotic coverage with ampicillin, 100 mg/kg, and gentamicin, 2.5 mg/kg.
6. The patient should not be transported until the airway is secure and oxygenation and ventilation are adequate.

C. Ongoing monitoring

1. Use pulse oximetry or transcutaneous monitor; cardiac monitor.
2. Remember to follow temperature and keep the patient warm.
3. Perform frequent clinical assessments of the patient with respiratory distress. Mechanical monitors may not be accurate, especially during transport.
4. An appropriate-size bag and mask, oxygen source, and endotracheal tube with laryngoscope should be at the patient's bedside at all times.
5. Prepare equipment for needle thoracentesis in the event of a pneumothorax.

VI. Meconium Aspiration Syndrome

The passage of meconium into the amniotic fluid is usually associated with a varying degree of perinatal asphyxia. If severe, the infant may gasp in utero and inhale particulate meconium into the lungs. This causes obstructive airway disease and interferes with gas exchange. The resulting hypoxia, hypercarbia, and acidosis may cause persistent pulmonary hypertension. Meconium aspiration syndrome (MAS) commonly occurs in postmature infants.

A. Clinical picture

1. History consistent with perinatal stress and passage of meconium.
2. Physical examination.
   a. Tachypnea, grunting, flaring, retracting, cyanosis, coarse breath sounds.
   b. Meconium staining of nails and umbilicus.
   c. Barrel-shaped chest.

3. Laboratory data.
   a. Chest x-ray film (hyperinflation of the lungs and/or bilateral patchy infiltrates).
   b. ABG values.
   c. Blood culture, urine culture.
   d. CBC count.
   e. Electrolyte, glucose, and calcium levels.
4. Persistent pulmonary hypertension is diagnosed by the combination of perinatal history (postmaturity, meconium-stained amniotic fluid, asphyxia), the physical examination, and the laboratory data. If the patient is profoundly cyanotic, obtain preductal and postductal ABG values to look for atrial and/or ductal shunting secondary to persistent pulmonary hypertension. In persistent pulmonary hypertension, the preductal Po_2 is ≥20 mm Hg greater than the postductal Po_2.

B. Therapy

1. Respiratory system.
   a. Most patients with MAS will require intubation for control of the airway, as well as adequate oxygenation and ventilation.
   b. Deliver sufficient oxygen to keep the arterial oxygen >100 mm Hg and the O_2 saturation >95%.
   c. A fractional concentration of oxygen (Fio_2) in inspired gas requirement of >0.60 or a Pco_2 of >60 mm Hg is an absolute indication for mechanical ventilation.
   d. If persistent pulmonary hypertension is suspected or documented, hyperventilate the infant to keep the Pco_2 <30 mm Hg.
2. Cardiovascular system.
   a. Treat hypotension with isotonic volume boluses and/or pressor agents.
   b. Dopamine and dobutamine infusions are most commonly used (see pp. 428, 429).
   c. Attempt to maintain a mean BP of >45 mm Hg to maximize pulmonary blood flow.
3. Acidosis: Treat metabolic acidosis with a volume bolus (10 mL/kg) of NS solution and/or 1–2 mEq/kg $NaHCO_3$.
4. For the patient with severe MAS or evidence of persistent pulmonary hypertension, use of neuromuscular relaxants and sedation will enhance therapy. The combination of pancuronium bromide (Pavulon) and fentanyl is often used.

5. Begin broad-spectrum antibiotic coverage with ampicillin, 100 mg/kg, and gentamicin, 2.5 mg/kg.
6. Neurologic system: If severe perinatal asphyxia has occurred or seizure activity has been noted by reliable observers, consider giving a loading dose of phenobarbital (20–30 mg/kg).
7. Do not transport the infant until the airway is secured and ABG determinations document adequate oxygenation and ventilation. The only possible exception to this rule is the patient who is a candidate for extracorporeal membrane oxygenation (ECMO). Certain ECMO candidates may not be able to be stabilized completely before transport. In that case the transport team should be highly skilled in the care of the critically ill neonate.

C. Ongoing monitoring

1. Use pulse oximeter and cardiac monitor.
2. Continually assess the infant's vital signs, with particular attention paid to the BP. Hypotension can augment hypoxia by increasing the atrial and/or ductal shunting. This will increase the metabolic acidosis, thereby raising pulmonary vascular resistance.
3. An appropriately sized bag and mask along with endotracheal tube and laryngoscope and oxygen source should be available at all times.
4. When in doubt about the performance of equipment, always hand ventilate while trying to evaluate the equipment failure.
5. Equipment for needle thoracentesis should be immediately available in the event of a pneumothorax. At least 10% of patients with MAS develop some type of air leak.

VII. Neonatal Surgical Emergencies

The newborn is subject to several surgical emergencies unique to the immediate neonatal period. Surgical problems in the neonate that will require care in a level 3 nursery include:

1. *Gastroschisis:* A defect in the abdominal wall at the base of the umbilicus through which a portion of the intestinal tract has escaped. There is no covering membrane.
2. *Omphalocele:* A herniation through the umbilicus of abdominal contents, which is usually covered by a translucent membrane.

3. *Tracheoesophageal fistula (TEF):* An anatomic malformation of the esophagus. It usually (85% of cases) ends in a blind pouch in the superior thorax, whereas the lower portion is connected to the trachea by a small fistula.
4. *Diaphragmatic hernia:* Incomplete development of the posterolateral portion of the diaphragm, leading to herniation of abdominal contents into the thoracic cavity. It usually occurs on the left side of the abdomen.

A. Clinical findings

1. Gastroschisis and omphalocele.
   a. Diagnosed by protruding abdominal contents.
   b. Defect may be covered by a translucent membrane.
2. TEF.
   a. Prenatal history of polyhydramnios.
   b. Inability of newborn infant to handle secretions. Coughing and choking are common.
   c. In the most common form of TEF, an NG tube cannot be passed to the stomach. It coils up in the blind esophageal pouch and is visible in that location on x-ray film.
   d. Respiratory distress is secondary to aspiration of oral secretions.
   e. Bowel distention is often seen.
   f. Diagnosis by NG tube in blind pouch or by seeing a wide air-filled pouch in the neck or superior mediastinum on chest x-ray film.
3. Diaphragmatic hernia.
   a. Usually manifests with immediate respiratory distress in the delivery room.
   b. Breath sounds decreased on the side of the hernia (usually left side).
   c. Bowel sounds may be appreciated in the chest.
   d. Heart sounds are best heard on the side opposite the hernia secondary to mediastinal shift.
   e. Scaphoid abdomen is secondary to lack of abdominal contents.
   f. ABG values show hypoxia, hypercarbia, and acidosis.
   g. Diagnosis by chest x-ray film showing abdominal contents in the chest.

B. Treatment

1. Respiratory system.
   a. Consider endotracheal intubation and mechanical ventilation for respiratory support.
   b. Nasal or mask continuous positive airway pressure (CPAP) is *contraindicated* because it may increase bowel distention.
   c. Respiratory failure can occur rapidly with high pressure in the abdomen. Elective intubation before transport is often prudent.
   d. Deliver sufficient oxygen to keep the arterial oxygen between 60 and 80 mm Hg for a premature infant and 80 and 100 mm Hg for a term infant.
   e. Oxygen requirement of >60% or P_{CO_2} >60 mm Hg are an absolute indication for mechanical ventilation.
2. Cardiovascular system.
   a. Assess perfusion by capillary refill, urine output, and BP.
   b. Aggressive treatment of hypertension with isotonic fluid boluses and/or pressor agents is mandatory.
      (1) Dopamine and dobutamine infusions are most commonly used (see pp. 428, 429).
3. Acidosis: Treat metabolic acidosis with a volume bolus (10 mL/kg) of NS solution and/or 1–2 mEq/kg $NaHCO_3$. Be sure the patient has adequate ventilation before $NaHCO_3$ administration.
4. Gastric emptying.
   a. All patients with abdominal acute conditions should have an indwelling NG tube.
      (1) Bowel decompression.
      (2) Removal of secretions that could be aspirated.
   b. Provide suction.
      (1) Continuous low wall suction is preferable.
      (2) If continuous suction is unavailable, provide intermittent suction with a syringe.
5. Infection.
   a. Obtain blood and urine cultures.
   b. Begin broad-spectrum antibiotic coverage with ampicillin, 100 mg/kg, and gentamicin, 2.5 mg/kg.
6. Evaluate the patient for hypoglycemia and hypocalcemia.
7. Cover a gastroschisis or omphalocele with a sterile dressing of warm saline solution soaked gauze. Then cover with plastic wrap.

8. Temperature control: Provide a warm environment, especially in view of the potential for heat and fluid losses from exposed organs or wet dressings.
9. Maintain patients with TEF prone with head up to help prevent aspiration of secretions.

C. **Ongoing monitoring**

1. Use pulse oximetry and cardiac monitor.
2. Follow vital signs closely. Patients with potential intra-abdominal fluid losses can become hypovolemic quickly.
3. Maintain aggressive temperature regulation.
4. A bag and mask of appropriate size with oxygen source and endotracheal tube with laryngoscope should be available at the patient's bedside at all times.
5. Equipment for needle thoracentesis should be immediately available in the case of a pneumothorax, especially for patients with diaphragmatic hernia.

PHYSIOLOGY OF AIR TRANSPORT 13

Transport team members are often asked to function in the aeromedical environment. Changes in altitude have potential adverse effects on both the patient and the team member, so it is important for the transport team member to have at least a basic understanding of altitude physiology.

I. Barometric Pressure and Dalton's Law

The sum of the partial pressures of individual gases in the atmosphere defines the barometric pressure. The partial pressures of both oxygen and nitrogen are the major contributors. An inverse relationship exists between altitude and barometric pressure.

Altitude (ft)	Barometric Pressure (mm Hg)
Sea level	760
2,000	706
5,000	632
8,000	565
10,000	523
18,000	379

Dalton's law states that the sum of the partial pressures of individual gases in a mixture is equal to the total pressure of that mixture.

Example: Partial pressure of oxygen (Po_2) at any altitude, given that it comprises 21% of the atmosphere, may be calculated as:

Sea level: 760 mm Hg × 0.21 = 160 mm Hg
8,000 ft: 565 mm Hg × 0.21 = 119 mm Hg

II. Alveolar Gas Equation

The expected partial pressure of oxygen in arterial blood (Pa_{O_2}) can be determined from the simplified alveolar gas equation. When there is no significant intrapulmonary shunting, alveolar oxygen pressure (P_{AO_2}) should approximate Pa_{O_2}:

$$P_{AO_2} = P_{IO_2} - \frac{P_{ACO_2}}{R} = (P_B - 47) \times F_{IO_2} - \frac{P_{CO_2}}{0.8}.$$

P_{AO_2} = Alveolar partial pressure of oxygen.
P_{IO_2} = (Barometric pressure − Partial pressure H_2O at 37°) × F_{IO_2}.
P_{ACO_2} = Alveolar partial pressure of carbon dioxide (use Pa_{CO_2}).
R = Respiratory quotient (generally 0.8).
P_B = Barometric pressure.

Example: You are traveling to Hawaii via commercial aircraft, which generally maintains a cabin altitude of 8,000 ft. What is your resultant Pa_{O_2}? P_B at a cabin altitude of 8,000 ft is 565 mm Hg. (Assume Pa_{CO_2} = 40 mm Hg.)

$$P_{AO_2} = P_{IO_2} - \frac{P_{ACO_2}}{R} = (565 - 47) \times 0.21 - \frac{40}{0.8}$$

$P_{AO_2} = 518 \times 0.21 - 50$
P_{AO_2} = 58 mm Hg
Therefore, as altitude increases, the resultant decrease in P_B will result in alveolar hypoxemia and increased pulmonary vascular resistance unless one adjusts the F_{IO_2} to compensate for the change.

III. Boyle's Law and Dysbarisms

Those disturbances in the body, exclusive of hypoxia, which result from a difference between ambient pressure and the pressure of gases within body cavities, tissues, and fluids are known as dysbarisms.

Boyle's law states that at constant temperature, the volume of a gas varies inversely with the pressure. Therefore, the volume of gas within closed spaces will change with changes in P_B. Clinically relevant situations would include pneumothorax, bowel obstruction, endotracheal tube cuffs, air splints, and military antishock trousers (MAST). This relationship can be described as follows:

Altitude (ft)	Atm	Gas Volume
Sea level	1.00	1.00
5,000	0.83	1.20
8,000	0.77	1.33
18,000	0.50	2.00

A balloon will double its volume on an ascent from sea level to 18,000 ft.

IV. Cabin Pressurization

Cabin pressurization reduces the effects of altitude by maintaining a preset P_B within the cabin. A cabin altitude of 8,000 ft simply means that the P_B within the cabin is equivalent to that at 8,000 ft above sea level, regardless of the assigned altitude of the aircraft. Cabin pressurization may be manipulated within limits by the flight crew. If the cabin is equipped with an altimeter, the transport team member should set this to read the field elevation before departure. The in-flight indication will then be the cabin altitude.

V. Potential Adverse Effects of Altitude Changes on Team Members and Patients

High-altitude conditions will potentiate the effects of drugs, sleep deprivation, fatigue, and eating habits (hypoglycemia). Night vision is impaired at cabin altitudes greater than 5,000 ft. Vibration and noise will enhance fatigue; use head sets when feasible. Changes in G-forces during climbs, descents, and banks may produce vertigo. Humidity is generally low during in-flight conditions; insensible water losses can be substantial. Table 13–1 provides the etiology and treatment for common problems related to air transport for both the patient and the team member.

VI. Case Problems in Aviation Physiology

A. A patient requires an F_{IO_2} of 0.40 at sea level

What F_{IO_2} would be required at 10,000 ft to deliver the same P_{AO_2} to the patient?

Solution: $(F_{IO_2})A \times (Alt)A = (F_{IO_2})B \times (Alt)B$

$$0.40 \times 760 = (F_{IO_2})B \times 523$$

$$(F_{IO_2})B = (0.40 \times 760)/523$$

$$= 304 \text{ mm Hg}/523$$

$$(F_{IO_2})B = 0.58, \text{ or } 58\%$$

TABLE 13–1.

Application of Effects of Aeromedical Principles*

	Condition	Cause	Treatment
Head			
Ears	Ear plugging	Pressure change	Yawn, swallow, blowing forcefully against pinched nostrils, oxymetazoline (Afrin); infant-sucking on pacifier; comatose patient bag with large volume
Sinuses usually frontal	Barosinusitis (dull-sharp pain)	Pressure change	Oxymetazoline, descent
Teeth	Aerodontalgia	Gas expansion	Ice inside mouth or over cheek
	Exploding filling	Gas expansion	Lower altitude if unable to relieve
	Pain	Gas expansion	
Face	Pain	Expansion of trapped air	Analgesics, descent if necessary
Eyes	Vitreous extrusion	Expansion of trapped air in penetrating eye injury	Sea level cabin pressure, immobilize head
	Torn sutures	Expansion of trapped air	Sea level cabin pressure
			Sea level cabin pressure, supplemental oxygen
	Retinal separation	Dilation of retinal blood vessels in response to hypoxia→ ↑ intraocular pressure → hemorrhage	Artificial tears
	Dry eyes	Lack of humidity	

CNS	Syncope	Decreased blood supply from G forces	Elevated FOB
	Seizures	Hypoxia, apprehension, hyperventilation	Anticonvulsants, sedation; have suction ready; supplemental oxygen
	Altered mental status	Hypoxia, G forces	Frequent neurologic checks, supplemental oxygen
	Pain	Expansion of trapped air from air embolus or skull fracture	Sea level cabin pressure
Mouth	Dry mouth	Lack of humidity	Glycerin swabs, ice or noncarbonated fluids
Pulmonary system			
Lungs	Pneumothorax	Expansion of trapped air; blebs, bullae	Chest tube, McSwain dart
	Hypoxia (consider altitude of receiving hospital)	Altitude, anemia, shock, sickle cell, peripheral vascular disease, obstructed artery, DM, Raynaud's disease, low Hgb, COPD	Supplemental oxygen
	Tracheal discomfort, pain necrosis	Expansion of air in airway cuff	Cuff pressure monitoring minimal leak
	Dry membranes	Lack of humidity	Humidification
Cardiovascular system			
Peripheral	Hypotension	G forces, pooling of blood in feet	Elevated FOB, increased fluids, vasopressors
	Fluid loss, dehydration (especially burns)	Lack of humidity	Increased fluids
	Nitrogen bubbles	Diving decompression sickness with pressure changes	Sea level cabin pressure
Heart	MI, angina	Hypoxia	Supplemental oxygen

(Continued.)

TABLE 13–1.—cont'd

	Condition	Cause	Treatment
Gastrointestinal system			
Stomach	Nausea; vomiting (wired jaws must have quick release)	Pressure changes	Antiemetics; if the patient is receiving tube feeding, hold 30 min before take-off and landing
Intestines	Pain, distention, labored respiration	Expansion of trapped air in hernia, volvus, incision, anastomoses, extralumen/intralumen	Position change, belching, NG/rectal tube, massaging abdomen left to right, descent
	Exploding colostomy bag	Gas expansion	Pin prick in top of bag
Urinary system			
Bladder	Ruptured balloon/bag	Expanding air	Fill balloon with water, vent out air in bag
Integument			
Skin	Breakdown	Vibration, narrow and hard stretcher	Position changes, padding, back rub
Times of useful consciousness without supplemental oxygen			
18,000 ft		30 min	
25,000 ft		4 min	
35,000 ft		45 sec	
>43,000 ft		<15 sec	

*FOB = foot of bed; DM = diastolic murmur; Hgb = hemoglobin; COPD = chronic obstructive pulmonary disease; MI = myocardial infarction; NG = nasogastric.

To determine the FiO_2 needed at 10,000 ft, one must first determine the patient's sea level PO_2. By multiplying 0.40×760, we find that the patient is getting 304 mm Hg oxygen pressure at sea level. At a 10,000 ft altitude, the P_B is 523 mm Hg. To get 304 mm Hg oxygen at 10,000 ft, the air P_B must be multiplied by a new FiO_2, which, after calculation, is 0.58. Therefore, at 10,000 ft, the patient must be given an FiO_2 0.58 to have the same PO_2 that was provided by an FiO_2 of 0.40 at sea level.

B. A patient at sea level has an FiO_2 of 0.50

What is the equivalent sea level FiO_2 delivered to the patient if this patient is taken to 5,000 ft (maintaining the actual FiO_2 at 0.50)?

$$\text{Solution: } (FiO_2)A \times (Alt)A = (FiO_2)B \times (Alt)B$$

$$(FiO_2)A \times 760 = 0.50 \times 632$$

$$(FiO_2)A = (0.50 \times 632)/760$$

$$(FiO_2)A = 0.42, \text{ or } 42\%$$

At 5,000 ft, the P_B is 632 mm Hg. The patient's FiO_2 remains at 0.50. Therefore, 0.50×632 is equal to 316 mm Hg of oxygen pressure at 5,000 ft. This 316 mm Hg at sea level would be 316/760, or 42%. If FiO_2 is maintained at only 0.50 during flight, it will be equivalent to the patient's receiving an FiO_2 of only 0.42 on the ground.

C. A plane has an operational pressurization of 5.0 psi

At what maximum altitude can it maintain a sea level cabin pressure?

$$\text{Solution: psi} \times 51.7 = \text{equivalent mm Hg}$$

One must first convert 5 psi into mm Hg ($5 \times 51.7 = 258.5$). The sea level pressurization of 760 mm Hg minus the 258 mm Hg that the plane can produce artificially gives a remainder of 502 mm Hg. Therefore, the aircraft can operate with a sea level cabin pressure until the outside pB is 502 mm Hg. Once the atmospheric (outside) pressure is less than 502 mm Hg, sea level cabin pressure cannot be maintained. 502 mm Hg corresponds to an altitude of 11,000 ft. If the plane is flown above 11,000 ft, cabin pressure will be above sea level.

D. Up to what altitude can the plane in C. maintain an 8,000 ft cabin altitude?

Solution: At 8,000 ft, P_B = 565 mm Hg.

Therefore, this is the pressure that we want to maintain in the cabin. The aircraft is capable of maintaining 258 mm Hg of artificial pressurization, so 565 minus 258 equals 307. This means that the aircraft can fly to an altitude that corresponds to 307 mm Hg of outside pressure and maintain an 8,000 ft cabin altitude. The altitude of 23,000 ft corresponds to a P_B of 307 mm Hg.

BIBLIOGRAPHY

Johnson A: Treatise on aeromedical evacuation. *Aviation Space Environ Med* 1977; 48:546.

U.S. Naval Flight Surgeon's Manual, ed 2. US Department of the Navy, Bureau of Medicine and Surgery, Washington, DC, US Government Printing Office, 1978.

MEDICOLEGAL ISSUES IN INTERHOSPITAL TRANSPORT

14

Interhospital transport lends itself to a number of medicolegal issues that are unique. Interhospital transport teams are usually hospital-based, employ different types of personnel, cross many political boundaries, and have a high level of physician supervision. The chief responsibility of the transport team base hospital is to be committed to a formal structure that will (1) provide a rapid response, (2) ensure safe and efficient transport, and (3) render appropriate care.

The purpose of this chapter is to alert the referring hospital personnel and the transport team member to potential medicolegal issues and is not to be used as a legal guide for the structuring of transport systems. It is the responsibility of each transport team to seek local counsel and consult with local authorities on legal matters.

I. Medical Control Officer

There must be a responsible physician to direct transport activities. Ideally this should be an attending physician who is trained in either emergency medicine or critical care. For teams who handle premature infants, a neonatologist should be involved. The medical control officer's responsibilities include (1) being available to the team during transport and responding to individual problems, (2) approving team protocols, (3) serving as a liaison to the referral community, (4) maintaining an active training program for team members to ensure safety and competence, and (5) making sure that equipment needs (including aircraft and ground units) are adequate and reliable.

II. Communications

The transport team base hospital is responsible for handling emergent calls efficiently and therefore should have an established communications network. Ideally this should function through a central dispatch center that is accessible to the referral community around-the-clock. Incoming calls should be taken by individuals who are trained in handling emergent calls and not by those who have other distracting duties. Mishandled calls are a potential liability to the base hospital. Therefore, an institution-wide protocol is needed for misdirected calls that were intended for the transport team. Incoming calls should ultimately be taken by a physician because it is the responsibility of the referring physician to secure a receiving physician.

III. Mobilization Time

Mobilization time (elapsed time from the initial incoming call until team departure) should be minimal. Critical care transport teams should be in a position to respond emergently. A lengthy response is a potential liability. Weather and topography often determine a region's expectation of a team response. However, for institutions who frequently do transport, a reasonable goal should be to have a dedicated team. A dedicated team will promote shorter mobilization and response times because it is acclimated to doing transport. This is difficult to accomplish when personnel are on-call from home or when they are being pulled from inpatient assignments.

IV. En Route Responsibilities for Team Members

The transport team member functions as an agent of the institution and therefore is responsible for conforming to the protocols defined and authorized by the institution. Team members may be liable if they do not perform within the scope of their employment or if they do not abide by team protocol. Team members are responsible for rendering appropriate care and therefore should be properly trained to manage critically ill patients. They should follow standard pediatric resuscitation guidelines. They should also ensure that equipment needs are adequate and reliable for each transport. There is never a *good* excuse for depleting the oxygen supply! The transport team should obtain parental consent and preferably a *written* order from the referring physician for transport. If the patient should require an emergency operative procedure before the parents' arrival at the base hospital, the parents should remain at the referring hospital until an operative permit can be obtained via telephone by the responsible surgeon. The transport team should then communicate with the base hospital before arrival to make sure that the admission unit is appropriately set up for the patient's needs.

V. Crossing Regional Boundaries

When a patient dies during transport, legally the coroner within the region where the patient is declared dead has jurisdiction. To avoid confusion, team members might consider continuing resuscitative efforts and pronouncing death on arrival at the receiving hospital.

VI. Licensure

Transport team members must be licensed to practice medicine within the state where the base hospital is located. Most transport teams function on the premise that the patient is admitted to the base hospital at the moment the team arrives at the referring hospital. Because the team members are functioning as agents of the base hospital, there should be no need to require licensure in each region where transports are done. Realistically, this is often an impossible task since many states require a minimum level of activity to maintain licensure.

VII. Insurance

There should be institutional verification that insurance policies (life, disability, workman's compensation, and malpractice) adequately cover transport team activities. Disability insurance always raises the issue of risk vs. loss to the insured. Insurance companies generally do not provide for the loss of potential earnings. However, transport team members are at an increased risk when compared with in-house employees and should have additional benefits. Institutional policies should be reviewed to make certain that there are no exclusion clauses for team members who are providing air medical transport.

When the team member acts as an agent of the institution and conforms to protocol, and because transport is an extension of the institution, malpractice policies should cover the individual. However, some insurance companies may not recognize transport as being within the scope of employment. Malpractice policies may be limited to what occurs during "training" and therefore may not cover individuals who are moonlighting on transport. The medical control officer should also be certain that his or her policy covers the additional administrative duties for transport.

VIII. Transporting Patients With "Do Not Resuscitate" Orders

Occasionally the transport team may be asked to transport a patient with a **no code** status back to the referring institution. A set of *written* orders from the patient's attending physician should accompany the team. These should include (1) the written "do not resuscitate" order, (2) an explanatory progress note supporting such an order, (3) an order to transport the child back to the referring institution, (4) explicit orders for patient care during the transport (oxygen therapy, IV lines, etc.), and (5) parental consent for transfer.

IX. What Are the Levels of Liability During the Transport Process?

The receiving hospital's responsibility begins with its availability to the referring physician. Liability begins to increase substantially once the patient is accepted for admission. At this juncture, it is extremely important to document the telephone conversation and the recommendations being given to the referring physician. Once the team arrives at the referring institution and begins to render care, it should be assumed that the patient has been admitted to the base hospital and that the transport team will assume full responsibility for patient care from this point on.

Liability for the referring hospital begins to diminish in proportion to the involvement of the receiving hospital. The referring institution is responsible for treatment before the receiving hospital's involvement and may assume responsibility for patient morbidity/mortality that could have resulted from not carrying out recommendations given over the telephone by the receiving physician. This includes recommendations about method of transport.

Under a new federal law, the Consolidated Omnibus Budget Reconciliation Act (COBRA), the transferring hospital also assumes liability for the medical integrity and adequacy of the receiving hospital, as well as the medical appropriateness of the patient's transfer. The Joint Commission for the Accreditation of Hospitals Organization also mandates that "a hospital is capable of instituting essential lifesaving measures and implementing emergency procedures that will minimize further compromise of the condition of any infant, child, or adult being transported." The transferring hospital and physician must ensure that the skills and equipment available during transport will meet the anticipated needs of the patient and not assume that everyone on board is adequately trained and adept at resuscitation. Transport teams well trained and highly experienced in the care of adult patients may not have comparable training and skills in the care of pediatric patients.

X. Who Is Liable When the Referring Hospital Refuses Transport Services When They Have Been Recommended?

The receiving hospital should document in writing (or recording) the reason for the refusal. The receiving hospital physician should share concern over the refusal and diplomatically remind the referring hospital that they will be entirely responsible for what happens en route until the patient arrives at the receiving institution. On rare occasions the receiving physician may refuse to accept a patient for whom the method of transport might be dangerous (i.e., if the receiving physician believes that the patient's care may be compromised by choice of an inappropriate transport team). Sometimes the referring institution would prefer to send personnel from their own hospital to accompany the patient during transport to "save time." It would be important at this point to query the referring physician about whether the accompanying personnel are comfortable and experienced in managing pediatric emergencies (**pediatric** airway skills, vascular access). With *proper* documentation, it is unlikely that the receiving hospital would be liable for the transport.

XI. How Should Conflicts With Referring Hospital Personnel Be Handled?

Occasionally a referring physician may disagree with a decision made by the team regarding a therapeutic intervention. If the intervention can wait, it may be prudent to perform it after leaving the premises to avoid further confrontation. For an urgent matter, the transport team should consult the receiving attending physician or the transport medical director. Conflicts of this kind are usually resolved when the referring physician and the receiving attending physician have an opportunity to discuss the issue over the telephone. This situation emphasizes the importance of having a medical control officer available to the team at all times.

BIBLIOGRAPHY

George JE: General legal principles, in *Law and Emergency Care,* St Louis, CV Mosby Co, 1980, pp 1–18.

Frew SA, Roush WR, LaGreca K: COBRA: Implications for emergency medicine. *Ann Emerg Med* 1988; 17:835–837.

Joint Commission for the Accreditation of Healthcare Organizations: *Accreditation Manual for Hospitals*. Chicago, JCAH, 1989, p 25.

15

TRANSPORT PROCESS: REFERRING AND RECEIVING HOSPITAL RESPONSIBILITIES

Stabilization of the critically ill child demands maximum utilization of tangible resources such as equipment and personnel and intangible resources such as knowledge and experience. When a critically ill child is seen in the emergency department, the most important and immediate concern is the medical stabilization of the child. As the stabilization process continues into the second stage, the child is transported from a facility without a pediatric intensive care unit (PICU) to a pediatric tertiary care center. This second stage of care is facilitated when a system for transport has been established in advance. A preexisting relationship between the referral center and community hospitals in the region, protocols for preparing children for transport, clear definitions of transport team member roles, and organization of transport equipment in both the community hospital and tertiary care center all will contribute to the health care providers' ability to use their intangible resources and to concentrate on patient care without administrative or technical distractions.

I. Preparation for Stabilization and Transport

In the community setting, a designated area, whether a drawer in the emergency cart or a plastic fishing tackle box, should contain equipment specific to the care of the pediatric patient (Appendix 15–1). In addition, easy to use reference

APPENDIX 15–1.
Pediatric Emergency Equipment

Intubation equipment
- 0.5 and 1 L 100% bag-valve resuscitation device with premature-, infant-, and child-size masks.
- Endotracheal tubes, sizes 2.5–6.0 uncuffed.
- Endotracheal tubes, sizes 5.0–8.0 cuffed.
- Laryngoscope blades, sizes 0, 1, 1.5 and 2.0.
- Suction catheters, sizes 6, 8, and 10 F.
- Pediatric sensor for pulse oximeter.

Lines
- Intravenous (IV) catheters, 22 and 24 gauge.
- Butterflies, 23 and 25 gauge.
- Pediatric volumetric set.
- Intraosseous needle.

Other Supplies
- Blood pressure cuff, premature, newborn, infant, and child sizes.
- Nasogastric tubes, 6, 8, and 10 F.
- Foley catheters, 6, 8, and 10 F.
- Restraints, infant and child sizes.
- Chest tubes, 8, 10, 12, and 16 F.
- Resuscitation medications and IV fluids.

NOTE: Standard adult sizes are used for adolescents.

materials such as code sheets and a chart of age-based normal vital signs (Appendix 15–2) should be kept here. This area must be easily accessed, and all staff, including temporary and registry nursing, must know of its location. An annual visit to the community hospital by the tertiary care center to review equipment, supplies, and medications and to discuss ways of facilitating transports will help to guarantee optimal care for the critically ill or injured child.

Similarly, in the tertiary care setting, a designated area should contain all equipment needed for transport. This includes patient care equipment, reference materials for the team's use, appropriate consent forms, documentation sheets, and other miscellaneous supplies. It is best if this equipment is organized and maintained in a closed system, so that objects are not "loaned" into other areas of the hospital.

II. Transport Call

Organization of information by the referring hospital before calling the tertiary care center will help to facilitate commu-

APPENDIX 15–2.
Normal Vital Signs*

Normal heart rates in children	
(beats/min)	
Infants (1 yr of age)	120–160
Preschoolers (1–4 yr of age)	90–140
School age	60–120
Normal respiratory rates in children	
(breaths/min)	
Infants	30–60
Preschoolers	20–40
School age	16–30
Normal blood pressures (BP) in children	
Infants	74–100/50–70
≥ 2 yr	Systolic BP = (2 × Age in yr) + 80; Diastolic BP = 2/3 systolic BP.

*Abnormal vital signs may not indicate pathologic condition but must be carefully evaluated to determine the cause of the variance.

nication and, therefore, patient care. The receiving critical care physician will need to know basic demographic information, a summary of the history and physical examination, and the current treatment of the child. Utilization of the same or a slightly modified transport form by both receiving and sending hospital will help with the transfer of clinical information and will prevent small oversights that may lead to major problems (i.e., no telephone number for return calls or misunderstandings about where the child is located in the hospital (Appendix 15–3). The responsible physician in the referral center should always be aware of both bed and transport team availability. If the center is unable to accomodate the patient, emergency stabilization information should be given and another institution recommended to the referring physician.

Depending on the referral center, transport team personnel may include specially trained physicians, nurses, and/or respiratory care practitioners. After consideration of variables such as severity of illness, distance, weather, travel time, and aeromedical physiology, the method of transport will be decided by the referring physician in consultation with the re-

APPENDIX 15–3.
Transport Initiation Information

Patient name
Patient's age
Referring physician's name
Referring hospital/facility's name
Patient's location
Telephone number
Patient information
- Pertinent history
- Current vital signs
- Weight
- Physical findings
- Laboratory values
- Current assessment
- Current therapy

ceiving physician. After the transport is arranged, the receiving physician should request that the referring hospital ask the parent/guardian of the ill child to wait at their hospital for the transport team's arrival. The team can then obtain necessary history and consent form signatures from the family and also provide them with updated assessment and plans.

III. Mobilization Time

Realistically, it may take approximately 30 minutes for the transport team to leave the referral center, except when using specialized helicopter services. If the team consistently takes much longer than 40 minutes to leave, the tertiary level hospital must reevaluate the design of the transport system in an effort to decrease that time period. This mobilization time, added on to the travel time between institutions, may mean a lengthy stay in the referral hospital emergency department, pediatric ward, adult ICU, or wherever the child is being cared for. During this time, all members of the referring hospital health care team should be encouraged to use via the telephone resources at the receiving hospital. Nurses and respiratory care practitioners, as well as physicians, may benefit from discussion with their counterparts. When possible, this time period should also be used by the referring hospital to complete and duplicate paperwork.

Before departure from their home hospital, the transport team should consider the specific needs of the child who will be transported. Any necessary equipment or medications not routinely carried can be added to the transport bags. The team may use the transit time to the referring hospital to review the patient's history and the plan for care. Medication doses should be calculated in advance. As much as possible, the team member roles should be clarified. The health care provider roles, which are generally well defined in the in-hospital setting, must have flexibility built in for the transport situation. This may lead to some unclear areas of practice. Open communication and trust between team members are essential so that these issues can be clearly resolved. A previously defined line of command going all the way to the attending physician should be used to mediate conflict between team members and avoid prolonged discussion and arguments during the transport. Posttransport conferences are used to review situations that led to conflict with the hope of avoiding similar problems in the future.

IV. Transfer of Care

Care of the child is assumed by the transport team after their arrival at the referring hospital, but the referring hospital team remains an invaluable resource. Although this is a very stressful time, basic courtesies such as introductions must be attended to immediately to establish a cooperative and collegial relationship between all individuals involved with the care of the child. By the time the transport team arrives, the referring hospital is often anxious for rapid transfer of the child so that the examination room and staff can be made available for the care of other patients. However, interfacility transport differs from field or emergency medical service transports in the emphasis on stabilization before moving the child ("stay and play" vs. "swoop and scoop") and in providing a mobile intensive care equipment. Some children, such as those who will be transported by air, have additional concerns that must be addressed (see Chapter 13). When the transport preparation checklist is complete the child will be moved (Appendix 15–4).

APPENDIX 15–4.

Transport Preparation Check List*

Patient status

( )Acceptable respiratory status: Po_2, pH, Pco_2.
( )Chest radiograph for ETT position in intubated airway.
( )Stable cardiovascular system: heart rate, rhythm, blood pressure, pulses, perfusion.
( )Adequate cerebral perfusion pressure.
( )Seizures controlled.
( )Reliable IV access.
( )Appropriate IV fluids and rates.
( )Major metabolic concerns assessed, treated: glucose, Na^+, K^+, HCO_3^- and Ca^{2+}.
( )Urine output established.
( )Adequate Hgb, Hct values.
( )Bleeding controlled: mechanical, coagulation.
( )Antibiotics for presumed infection.
( )Antipyretics for fever.
( )Warmth for hypothermia.
( )NG tube in all intubated airways.
( )Cervical spine precautions for potential spinal injury.
( )Appropriate restraints, analgesia, sedation.
( )Air transport considerations: air-filled cavities emptied: NG (GI); chest tube (pneumothorax).

Equipment, supplies status

( )Monitor(s) for patient evaluation: cardiorespiratory, pressure monitors; pulse oximeter.
( )Ventilator, IV pumps, suction.
( )Anticipated medications, supplies available.

Records, communication

( )Face sheet.
( )Copy of history, PE, laboratory values, nursing notes.
( )Radiographs.
( )Laboratory specimens.
( )Signed consents.
( )Receiving facility notified before departure.
( )Exposure to communicable disease.

*For both referring hospital and transport team. PO_2 = partial pressure of oxygen; PCO_2 = partial pressure of carbon dioxide; ETT = endotracheal tube; IV = intravenous; Hgb = hemoglobin; Hct = hematocrit; NG = nasogastric; GI = gastrointestinal; PE = physical examination.

V. Evaluation and Follow-up

Evaluation of the stabilization and transport process and follow-up of problems that may have occurred is essential to improve patient care services and for personal development of all involved staff. A case study or didactic presentation by the tertiary hospital staff to the referring hospital, informal discussion between hospitals concerning administrative issues, follow-up regarding the status of the patient, and quality assurance processes in each institution all serve to strengthen ties between institutions who share the ultimate goal of improving patient care.

PROCEDURES 16

I. Endotracheal Intubation

A. Differences in the pediatric airway

1. Relatively cephalad and anterior larynx in the young child.
2. Narrowest part of trachea, and therefore diameter for endotracheal tube (ETT) size, is the subglottic area, not at the vocal cords.
3. Relatively large tongue.
4. Hyperextension of the neck may occlude airway rather than assisting visualization.

B. Equipment

1. Bag and mask device connected to oxygen source.
2. Laryngoscope with extra battery and light bulb.
3. ETTs: size for age + one half size larger and smaller.
4. Stylet for ETT.
5. Suction source, tubing, and tonsil (Yankauer) tip.
6. Endotracheal suction catheters.
7. Syringe to inflate ETT cuff (if appropriate).
8. Tape.
9. Benzoin.
10. Stethoscope.
11. Nasogastric tube.
12. Cardiac monitor.
13. Pulse oximeter.
14. Latex gloves.
15. Intubation medication, if needed.

C. Procedure

1. Preparation.
   a. Check equipment.
   b. Connect cardiac monitor and pulse oximeter.
   c. Empty stomach with nasogastric tube, if gag present.

d. Insert stylet, if needed (stop 1 cm from distal end of ETT and bend over top of proximal end).
e. Give medications if needed.

2. Intubation.
   a. Ventilate with 100% oxygen via bag and mask.
   b. Have assistant apply cricoid pressure (Selleck maneuver) both to prevent aspiration and for improved visualization.
   c. Insert ETT.
   d. Check breath sounds.
   e. Tape ETT securely, keeping lip marker in place; recheck breath sounds.
   f. Obtain chest x-ray film to determine ETT placement. Tip of tube should be 1–2 cm above carina.

   Stop intubation attempt if O_2 saturation drops to <90% or heart rate drops. Ventilate patient with 100% oxygen via bag and mask before reattempting intubation.
3. After intubation, if patient fails to respond clinically to ventilation:
   a. Reassess breath sounds.
      (1) ETT may be down right main stem bronchus. If breath sounds are greater on the right, slowly pull tube back until breath sounds are equal. Have bag and mask apparatus at hand in case ETT is dislodged from trachea.
      (2) ETT may have dislodged into esophagus. Breath sounds should be distant bilaterally and sounds increased over the stomach. Using laryngoscope, check to see if ETT goes through cords. If not, remove ETT, ventilate with 100% oxygen via bag and mask and reattempt intubation.
      (3) ETT may be obstructed by blood or secretions. Suction tube with normal saline (NS) solution to attempt to remove obstruction. If unsuccessful, remove ETT, ventilate with 100% oxygen via bag and mask, and reattempt intubation.
      (4) Patient may have developed pneumothorax from disease process or ventilation attempts. Insert 20-gauge angiocatheter attached to syringe (or butterfly needle with distal portion in sterile water) into right second interspace in the midclav-

icular line. If air is aspirated into syringe (or bubbles appear in sterile water), prepare to place chest tube (see p. 346). If unsuccessful, repeat procedure on left side.

I. Needle Cricothyroidotomy

Open cricothyroidotomy is difficult and dangerous in the young child and should therefore be attempted only by providers with substantial experience, if at all. Needle cricothyroidotomy (NCT) is a technique that can be lifesaving when intubation or bag and mask ventilation are unsuccessful (e.g., in the case of a foreign body aspiration or epiglottitis). NCT will buy time during preparation for establishment of a definitive airway (i.e., surgical tracheostomy).

A. Equipment

1. Gloves.
2. 14-gauge (or 16-gauge) over the needle catheter (angiocatheter).
3. 10-mL syringe: Attach to angiocatheter.
4. Oxygen tubing and source.
5. Jet ventilation apparatus if available.
6. Adapter removed from a 3.0 ETT.

B. Procedure

1. Preparation.
   a. Sterile preparation of trachea with antiseptic solution.
   b. Locate the cricothyroid membrane: the small midline indentation just below the protuberance of the thyroid cartilage (Adam's apple).
   c. With an assistant holding the trachea stable, insert the 14-gauge angiocatheter with the syringe attached into the middle of the cricothyroid membrane, with the needle at a 45-degree angle (pointed caudally). Aspirate with the syringe as the needle is inserted. Enter the trachea carefully so as to avoid perforating the posterior wall.
   d. Return of air in the syringe indicates that the trachea has been entered. Advance the catheter gently down the trachea and remove the needle from the catheter.
   e. Connect the catheter to a high-flow oxygen source at a minimum of 15 L/min. Use of a jet ventilator is

optimal. Intermittently ventilate by applying the high-flow oxygen source to the catheter every 2–4 seconds or by cutting a side hole in the oxygen tubing and occluding it with a finger every 2–4 seconds.

f. If no other form of connector is available, attach the hub of the 3.0 ETT into the angiocatheter and ventilate with the bag connected to the ETT hub.

g. Proceed with preparation for a surgical airway or intubation in the operating room. This method of providing an airway will allow oxygenation but does not allow appropriate ventilation (CO_2 removal via exhalation) to maintain the patient's pH for longer than 20–30 minutes.

II. Thoracentesis

A. Needle thoracentesis

1. Equipment.
   a. 20-gauge angiocatheter or 23-gauge butterfly needle with 12 in. tubing.
   b. 10 or 20 mL syringe or bottle of sterile water.
   c. Antiseptic solution.
2. Procedure.
   a. Prepare skin overlying anterior first 3 ribs with antiseptic.
   b. Attach syringe to angiocatheter.
   c. Insert the angiocatheter over the top of the second rib in the midclavicular line, aspirating with the syringe during insertion.
   d. If air is aspirated into the syringe, leave the angiocath (minus its needle) in the chest and prepare to insert a chest tube (see below).
   e. To use butterfly needle: Place tubing in container of sterile water (below level of patient's ribcage).
   f. Insert needle as above-over top of second rib in midclavicular line. If bubbles come from underwater tubing, proceed with chest tube placement (below). Alternatively, air can be aspirated from the butterfly tubing into a syringe.

B. Tube thoracostomy (chest tube placement)

1. Equipment.
   a. Sterile gloves.
   b. Antiseptic preparation.

   c. Local anesthetic (1% lidocaine).
   d. Chest tube (8–10 F for neonates; up to 28–32 F for adolescence).
   e. 4 by 4 in. gauze.
   f. Scalpel blade and handle.
   g. Small curved hemostat.
   h. Large curved hemostat.
   i. Water seal drainage system or Heimlich valve.
   j. 3-0 or 2-0 suture material.
   k. Tape.
   l. Heavy scissors.
2. Procedure.
   a. Identify the affected side of the chest. Restrain or have an assistant hold the patient's arm above the patient's shoulder.
   b. Prepare the lateral aspect of the chest from the axilla to the abdomen with antiseptic solution.
   c. The skin incision should be made over the fifth, sixth, or seventh intercostal space in the anterior axillary or midaxillary line. The skin incision should be made well away from the areola of the breast. The skin incision site should be anesthetized with locally infiltrated anesthetic if appropriate.
   d. Make a 2–3 cm long skin incision using the scalpel blade.
   e. Tunnel the tip of the hemostat under the skin and over the top of the rib which is 1–2 interspaces cephalad to the skin incision. Tunnel the hemostat anteriorally if the chest tube is being placed to drain a pneumothorax. Direct the hemostat posteriorally if the chest tube will drain fluid.
   f. Using the tip of the hemostat, bluntly puncture through the intercostal muscles and the pleura. This may require a lot of force. Firmly grasp the hemostat near its tip with your free hand to better direct the applied force and to control the tip when the pleura is punctured. Spread the blade of the hemostat forcefully to create an opening for passage of the tube into the chest.
   g. Pass the chest tube between the blades of the hemostat into the pleural cavity. Advance the chest tube far enough into the chest so that none of the side

holes of the tube lies outside the chest cavity. If for some reason the hemostat is removed from the newly created hole in the musculature, use a finger to mark the location of the hole (otherwise it may be difficult to locate subsequently).

h. Fog or fluid will be seen in the chest tube when it is positioned in the pleural space.
i. Attach the chest tube to a water seal device set at 15–20 cm H_2O of negative pressure. Alternatively a Heimlich flutter valve can be used.
j. Secure tube in place with suture and tape.
k. Obtain a chest x-ray film to check tube position.
l. Dysfunction of the chest tube should be suspected as the cause of any deterioration in a patient with a chest tube.

III. Periocardiocentesis

In the presence of suspected pericardial fluid, drainage is required emergently only if hemodynamic compromise is present from pericardial tamponade.

A. Equipment

1. Antiseptic solution.
2. Sterile gloves.
3. 18-gauge angiocatheter.
4. Syringe.

B. Procedure

1. Prepare the subxyphoid and xiphoid areas with antiseptic solution.
2. Attach syringe to angiocatheter.
3. Insert the angiocatheter in the skin just below the notch between the left side of the xiphoid and the left costal margin. Aim the needle toward the inferior tip of the left scapula 45 degrees laterally and 45 degrees superiorally. Advance the angiocatheter while aspirating on the syringe.
4. Monitor the electrocardiogram (ECG) while advancing the angiocatheter. Dysrhythmias and injury currents (i.e., marked ST-wave changes or wide QRS complexes) suggest that the angiocatheter has impacted or entered one of the ventricles of the heart. Withdraw the angiocatheter slowly until the ECG normalizes. Dysrythmias usually will disappear when the angiocatheter

is withdrawn. Persistent ventricular dysrhythmias should be treated with lidocaine and/or defibrillation as appropriate.

5. Following puncture of the pericardium, aspirate as much fluid as possible. The patient should improve after fluid aspiration if cardiac tamponade was present. The inability to withdraw fluid from the pericardium indicates that there is no fluid present in the pericardium, that the angiocatheter is not actually in the pericardium, or that the pericardial fluid is clotted, loculated, or too viscous to aspirate. Further aspiration attempts should be made if the suspicion of cardiac tamponade is very high and the patient is hemodynamically unstable. Otherwise one should consider and address any other potential causes for the patient's condition.
6. If fluid is aspirated from the pericardium, leave the angiocatheter in place and withdraw the needle. Cap the angiocatheter with a Luer lock syringe. This permits easy aspiration of any fluid that subsequently accumulates that could lead to further cardiovascular compromise.
7. Secure the pericardial catheter to the skin with suture and/or tape.
8. If signs of hemodynamic compromise recur, aspirate the pericardial catheter.

   NOTE: To perform pericardiocentesis for patients with dextrocardia, the angiocatheter should be inserted at the right xyphochondral junction and advanced toward the inferior tip of the right scapula.

IV. Intraosseous Infusion

Placement of an intraosseous line is an excellent means of establishing vascular access in a young child for whom peripheral intravenous (IV) cannulation is impossible or is too time consuming in view of a need for urgent administration of medication.

A. Equipment

1. Gloves.
2. Antiseptic preparation.
3. Large-gauge needle (styleted bone marrow needles are best, followed by any large-bore styleted needle, followed by a regular needle).

4. Syringe.
5. Saline flush.

B. Procedure

1. Prepare the field in a sterile manner.
2. Select an insertion site. The best site is the anteromedial aspect of the tibia 2 cm below the tibial tubercle. The bone is just below the skin and is flat, and there are no important structures that can be injured at this site. Other potentially useful sites are the distal femur and the anterior iliac spine. The insertion site should be free of infection. Do not use a bone that is fractured, infected, involved with tumor, or that has had a previous intraosseous attempt.
3. Administer local anesthetic if appropriate.
4. Insert the needle through the skin into the cortex of the bone, angled slightly caudally to avoid the epiphysis. Use a twisting motion to drill through the bone cortex. Apply firm pressure to the needle to facilitate drilling into the bone. Be careful not to bend the needle. Do not put your hand on the other side of the bone to stabilize.
5. A loss of resistance is felt when the marrow cavity is entered. Marrow can often be aspirated through the needle and can be sent for laboratory analysis (except complete blood cell count). In a child in severe shock, marrow may not be aspirated, even if the needle is in place.
6. Infuse 3–10 mL of NS solution to assure that flow is without significant resistance and that the fluid does not extravasate.
7. Infuse whatever fluid, blood products, or drugs are required by the patient. Some resistance to infusion will be encountered. Watch periodically for severe soft tissue swelling, which may indicate that the needle has become dislodged.

   NOTE: (1) When one is using a needle without a stylet, the needle may become plugged with bone during insertion. Forceful injection of fluid may be required to clear the needle. (2) Clearly document all intrasosseous needle sites so that the receiving health care providers are aware of them and can monitor them.

V. Central Venous Cannulation: Femoral and External Jugular

A. Seldinger technique

During initial stabilization and transport, central venous pressure measurement is rarely available or practical. However, catheter placement in the femoral and external jugular areas (two of the sites used for central venous access) can be quite useful. When peripheral veins are too small or too constricted for rapid access, these two large, easily accessible veins can be used to great benefit. Later, if desired in the pediatric intensive care unit, central venous pressure monitoring can be accomplished via the exiting catheter sites.

Either vein can be accessed with a regular catheter over the needle system (angiocatheter)—although many of these catheters are too short for stabilization in the femoral area—or with a longer catheter via the Seldinger technique.

During an acute resuscitation when activity may be focused about the patient's head and chest, the femoral vein is easier to reach than the external jugular. External jugular catheterization carries a risk of pneumothorax, making the femoral route preferable in most cases. The external jugular vein is, however, easier to see.

1. Equipment.
   a. Gloves.
   b. Syringe with saline flush.
   c. Tape.
   d. Benzoin.
   e. Suture.
   f. Catheter with guidewire system (Cook catheter, 3.0–4.0 F).
   g. Antiseptic solution.
   h. Sterile gauze pads.
   i. Scalpel blade and handle.
   j. 1% Lidocaine solution.
2. Procedure.
   a. Attach syringe to metal catheter (thin-walled needle).
   b. Advance metal catheter into vein, aspirating with syringe.
   c. When blood return is achieved, insert guidewire (end with soft tip) through metal catheter well into

vein (several cms. beyond catheter tip). If guidewire does not pass freely, reposition metal catheter in vein.

d. Stabilize the guidewire against the skin and remove the metal catheter over the end of the guidewire, leaving the guidewire in place in the vein (do not let go of the guidewire).
e. If the plastic catheter is of a large bore, make a small incision where the guidewire enters the skin. This will facilitate passage of the catheter over the guidewire.
f. Advance the infusion catheter over the guidewire into the vein. A gentle twisting motion should aid entry through the skin incision site.
g. Hold the infusion catheter in place and withdraw the guidewire through it.
h. Attach the saline filled syringe to the catheter and aspirate. If blood returns easily, flush with saline solution.
i. Suture catheter to skin.

NOTE: Once the guidewire is inserted into the vein, do not let go of it until it is withdrawn. Otherwise it may slip forward and be lost into the vein.

1. Femoral vein access.
   a. Prepare inguinal area in sterile fashion.
   b. Palpate the femoral artery 1–2 cm below the inguinal ligament, approximately half way between the symphysis pubis and anterior superior iliac spine. Maintain a finger over the artery for orientation. The femoral vein is located approximately 0.5 cm medial to the artery. For the right-handed operator, it is usually easier to stand on the patient's right side and use the right leg, keeping the left hand on the femoral artery.
   c. Enter the vein at a 30–45 degree angle, using an over-the-needle catheter or via the Seldinger technique.
   d. If the femoral artery is accidentally entered, withdraw the catheter and apply pressure for 5–10 minutes before reattempting cannulation on that side.
   e. Stabilize the catheter well with tape, bio-occlusive dressing (Op-site), and/or suture, because leg movement will tend to dislodge it.

2. External jugular access.
   a. Place the patient in Trendelenburg position or with a towel roll under the shoulder. Hold the head turned to the opposite side from the vein to be cannulated.
   b. Prepare the site in a sterile fashion.
   c. Pierce the skin one half to two thirds of the way between the angle of the jaw and the clavicle, and advance into the vein. Either an over the needle catheter or the Seldinger technique may be used. Generally the former is preferred in the infant with a short neck, especially if the goal is venous access rather than central access.
   d. Stabilize the catheter well with tape, bio-occlusive dressing (Op-site), and/or suture.
   e. If the patient's respiratory or cardiovascular status deteriorates during or after the procedure, consider the possibility of a pneumothorax secondary to needle contact with the apex of the lung.

VII. Saphenous Vein Cutdown

With the reintroduction of the technique of intraosseous infusion, use of a venous cutdown is rarely needed during the most acute phase of a resuscitation. Occasionally an operator will be present who can perform a cutdown within a very few minutes, and in that case the line is certainly useful. Otherwise, saphenous vein cutdown can be reserved for the postresuscitation phase, either before removal of an intraosseous line or for an easier to maintain line for transport.

In the patient with major abdominal injury, any line placed below the diaphragm may result in medication infusion out the inferior vena cava into the abdomen instead of into the cardiovascular system. The cutdown technique can be used on several other veins, including the femoral, the external jugular, and the basilic vein in the antecubital fossa. Performing a cutdown on the saphenous vein has several advantages over other veins, most notably that there are no other major structures in the immediate area to accidentally damage and the area of the distal leg is far removed from the often crowded area at the head and chest.

A. **Equipment**

1. Sterile gloves.
2. Antiseptic preparation.
3. Local anesthetic (1% lidocaine).
4. Sterile gauze.
5. Scalpel blade and handle.
6. Small hemostats.
7. Iris scissors.
8. Catheter.
9. Suture.
10. Small forceps.
11. Sterile drapes.
12. Saline flush.
13. Catheter introducer if available.

B. **Procedure**

1. Prepare medial malleolus in sterile fashion with sterile drapes.
2. Location of the saphenous vein: superficial vein, just anterior and superior to the medial malleolus of the ankle.
3. Infiltrate skin with lidocaine. Make a 1–2 cm transverse skin incision.
4. Dissect the vein (usually blood filled) free with a curve hemostat. Expose 1–2 cm of vein.
5. Pass absorbable suture ligatures proximally and distally around the exposed vein. Do not tie initially.
6. Two methods for cannulation exist:
   a. Using the proximal and distal ligatures for traction and stabilization, puncture the vein carefully with an over-the-needle catheter device (angiocatheter). Slide the catheter over the needle into the vein. This method is easier and faster and will preserve the vein for future use.
   b. Traditional method: Tie the distal ligature around the vein. Make a transverse venotomy in the mid-portion of the exposed vein using a no. 11 blade or iris scissors. Advance the catheter (without a needle) through the venotomy into the vein. Tie the proximal ligature over the catheter. Note that the vein can easily be transsected accidentally during the venotomy. Also insertion of the catheter into the venotomy hole may be technically difficult (like

threading a bleeding needle). If a catheter introducer is available, it can be extremely helpful.

7. Attach saline syringe and assure free flow of blood and saline solution.
8. Suture the skin incision closed. Secure the catheter using tape, bio-occlusive dressing (Op-site), and/or suture. Cover with a sterile dressing.

II. Umbilical Catheter Placement

The umbilical vessels provide a unique opportunity for vascular access in the neonatal patient for whom peripheral access has been unsuccessful.

The umbilical vein, identified by its relatively large lumen and thin wall, can be used for administration of fluids and medication. It can be accessed very quickly, even when the operator has little experience with the technique.

The umbilical arteries (usually 2, occasionally only 1) are relatively thick walled with a small lumen. An umbilical artery catheter (UAC) can be used for fluid administration, for blood pressure monitoring, and for arterial blood gas determinations. Extreme caution must be used if medications are to be administered, because the vessel provides access to the *arterial* circulation. A UAC takes longer to place and is more difficult for those not experienced in the procedure.

A. Equipment

1. Sterile gloves and gown.
2. Face mask.
3. Antiseptic preparation.
4. Sterile drapes.
5. Sterile gauze.
6. Cloth umbilical cord tape.
7. Scalpel blade and handle.
8. Blunt iris forceps.
9. Small blunt hemostats.
10. Suture.
11. Tape.
12. 3.0 and 5.0 F umbilical catheter (sterile feeding tube if umbilical catheters not available).
13. 3-way stopcock.
14. Sterile syringe.
15. Saline flush.

B. Procedure

1. General:
   a. Remove cord clamp. Prepare cord and surrounding skin with antiseptic. Tie the cloth umbilical tape loosely around the base of the cord (may be tightened if bleeding occurs).
   b. Don sterile gloves, face mask, and gown.
   c. Prepare and drape area in sterile fashion.
   d. Transect or trim cord horizontally to obtain fresh access to vessels.
2. Umbilical vein catheterization:
   a. If necessary, use a small blunt forceps or hemostat to dilate the lumen of the vein.
   b. Advance the catheter into the vein. If resistance is encountered, withdraw the catheter a few centimeters, rotate it, and advance again (the catheter may have tracked into a branch of the vessel).
   c. Aspirate with a syringe to ascertain blood flow. Flush with saline solution.
   d. Obtain an x-ray film to confirm proper placement. The tip of the catheter should be in the umbilical vein or the inferior vena cava and should not be in the liver or a branch vein.
   e. Secure catheter with suture and tape.
3. Umbilical artery catheterization:
   a. It is very helpful to have an assistant, outfitted in a sterile fashion.
   b. Fill the catheter to be used with saline solution.
   c. Mark or note the distance on the catheter that represents 60% of the shoulder to umbilicus distance.
   d. Dilate the artery with a small curved forceps or blunt probe. Dilatation via gentle repetitive stretching is most effective. The artery should be dilated for a distance of 1 cm. This procedure may take up to several minutes. Rushing insertion of the catheter into an incompletely dilated artery will result in failure of the procedure.
   e. Advance the catheter tip into the artery. Resistance will be met at the undilated portion of the artery and at the abdominal wall and can be overcome with gentle steady pressure. Continued resistance gener-

ally means the catheter is in a false lumen. Do not force the catheter. If a false lumen is encountered:

(i) Remove the catheter and reintroduce. Unfortunately, often the same false lumen will be encountered.

(ii) Trim the umbilical stump, and reinitiate dilatation of the artery. If the false lumen was close to the insertion site of the catheter, it may be excised.

(iii) Remove the catheter and attempt cannulation of the other artery. If the UAC is not absolutely necessary, consider saving the other artery for the receiving hospital to cannulate.

(iv) Insert the catheter into the false lumen, then insert a second catheter into the artery *beside* the first one. This technique may have remarkable success if the first catheter blocks the false lumen.

(f) Advance the catheter to the predetermined distance. Assure back and forth flow into the saline-filled syringe. Avoid introduction of air bubbles into the arterial circulation.

(g) Suture and tape the catheter in place.

(h) Obtain an x-ray film to assess the catheter position.

(i) The catheter tip should be below the level of the third lumbar vertebral body. Alternatively it may be at the level of T10 to T11. Avoid catheter placement in between those areas, because microemboli may be thrown into the renal vasculature.

(j) The infant should remain on his or her back while the catheter is in place, because fatal, unnoticed hemorrhage may occur if the catheter comes out while the infant is on his or her stomach.

PHARMACOLOGY 17

I. Drug Formulary.

A formulary of drugs needed for pediatric emergencies is provided in this chapter. To further help the reader select and use medications, the following organization has been employed.

1. **Brand name listing:** Drugs are listed by their brand names; the corresponding generic names follow.
2. **Drug groups:** Drugs belonging to recognized therapeutic groups are listed by generic name to offer the user a quick glance at available therapeutic options.
3. Commonly used medications in critical care pediatrics:
   a. Nonantibiotic drugs.
   b. Antibiotic drugs.

A. Brand name listing.

Asterisk (*) indicates listing is under the antibiotic section of formulary.

Brand name:	**Generic name:**
Adenocard	Adenosine
Alprostadil	Prostaglandin E_1
Alupent	Metaproterenol
Amphojel	Aluminum hydroxide and magnesium hydroxide
Ancef	Cefazolin*
Anectine	Succinylcholine
Antilirium	Physostigmine
Apresoline	Hydralazine
AquaMEPHYTON	Vitamin K_1
Aspirin	Acetylsalicylic acid
Ativan	Lorazepam
Bactocill	Oxacillin*
Bactrim	Trimethoprim-sulfamethoxazole*
Benadryl	Diphenhydramine
Brethine	Terbutaline

Bretylol	Bretylium
Bricanyl	Terbutaline
Bronkosol	Isoetharine
Calan	Verapamil
Capoten	Captopril
Chloromycetin	Chloramphenicol*
Claforan	Cefotaxime*
Cortef	Hydrocortisone
Dantrium Intravenous	Dantrolene
DDAVP	Desmopressin acetate
Decadron	Dexamethasone
Demerol	Meperidine
Depakene	Valproic acid
Depakote	Valproic acid
Desferal	Deferoxamine
Digibind	Digoxin immune FAB
Dilantin	Phenytoin
Diuril	Chlorothiazide
Dobutrex	Dobutamine
Edecrin	Ethacrynic acid
Flagyl	Metronidazole*
Fortaz	Ceftazidime*
Fungizone	Amphotericin B*
Garamycin	Gentamicin*
Hexadrol	Dexamethasone
Hyperstat	Diazoxide
Inapsine	Droperidol
Inderal	Propanolol
Inocor	Amrinone (see p. 70)
Intropin	Dopamine
Isoptin	Verapamil
Isuprel	Isoproterenol
Kayexalate	Sodium polystyrene sulfonate
Kefzol	Cefazolin*
Ketalar	Ketamine
Lanoxin	Digoxin
Lasix	Furosemide
Levarterenol	Norepinephrine
Levophed	Norepinephrine
Luminal	Phenobarbital
Maalox	Aluminum hydroxide and magnesium hydroxide

Medipren	Ibuprofen
Mephyton	Vitamin K_1
Metaprel	Metaproterenol
microNefrin	Epinephrine, racemic
Motrin	Ibuprofen
Mucomyst	Acetylcysteine
Narcan	Naloxone
Nebcin	Tobramycin*
Nipride	Nitroprusside
Noctec	Chloral hydrate
Norcuron	Vecuronium
Normodyne	Labetalol
Osmitrol	Mannitol
Pavulon	Pancuronium
Pediaprofen	Ibuprofen
Pentothal	Thiopental
PGE_1	Prostaglandin E_1
Phenergan	Promethazine
Phytonadione	Vitamin K_1
Pitressin, Aqueous	Vasopressin
Pronestyl	Procainamide
Prostaphlin	Oxacillin*
Prostigmin	Neostigmine
Prostin VR	Prostaglandin E_1
Protopam	Pralidoxime (2-PAM)
Proventil	Albuterol
Regitine	Phentolamine
Reglan	Metoclopromide
Rifadin	Rifampin*
Rimactane	Rifampin*
Rocephin	Ceftriaxone*
Septra	Trimethoprim-sulfamethoxazole*
Solu-Cortef	Hydrocortisone
Solu-Medrol	Methylprednisolone
Somnos	Chloral hydrate
Sublimaze	Fentanyl
Tagamet	Cimetidine
Tazidime	Ceftazidime*
Trandate	Labetalol
Unipen	Nafcillin*
Valium	Diazepam
Vancocin	Vancomycin*

Vaponefrin	Epinephrine, racemic
Ventolin	Albuterol
Versed	Midazolam
Vitamin B_6	Pyridoxine
Xylocaine	Lidocaine
Zantac	Ranitidine
Zinacef	Cefuroxime*
Zovirax	Acyclovir*

B. Drug groups.

1. Airway edema.
2. Analgesics.
3. Antiarrhythmics.
4. Anticonvulsants.
5. Antiemetics.
6. Antihypertensives/afterload reducers.
7. Antipyretics.
8. Bronchodilators.
9. Cerebral edema.
10. Chronotropes.
11. Corticosteroids.
12. Diuretics.
13. Gastrointestinal drugs.
14. Hormones, synthetic substitutes.
15. Inotropes.
16. Neuromuscular blockers.
17. Sedatives, hypnotics.
18. Vasoconstrictors.

Airway edema:
Corticosteroids
Epinephrine, racemic

Analgesics:
Acetaminophen
Acetylsalicylic acid
Fentanyl
Ibuprofen
Meperidine
Morphine sulfate

Antiarrhythmics:
Adenosine
Bretylium
Digoxin
Lidocaine
Procainamide
Propanolol
Phenytoin
Verapamil

Anticonvulsants:
Diazepam
Lorazepam
Phenobarbital
Phenytoin

Pyridoxine
Paraldehyde
Thiopental
Valproic acid

Antiemetics:
Droperidol
Metoclopramide
Promethazine

Antihypertensives/afterload reducers:
Captopril
Diazoxide
Hydralazine
Labetalol
Nitroprusside
Propanolol

Antipyretics:
Acetaminophen
Acetylsalicylic acid
Ibuprofen

Bronchodilators:

Aerosol bronchodilators:
Albuterol
Isoetharine
Isoproterenol
Metaproterenol
Terbutaline

Oral bronchodilators:
Corticosteroids
Metaproterenol
Terbutaline
Theophylline

Intravenous bronchodilators:
Corticosteroids
Isoproterenol
Theophylline

Subcutaneous bronchodilators:
Epinephrine
Terbutaline

Cerebral edema:
Corticosteroids
Furosemide
Mannitol

Chronotropes:
Atropine
Epinephrine
Isoproterenol
Norepinephrine

Corticosteroids:
Dexamethasone
Hydrocortisone
Methylprednisolone
Prednisone

Diuretics:
Chlorothiazide
Ethacrynic Acid
Furosemide
Mannitol

Gastrointestinal drugs:
Aluminum hydroxide
Aluminum hydroxide and magnesium hydroxide
Cimetidine
Metoclopramide
Ranitidine

Hormones, synthetic substitutes:
Corticosteroids
Desmopressin acetate
Insulin
Vasopressin

Inotropes:
Amrinone (see p. 70)
Calcium chloride
Calcium gluconate
Digoxin
Dobutamine
Dopamine
Epinephrine
Isoproterenol
Norepinephrine

Neuromuscular blockers:
Pancuronium
Succinylcholine
Vecuronium

Sedatives, hypnotics:
Chloral hydrate
Diazepam
(Fentanyl)
Ketamine
Lorazepam
(Meperidine)
Midazolam
(Morphine sulfate)
Thiopental sodium

Vasoconstrictors:
Epinephrine
Norepinephrine

C. Commonly used medications in critical care pediatrics.

Nonantibiotic Drugs*

Name	Dose	Route	Notes
Acetaminophen	10–15 mg/kg/dose q4h.	po, pr.	
Acetylcysteine (Mucomyst)	For acetaminophen poisoning: 140 mg/kg loading dose; follow with 70 mg/kg q4h × 17 doses.	po.	May be administered undiluted or diluted 1:3 with water, saline solution, cola, or orange or grapefruit juice.
Acetylsalicylic acid (aspirin)	Antipyretic: 10–15 mg/kg/dose q4h; up to total 60–80 mg/kg/day.	po, pr.	May increase risk for Reye's syndrome following acute febrile illness, especially influenza and varicella.
Adenosine (Adenocard)	Adults: initial dose 6 mg; if not effective in 1–2 min, may try 12 mg × 2. Infants, children: 1–6 mg have been used.	IV.	*Rapid administration is essential* for effectiveness because its one-half life in blood is several seconds. Push rapidly, follow immediately with NS flush. The closer the IV site is to the heart, the more effective the dose.
Albumin, 5% and 25%	*5% albumin:* used primarily for volume expansion in patients with low albumin levels; usual dose 10–20 mL/kg (provides 0.5–1.0 g/kg albumin).	IV.	

(Continued.)

Nonantibiotic Drugs* (cont'd.).

Name	Dose	Route	Notes
	25% albumin: used primarily to correct hypoalbuminemia without hypovolemia; usual dose 2–4 mL/kg (0.5–1.0 g/kg albumin)		Prefer to infuse over 2–4 hr but may be infused over 10–30 min. Correction of hypoalbuminemia with IV albumin is temporary.
Albuterol (Proventil, Ventolin)	Inhalant solution 0.5% = 5 mg/mL. 0.05–0.20 mg/kg/dose, maximum 4.0 mg/dose, q4–6h; add NS solution to 3–5 cc volume, administer over 10–15 min. Severe bronchospasm: up to q15 min.	Aerosol.	Monitor HR and rhythm.
Aluminum hydroxide (Amphojel)	*Antacid:* 0.5–1.0 mL/kg, up to 30 mL/dose q2–4h.	po.	
Aluminum hydroxide and magnesium hydroxide (Maalox)	*Antacid:* 0.5–1.0 ml/kg, up to 30 mL/dose q2–4h.	po.	Avoid magnesium hydroxide in renal failure.
Atropine	*Bradycardia:* 0.01–0.03 mg/kg q2–5 min × 2–3 doses prn. Maximum dose 1 mg for children, 2 mg for adolescents. Doses <0.1 mg may paradoxically worsen bradycardia.	IV, IM, ETT.	Dose by ETT may need to be 2–3 times higher than IV, IM dose. Antidote for atropine overdose is physostigmine.

	Bronchodilation: 0.02–0.05 mg/kg tid, qid.	Aerosol.	
	Organophosphate or carbamate poisoning: Children: 0.02–0.05 mg/kg/dose q10–20min until anticholinergic effects observable, then q1–4h prn to maintain effect for at least 24h.	IV.	
	Organophosphate or carbamate poisoning: Adolescents: 1–2 mg/dose q10–20min until anticholinergic effects observable, then q1–4h prn to maintain effects for at least 24 hr.	IV.	
	Neuromuscular blockade reversal: 0.025–0.03 mg/kg 30 sec before neostigmine dose.	IV.	
Bretylium tosylate (Bretylol)	*Ventricular fibrillation:* 5 mg/kg/dose over 1 min, undiluted; follow with additional doses of 10 mg/kg prn at 15–30 min intervals to a maximum total dose of 30 mg/kg.	IV.	May cause hypotension, aggravation of digitalis toxicity. Rapid administration in awake patient (i.e., patients with ventricular dysrhythmias other than ventricular fibrillation) produces nausea, vomiting.

(Continued.)

Nonantibiotic Drugs* (cont'd.).

Name	Dose	Route	Notes
	Other ventricular dysrhythmias and maintenance for ventricular fibrillation: 5–10 mg/kg over 10 min q6h, preferably diluted to 10 mg/mL.		
Calcium chloride	*Cardiac resuscitation:* 10–25 mg/kg (0.1–0.25 mL/kg of 10% CaCl); maximum dose 1 g.	IV.	Dilute dose at least 1:1 with sterile water to reduce irritation (not necessary during cardiac resuscitation). Administer in central vein. Administer *slowly* (minimum time 5–10 min) to avoid cardiac tetany, bradycardia; monitor patient's heart rate, rhythm during administration.
	IV maintenance or hypocalcemia: neonate 20–67 mg/kg/dose; infants, young children 15–33 mg/kg/dose; older children 10–15 mg/dose; q8h. Maximum dose 1 g/dose. For maintenance, calcium gluconate is preferred because it is less irritating.		

Calcium gluconate	*IV maintenance or hypocalcemia:* neonate 66–200 mg/kg/dose; infants, young children 50–100 mg/kg/dose; older children 20–50 mg/kg; q8h. Maximum dose 2 g/dose. *As antidote for poisoning:* Children: 100 mg/kg over 5 min. Adults: 5–8 mL over 5 min.	IV.	Administer slowly (minimum time 5–10 min) to avoid cardiac tetany, bradycardia; monitor patient's heart rate, rhythm during administration.
Captopril (Capoten)	0.1–0.5 mg/kg q6–12h. Increase dose slowly as needed up to 1–2 mg/kg q6–24h.	po.	Monitor patient closely for hypotension. May cause hypotension, renal dysfunction, hyperkalemia.
Charcoal, activated	*Prevention of drug adsorption:* optimal 5–10 g/g of ingested poison. Estimated dose: 1–2 g/kg patient weight. *Enhancement of drug elimination:* 5–10 g/dose.	po.	Charcoal should not be given before ipecac. Sorbitol-containing charcoal suspensions are preferred to prevent constipation.
Chloral hydrate (Noctec, Somnos)	*Hypnotic:* 20–40 mg/kg/dose. May be repeated in 1 h at 1/2 the initial dose for a total up to 50 mg/kg. *Sedation for procedures:* may give a single dose up to 50–100 mg/kg.	po, pr.	Watch for respiratory depression.

(Continued.)

Nonantibiotic Drugs* (cont'd.).

Name	Dose	Route	Notes
Chlorothiazide (Diuril)	20–40 mg/kg/day po in 2 divided doses. IV dose not well established, but 10–30 mg/kg/day in 2 divided doses has been used.	po, IV.	
Cimetidine (Tagamet)	20–40 mg/kg/day in 4 divided doses.	po, IV.	Neonates and patients with impaired renal excretion should receive 20 mg/kg/day in 2–3 doses. It can be given continuously.
Dantrolene (Dantrium Intravenous)	*For malignant hyperthermia (MH): crisis:* 1 mg/kg/dose by rapid IV infusion; repeat immediately up to total dose 10 mg/kg until signs of MH (tachycardia, dysrhythmias, muscle rigidity, elevated temperature, cyanosis, mottling are gone. Mean effective dose is 2.5 mg/kg). *After crisis:* 4–8 mg/kg/24 hr divided qid for up to 3 days.	Crisis: IV. After crisis: IV, po.	

Deferoxamine (Desferal)	*Challenge test:* 50 mg/kg IM. *Chelation therapy:* 10–15 mg/kg/hr IV by continuous infusion.	IM, IV.	IV administration may produce hypotension; treat hypotension with fluid boluses and inotropes as needed.
Desmopressin acetate (DDAVP)	*For diabetes insipidus:* Intranasal route (preferred): 1–30 μg/day (up to 40 μg/day in adult) divided into 1–2 doses. IV/SC route: 2–4 μg/day divided into 2 doses in adults.	Intranasal; IV, SC.	Intranasal bioavailability is 10%–20%. Antidiuretic effects after intranasal administration occur within 1 hr (slightly faster after IV/SC administration), peak in 1–5 hr, persist 8–20 hr, then abruptly end over 60–90 min. Dose should be repeated when breakthrough diuresis recurs.
Dexamethasone (Decadron, Hexadrol)	*Airway edema:* 0.25 mg/kg/dose q6h as needed. *Anti-inflammatory or immunosuppressive:* 0.03–0.2 mg/kg/day (1–5 mg/m^2/day) divided q6–12h.	IV, IM, po.	

(Continued.)

Nonantibiotic Drugs* (cont'd.).

Name	Dose	Route	Notes
	Cerebral edema or septic shock: 1–2 mg/kg × 1 (usual maximum dose 40 mg) followed by 1–2 mg/kg/day, usual maximum of 16 mg/day (higher doses may be used in septic shock) in 4 divided doses.		
Dextrose	*Hypoglycemia:* Neonates, young infants: 1–2 mL/kg D_{10} (0.1–0.2 g/kg). Older neonates, children: 1–2 mL/kg D_{50} (0.5–1.0 g/kg).	IV.	Dilute D_{50} 1:1 with sterile water to make D_{25} solution. D_{10} solution should be used in neonates.
Diazepam (Valium)	*Status epilepticus:* 0.1–0.5 mg/kg q15–20min for 2–3 doses. Maximum dose is 10 mg (5 mg in children 5 yr of age). If parenteral administration is not possible, 0.2–0.5 mg/kg pr, maximum dose 10 mg pr.	IV, Deep IM; pr.	Can cause respiratory depression, hypotension.
	Sedation or muscle relaxation: 0.05–0.2 mg/kg/dose IV, deep IM q6–12h or 0.4–1.6 mg/kg/day po in 2–4 divided doses.	po, IV, deep IM.	May produce respiratory depression, hypotension.

Diazoxide (Hyperstat)	*Hypertension:* 1–5 mg/kg/dose, maximum dose 150 mg. Push over 15–30 sec. May repeat in 5–15 min until adequate BP reduction achieved, then q2–4h prn.	IV.	Must push rapidly to achieve antihypertensive effect. Can cause hyperglycemia, salt and water retention.
Digoxin (Lanoxin)	*Total digitalizing dose* (IM, IV*) Preterm infant: 0.01–0.03 mg/kg. Term infant–2 mo: 0.02–0.04 mg/kg. 2 mo–2 yr: 0.03–0.05 mg/kg. 2–10 yr: 0.02–0.04 mg/kg. 10 yr–adult: 0.01–0.015 mg/kg, up to 0.5–1.0 mg. **Oral doses should be 20% higher than IV/IM doses. Doses based on ideal body weight.*	IM, IV; po.	The *total digitalizing dose (TDD)* is usually given in divided doses as follows: 1/2 TDD, 1/4 TDD, 1/4 TDD at 6–12 hr intervals. An alternative schedule is to give 1/3 TDD × 3 at 8 hr intervals.
	Maintenance digoxin: Daily maintenance digoxin dose is usually 1/4 TDD given in 2 divided doses on q12h basis. Usually started 16–24 hours after last fraction of TDD.	IM, IV; po.	

(Continued.)

Nonantibiotic Drugs* (cont'd.).

Name	Dose	Route	Notes
Digoxin immune FAB (Digibind)	*Amount ingested known:* Dose (mg Digibind) = $\frac{\text{amount digoxin ingested (mg)}}{\text{0.015 (mg digoxin/mg FAB)}}$.	IV.	Indications for use: *Serious dysrhythmias:* i.e., ventricular tachycardia, fibrillation; blocks unresponsive to atropine, pacers. *Poor prognostic factors:* underlying cardiac disease; digoxin level >15 μg/mL or digitoxin level >150 μg/mL; initial hyperkalemia, the result of release of intracellular K^+ from digitalis toxicity.
Diphenhydramine (Benadryl)	1–1.25 mg/kg q4–6h prn up to total 5 mg/kg/day.	IV, po.	
Dobutamine (Dobutrex)	2–20 μg/kg/min.	IV.	See Appendix II (p. 429) for preparation, administration.
Dopamine (Intropin)	2–30 μg/kg/min.	IV.	See Appendix II (p. 428) for preparation and administration.
Droperidol (Inapsine)	*For nausea, vomiting:* 0.01–0.1 mg/kg/dose; begin with small dose, increase prn. Adults: 1.25–2.5 mg IV or 2.5–10 mg IM.	IV, IM.	Potent antiemetic. Sedative effects are prominent. Tachycardia and hypotension secondary to vasodilatation is common.

Epinephrine	*Asystole, bradycardia:* 0.01 mg/kg (0.1 cc/kg of 1:10,000 solution) q3–5 min until rhythm restored. Neonatal resuscitation dose: 0.01–0.03 mg/kg/dose.	IV; ETT.	ETT dose may need to be 2–3 times the IV dose.
	Anaphylaxis: 0.01 mg/kg, maximum single dose 0.4–0.5 mg. Usually given as 0.01 cc/kg of 1:1,000 solution SC; 0.1 cc/kg of 1:10,000 solution IV used when circulation is impaired. May repeat dose q15–20min.	SC, IV.	
	Asthma, bronchospasm: 0.01 mg/kg SC (0.01 cc/kg of 1:1,000 solution). Maximum dose 0.4–0.5 mg (0.4–0.5 cc). SC Terbutaline or aerosolized β_2-agonist is preferable.	SC.	Monitor heart rate and rhythm.
	Hypotension: 0.05–1.0 μg/kg/min by continuous infusion.	IV.	See Appendix II (pp. 431, 432) for preparation and administration.
Epinephrine, racemic (Vaponefrin, microNefrin)	*Upper airway obstruction:* 0.25–0.5 cc of 2.25% solution mixed with NS solution to 2–3 mL total. Administer over 10–15 min. Repeat q4–6h; administer up to q15–30min in emergency.	Aerosol.	Monitor heart rate and rhythm.

(Continued.)

Nonantibiotic Drugs* (cont'd.).

Name	Dose	Route	Notes
Ethacrynic acid (Edecrin)	1 mg/kg/dose as a single daily dose, maximum dose 50 mg. Repeat dose is not recommended.	IV.	
Ethanol	*Antidote for poisoning:* IV therapy: 0.7 g/kg loading dose; follow with 110 mg/kg/hr to maintain EtOH level 50–100 mg/dL. Or po therapy: 400–500 mg/kg q4–5h.	IV, po.	Avoid EtOH concentrations >10% in peripheral veins. ≥20-gauge IVs are preferred because of the high osmolality of EtOH.
Fentanyl (Sublimaze)	1–3 μg/kg/dose q½–lh. Tolerance develops rapidly on chronic use and patient may require 5–10 μg/kg/dose.	IM, IV.	Rapid IV injection may cause apnea and chest wall rigidity that prevents respiratory movements; latter may be treated with naloxone or neuromuscular blocker (i.e., pancuronium or vecuronium; intubation, ventilation required when latter drugs are used).
Furosemide (Lasix)	Start at 0.5 mg/kg/dose IV q6–24h; usual maximum dose is 6 mg/kg/day. Start oral dose at 1–2 mg/kg/dose q6–24h.	IV, IM, po.	Oral bioavailability averages 50%, but a range of 13%–100% has been reported.

Glucagon	Neonates: 0.03 mg/kg, up to a maximum of 0.5 mg. Children: 0.1 mg/kg, maximum dose 1 mg; repeat dose q20min prn.	IM, IV.	
Heparin	*Heparinization:* 50–100 units/kg q4–6h; or 50–100 units/kg bolus followed by continuous infusion of 15–25 units/kg/hr. Titrate to achieve PTT 1.5–2.5 times control. *Heparinized IV solutions for lines (e.g., arterial, CVP) running ≤5 mL/hr:* 0.5–1.0 units heparin/mL. *Heparin flush solutions to "lock" IV lines:* 10–100 units heparin/mL of NS solution.	IV.	Heparin antidote: 1–1.5 mg protamine for approximately 100 units of heparin.
Hydralazine (Apresoline)	0.1–0.5 mg/kg/dose q4–6h. Up to 3.5 mg/kg/day in older infants and children.	IV.	Slow IV push over 3–5 mins; in neonates give over 15–20 min. Monitor HR and BP during administration and for 30–60 min after dose.
Hydrocortisone (Cortef, Solu-Cortef)	*Anti-inflammatory or immunosuppressive:* 0.8–4.0 mg/kg/day (25–120 mg/M^2/day) in 4 divided doses.	po, IM, IV.	

(Continued.)

Nonantibiotic Drugs* (cont'd.).

Name	Dose	Route	Notes
	Status asthmaticus: 2–5 mg/kg/dose q6h. Methylprednisolone or dexamethasone is preferred.	IV, IM.	
	Physiologic replacement (e.g., hypopituitarism, congenital adrenal hyperplasia): Maintenance dose 10–15 mg/m^2/day po in 3 divided doses.	po, IV, IM	
	Septic shock: 50 mg/kg × 1, followed by 20–50 mg/kg q6h.	IV, IM.	
Ibuprofen (Motrin, Medipren, Pediaprofen)	*Antipyretic:* 5–10 mg/kg/dose q8h.	po.	
Insulin, regular	*Diabetes mellitus:* 0.5–1.0 unit/kg/day divided into q4–6h SC injections; titrate dose.	SC.	Must closely monitor glucose. In addition, electrolytes, ECG must be closely monitored in DKA and hyperkalemia.
	Diabetic ketoacidosis (DKA): Continuous infusion: initiate at 0.1 unit/kg/hr (see p. 210).	IV.	
	Hyperkalemia: 1 unit insulin for every 3–5 g of glucose; infuse over 1–2 hr.	IV.	

Ipecac	6 mo–1 yr: 5–10 mL. 1–12 yr: 15 mL. >12 yr: 15–30 mL. May repeat dose × 1 if emesis has not occurred after 20 min.	po.	The dose should be followed with water, juice, or milk, if possible. Because activated charcoal absorbs ipecac, after ipecac is administered, activated charcoal should not be administered until after vomiting has taken place. *Precaution:* 1. Do not use ipecac in the unconscious or semicomatose patient, the convulsing patient. 2. Remove the dose with lavage if the patient has not vomited 30 min after a second dose of ipecac: Ipecac is potentially cardiotoxic in high doses.
Isoetharine (Bronkosol)	1% solution = 10 mg/ml. 0.1–0.2 mg/kg; add NS solution to 3–5 mL volume. Administer q4–6h. May be used up to q30–60min in critical situation.	Aerosol.	Monitor HR and rhythm.

(Continued.)

Nonantibiotic Drugs* (cont'd.).

Name	Dose	Route	Notes
Isoproterenol (Isuprel)	*Hypotension and/or bradycardia:* 0.05–1.0 μg/kg/min by continuous infusion. See Appendix II (p. 430).	IV.	Must be used with tremendous caution: Some patients are exquisitely sensitive to isoproterenol and will respond with profound tachycardia and possible dysrhythmias at very low doses. Therefore, start with a low dose; closely monitor HR, heart rhythm, BP, and oxygen saturation and titrate the dose according to these parameters.
	Bronchodilation (asthma) IV: 0.1–2.0 μg/kg/min by constant infusion. (see p. 51).		
	Bronchodilation (aerosol): Inhalant solution = 0.5%. 0.25 mL for infants/young children, 0.5 mL for older children; add NS solution to 3–5 mL volume. Administer by aerosol over 10–15 min.	Aerosol.	Monitor HR, rhythm, BP, and oxygen saturations closely. Stop aerosol if dysrhythmia develops.
Ketamine (Ketalar)	*Sedation:* 0.5–3.0 mg/kg/dose.	IV.	May elevate ICP, produce tachycardia and hypertension, laryngospasm. May be useful for

			facilitated intubation (see p. 413).
Labetalol (Normodyne, Trandate)	*Severe hypertension, hypertensive emergency:* Adults: Start with 20 mg IV over 2 min; follow with 20–80 mg q10–60min until desired BP is achieved; maximum total dose 300 mg. Children: Start at 0.25 mg/kg IV over 2 min; repeat prn, increase doses to a maximum of 40 mg.	IV.	Limited pediatric experience. Avoid in asthmatics because of β-blockade.
Lidocaine (Xylocaine)	*Ventricular dysrhythmia:* 1 mg/kg bolus; repeat dose prn q5–10min. Follow bolus dose with continuous IV infusion at 20–50 μg/kg/min (see Appendix II, p. 436).	IV, ETT.	Large doses of lidocaine can produce CNS toxicity, seizures. A lidocaine infusion controls dysrhythmias with a lower total lidocaine dose than do repeated lidocaine boluses; an infusion should be started as soon as possible after a bolus dose is given. An ETT dose may need to be 2–3 × higher than the IV dose.

(Continued.)

Nonantibiotic Drugs* (cont'd.).

Name	Dose	Route	Notes
Lorazepam (Ativan)	*Sedation:* 0.05–0.1 mg/kg/dose q6–12h. Usual maximum dose 2–4 mg.	po, IM, IV.	Administer by slow IV push over at least 2–5 min. It is preferable to dilute it 1:1 with sterile water, NS solution, or D_5W because it is very thick, and because small doses may have to be diluted for accurate administration. Give IM dose undiluted.
	Status epilepticus: 0.05–0.1 mg/kg; may use up to 8 mg/dose. May repeat dose × 1 if needed in 15–20 min.	IM, IV.	
Magnesium sulfate	*Cathartic:* 250 mg/kg/dose q4–6h.	po.	Do not use a magnesium cathartic in renal failure.
	Hypomagnesemia or refractory hypocalcemia: 25–50 mg/kg $MgSO_4$ q4–6h for 3–4 doses as needed. Neonates: 50–100 mg $MgSO_4$/kg q8–12h.	IV, IM.	IV administration: It is recommended that $MgSO_4$ be diluted to 10 mg/mL and administered over 1–2 hr, but it may also be given as a bolus diluted to 100 mg/mL at a maximum rate of 2–3 mg/kg/min. Monitor for hypotension or loss of deep tendon reflexes.

Mannitol (Osmitrol)	*Diuretic:* Usually begin with 0.2 g/kg over 5 min as a test dose; increase to 0.25–1.0 g/kg over 20–60 min.	IV.	Must be administered with an 0.8 μm filter. Place an indwelling bladder catheter in the patient. Massive diuresis may produce hypovolemic circulatory compromise; treat circulatory compromise with push of plasma volume expander (LR, NS solution) to restore circulation.
	Cerebral edema: 0.25–1.0 gm/kg over 5–10 min		
Meperidine (Demerol)	0.5–2.0 mg/kg/dose q3–4h.	IM, IV.	May produce respiratory depression, hypotension.
Metaproterenol (Alupent, Metaprel)	*Aerosol:* 5% inhalant solution = 50 mg/mL. 0.2–0.6 mg/kg/dose, maximum dose 15 mg; add NS solution to 3–5 mL volume. Administer by aerosol over 10–15 min.	Aerosol.	Monitor HR and rhythm during administration.
	Oral: 0.3–0.5 mg/kg/dose, maximum dose 20 mg, q6–8h.	po.	
Methylene blue	*Antidote for methemoglobinemia: 1–2 mg/kg IV over 5 min. Repeat in 20–30 min prn.*	IV.	Use 1% solution (10 mg/mL).
Methylprednisolone (Solu-Medrol)	*Anti-inflammatory or immunosuppressive:* 0.16–1.6 mg/kg/day (5–50 mg/M^2/day) in 2–4 divided doses.	IM, IV.	

(Continued.)

Nonantibiotic Drugs* (cont'd.).

Name	Dose	Route	Notes
	Status asthmaticus: 2–8 mg/kg/day in 4 divided doses. *Septic shock:* 30 mg/kg initially; controversial.		
Metoclopromide (Reglan)	*Antiemetic:* Children: 2 mg/kg. Adults: 20 mg.	IV.	Can produce extrapyramidal reactions (dystonia), which can be treated with diphenhydramine.
Midazolam (Versed)	*Sedation:* 0.1–0.2 mg/kg IV over 2–5 min or deep IM; repeat q30–60min prn. In patient with intubated airway, may alternatively follow initial dose with constant infusion at 0.05–0.1 mg/kg/hr.	IV, IM.	May produce respiratory depression, hypotension, bradycardia. Dose needs to be lowered when given in conjunction with narcotics.
Morphine sulfate	0.1–0.2 mg/kg/dose q2–4h prn. Can also be provided as a continuous IV infusion after a bolus dose. Constant infusion dose: 0.006–0.02 mg/kg/hr for neonate; 0.025–0.1 mg/kg/hr.	IM, IV, SC.	May produce respiratory depression, hypotension.
Naloxone (Narcan)	*Narcotic reversal:* 0.01 mg/kg. Usual maximum dose 0.4–0.8 mg.	IM, IV.	*Propoxyphene overdose:* Higher than usual doses of naloxone are needed to reverse toxicity.

	Acute narcotic overdose: The AAP recommends an initial dose of 0.1 mg/kg when impending respiratory failure is present, where mechanical airway support cannot be immediately provided.	IM, IV.	Because naloxone's half-life is shorter than many opiates, repeated doses or a continuous infusion of naloxone may be needed. The naloxone dose needs to be titrated against the clinical picture.
Neostigmine (Prostigmin)	*Reversal of neuromuscular blocking agent:* 0.025–0.08 mg/kg (use lowest dose for neonates) to a maximum of 5.0 mg/dose. Give as IV push. *Must give this along with atropine, 0.03 mg/kg.*	IV.	A partial antidote is atropine 0.01–0.04 mg/kg.
Nitroprusside (Nipride)	0.5–8.0 μg/kg/min as constant IV infusion.	IV.	See Appendix II (p. 435) for preparation and administration. Manufacturer recommends dilution with only D_5W. Solution is photosensitive and must be protected from light. Freshly prepared solutions are normally brownish; solution should be discarded if it is blue, green, bright orange, or red.
Norepinephrine (Levarterenol, Levophed)	0.02–1.0 μg/kg/min by continuous IV infusion.	IV.	See Appendix II for preparation and administration.

(Continued.)

Nonantibiotic Drugs* (cont'd.).

Name	Dose	Route	Notes
Pancuronium bromide (Pavulon)	Neonates: 0.05–0.15 mg/kg q2–4h prn. Infants and children: 0.1–0.15 mg/kg/dose q1–2h prn.	IV.	Side effects include tachycardia, increased ICP, hypertension or hypotension; side effects are lessened by giving medication as slow, rather than rapid, IV push. Renal elimination is enhanced by diuretics (furosemide, theophylline); therefore, effects may be shorter in the presence of these drugs. Tachyphylaxis develops rapidly. Give sedation and/or analgesis in conjunction.
Paraldehyde	*Anticonvulsant:* 0.3 mL/kg/dose q4–6h prn.	pr.	Mix with an equal volume of olive oil or cottonseed oil.
Phenobarbital (Luminal)	*Anticonvulsant loading dose:* Neonate: 20–30 mg/kg in 1–4 doses. Infants and children: 20 mg/kg in 1–4 doses; may give additional doses of 5 mg/kg q20min prn to a maximum of 40 mg/kg/day. Oral doses are acceptable for prophylaxis.	IV, IM, po.	Maximum IV administration rate of 1–2 mg/kg/min (up to 50 mg/min) is recommended to avoid serious respiratory and myocardial depression.

	Anticonvulsant maintenance dose: 5–8 mg/kg/day in 1–2 doses.		
Phentolamine (Regitine)	Children: 0.05–0.1 mg/kg/dose; repeat q5min until hypertension is controlled, then q2–4h prn. Adults: 2.5–5.0 mg/dose; repeat q5min until hypertension is controlled, then q2–4h prn.	IM, IV.	
Phenytoin (Dilantin)	*Anticonvulsant loading dose:* 18–20 mg/kg IV in ≥1 doses.	po, IV.	*Precautions:* 1. Phenytoin crystallizes when it contacts dextrose; to prevent permanent IV occlusion, the IV must be cleared of dextrose with NS flushes before and after phenytoin administration. 2. IV administration rate should not exceed 1–2 mg/kg/min (50 mg/min) to avoid significant hypotension and dysrhythmias; monitor HR, heart rhythm and BP during IV administration. 3. Phenytoin is very caustic: Do not administer IM; IV administration may produce tremendous pain in the awake patient.
	Anticonvulsant maintenance dose: Usual dose is 5–8 mg/kg/day in 2 divided doses. Infants may require up to 2–3 mg/kg IV q6–8h to maintain therapeutic levels.	po, IV.	
	Antidysrhythmic: 1–5 mg/kg IV over 5 min; occasionally may require 10 mg/kg.	IV.	

(Continued.)

Nonantibiotic Drugs* (cont'd.).

Name	Dose	Route	Notes
Physostigmine (Antilirium)	*Antidote for overdose:* Children: 0.01–0.03 mg/kg/dose, repeat q10min prn up to a maximum total dose of 2 mg. Adults: 0.5–2.0 mg/dose, repeat q10min prn up to a maximum dose of 4 mg in 30 min.	IM, IV.	No longer recommended for tricyclic overdose because asystole has been reported. If used, however, the infusion rate should not exceed 0.01 mg/kg/min or 0.5 mg/min, whichever is slower. Pretreat with atropine or have atropine ready for bradycardia or seizures that result from parasympathomimetic stimulation
Potassium salts	*Hypokalemia:* 0.5–1.0 mEq K^+/kg/dose up to 20 mEq/dose. Administer over 60 min.	IV.	Must be infused no faster than over 1 hr. Monitor HR and rhythm on cardiac monitor during administration. Serum K^+ value should generally be <3 mEq/L. Administered solution: Dilute to 0.33 mEq K^+/mL. Recheck serum K^+ several hours after K^+ bolus infusion is completed.
Pralidoxime (2-PAM) (Protopam)	*Antidote for organophosphate poisoning:* 20–50 mg/kg/dose	IV.	Indications: tachycardia and hypertension. Rapid

	IV over 5 min or in NS solution IV over 15–20 min. Repeat in 1–2 hr, then at 10–24 hr intervals if cholinergic signs recur. Adult dose 1–2 g administered in same way.		administration can cause hypertension, laryngospasm, and muscle rigidity.
Prednisone	*Anti-inflammatory or immunosuppressive:* 0.2–1.0 mg/kg/day (or 6–30 mg/m^2/day) divided q8–24h. *Asthma exacerbation, nephrotic syndrome:* 1–2 mg/kg/day in 1–3 divided doses; may be provided qod for chronic therapy.	po.	
Procainamide (Pronestyl)	*IV therapy:* loading dose: 15 mg/kg IV (maximum 600–1,000 mg) over 30–60 min. Follow with continuous IV infusion: 2–5 mg/kg/hr (maximum total 2 g/day); prepare infusion in NS or 0.50 NS.	IV, IM.	Used for treatment of SVT, as well as ventricular dysrhythmias. Effective within minutes after IV administration. Widened QRS, prolonged QT, and PR intervals suggest toxicity. It has been associated with a lupus-like syndrome. Dilution in dextrose-containing solutions may partially inactivate procainamide.

(Continued.)

Nonantibiotic Drugs* (cont'd.).

Name	Dose	Route	Notes
	IM therapy: Alternative therapy: 20–30 mg/kg/day IM divided q3–6h; maximum dose 4 g/day.	IM.	
Promethazine (Phenergan)	*Antiemetic:* 0.25–0.5 mg/kg/dose q4–6h prn.	IM, pr.	
Propanolol (Inderal)	*Dysrhythmias:* 0.01–0.1 mg/kg/dose by slow IV push q6–8h; maximum 1 mg/dose. (po: 0.5–1.0 mg/kg/day divided q6–8h; maximum dose 60 mg/day). Cardiology consultation recommended.	IV, po.	*It is critical to note that IV and po doses of propanolol are not equivalent:* The IV dose is much more potent than the same dose given orally. Therefore, great care must be taken in calculating and administering propanolol doses. Propanolol is not recommended in the presence of renal or hepatic failure, heart failure, asthma, severe lung disease, or diabetes.
	Hypertension: po: 0.5–4.0 mg/kg/day divided q6–12h. Begin with low dose, increase slowly as needed.		
	Thyrotoxicosis: po: 2 mg/kg/day divided q6h.		

	Tetralogy spells: 0.15–0.25 mg/kg/dose slow IV push; may repeat once after 15 min. Maintenance po dose: 0.5–1.5 mg/kg/dose q6h.		
Prostaglandin E_1 (Alprostadil, PGE_1, Prostin VR)	0.01–0.4 μg/kg/min by continuous IV infusion. Usual starting dose is 0.05 μg/kg/min.	IV.	See p. 93 for preparation and administration. 10%–12% of infants become apneic; hypotension, cutaneous flushing, fever, hypokalemia, hypoglycemia, bradycardia, tachycardia, or seizures may also occur.
Pyridoxine (vitamin B_6)	*Neonatal seizures:* 50–100 mg/dose. *INH overdose:* 1 g/g INH ingested. Can give 5 g empirically if amount ingested is unknown.	IV, IM.	
Racemic epinephrine	See Epinephrine, racemic.		
Ranitidine (Zantac)	Children: 1–2 mg/kg/day IV divided q6–8h; 2–4 mg/kg/day po divided q12h. Adults: 50 mg IV q6–8h; 150 mg po bid.	po, IV.	
Sodium bicarbonate	*Resuscitation:* 0.5–1.0 mEq/kg, maximum dose 1–2 mEq/kg; repeat prn, not recommended more frequently than q10min.	IV.	

(Continued.)

Name	Dose	Route	Notes
	Metabolic acidosis: 1–2 mEq/kg over 20–60 min; reevaluate acid-base status.		
	Rapid urinary alkalinization: Start with 1–2 mEq/kg bolus over 20–30 min. Follow with IV solution: 100–150 mEq $NaHCO_3$ in 1 L D_5W; run at 1–2 times maintenance rate. If desired urine pH is not attained in 1 hr, may give another $NaHCO_3$ bolus IV; then increase the IV $NaHCO_3$ concentration and/or increase the IV rate.	IV.	Desired urine pH is usually >6.5.
Sodium chloride	*Hyponatremia:* 6 mEq Na/kg IV over 30–60 min will raise serum Na value by 10 acutely. Volumes of various Na-containing solutions that will provide 6 mEq Na/kg are as follows: 0.9 NS (154 mEq/L): 38 mL/kg; 3% NaCl (513 mEq/L): 12 mL/kg; 5% NaCl (855 mEq/L): 7 mL/kg; NaCl additive (4 mEq/mL): 1.5 mL/kg.	IV.	It is desirable to dilute the NaCl to a concentration of 0.5 mEq/mL for administration; it is acceptable to use a concentration of 2 mEq NaCl/mL for a central line. It is important to accurately calculate and administer the correct dose over an appropriate time to avoid iatrogenic problems.

Sodium polystyrene sulfonate (Kayexalate)	1 g/kg/dose po or as a retention enema q2–6h as needed.	po, pr.	Suspension contains sorbitol (powder does not), which helps prevent constipation. 1 g/kg should remove 1 mEq K^+. Retention enema should be retained for at least 60 min; elevate buttocks.
Succinylcholine (Anectine)	1–2 mg/kg/dose IV or 1–4 mg/kg/dose IM. May repeat 0.3–0.6 mg/kg/dose q5–10min prn. Premedicate with atropine 0.3 mg/kg.	IM, IV.	*Precautions:* 1. May produce bradycardia; therefore, precede with atropine. 2. May cause significant *hyperkalemia, cardiac dysrhythmias,* and should be avoided in the following patients (with): hyperkalemia; muscular dystrophies; several days to weeks after severe burns, trauma; cardiac glycoside toxicity. 3. It initially produces *muscle fasciculations,* which can be prevented by administering a small dose of a nondepolarizing agent, e.g., pancuronium, 0.01 mg/kg, before giving the succinylcholine. An alternative drug for these complex situations is high dose vecuronium.

(Continued.)

Nonantibiotic Drugs* (cont'd.).

Name	Dose	Route	Notes
Terbutaline (Brethine, Bricanyl)	po: Infants and children: 0.05–0.15 mg/kg/dose 3–4 times/day; maximum dose 5 mg/day. Adolescents, adults: 2.5–5.0 mg/dose 3–4 times/day. SC: Children <12 yr old: 0.005–0.01 mg/kg/dose, maximum dose 0.4 mg/dose q15–20 min × 3. Children >12 yr old to adults: 0.25 mg/dose, repeat in 15–30 min prn × 1 only; total dose should not exceed 0.5 mg in 4 hr.	po, SC.	Monitor HR, rhythm during SC and aerosol administration. Tremors commonly accompany administration.
	Aerosol: Use injectable preparation: 0.1% solution = 1 mg/mL. Dose 0.05–0.3 mg/kg, maximum dose 3 mg; add NS solution, if needed, to make 3–5 mL solution. Administer by aerosol over 10–15 min q4–6h. Administer up to q15–30min in critical situation.	Aerosol.	Same precautions as previously listed.

Theophylline	*Apnea:* Loading dose 5–7 mg/kg. Maintenance dose 1–2 mg/kg/dose q6–12h. *Bronchodilation: Children >12 mo:* Loading dose 5–8 mg/kg; maintenance dose: 20–24 mg/kg/day in 4 divided doses or as a continuous IV infusion. *Infants <12 mo:* Loading dose 5 mg/kg; daily mg/kg maintenance dose = age in mo + 8; give maintenance dose in 3–4 divided doses.	po, IV.	See p. 45 for more information on theophylline.
Thiopental (Pentothal)	*Emergency intubation:* 1–5 mg/kg. *Status epilepticus:* 3–9 mg/kg.	IV.	Must be used only by persons familiar with the medication, able to provide life support. Will depress cardiovascular function; therefore, it should be avoided in patient with circulatory compromise. Larger doses will produce respiratory depression, apnea; must be prepared to intubate, ventilate.
Valproic acid (Depakene, Depakote)	**Status epilepticus:** Alternative when parenteral access is not available. 20 mg/kg pr; mix with equal volume of water.	pr.	Administer as a retention enema.

(Continued.)

Nonantibiotic Drugs* (cont'd.).

Name	Dose	Route	Notes
Vasopressin (Pitressin, Aqueous)	*Diabetes insipidus:* 2.5–10 units IM/SC; repeat prn breakthrough diuresis. Another recommendation for initial dose: 0.05–0.1 unit/kg IM/SC; titrate.	IM, SC.	Effect usually lasts 2–8 hr but will vary with the individual. Administer next dose when breakthrough diuresis recurs.
Verapamil (Calan, Isoptin)	0.1–0.3 mg/kg IV (maximum of 2 mg/dose for <1 yr old or 5 mg/dose >1 yr old) over at least 2–3 min. May repeat 1–2 times after 15–30 min.	IV.	Contraindicated in the presence of any signs or symptoms of congestive heart failure. Calcium chloride, 10 mg/kg IV, has been effective in reducing (but not eliminating) cardiovascular toxicity. Follow with 0.01 mg/kg atropine and fluid if necessary.
Vecuronium (Norcuron)	0.1–0.2 mg/kg/dose q45–60min or as needed. May be given as continuous infusion at 0.05–0.1 mg/kg/hr; titrate dose.	IV.	Lower incidence of reactions associated with histamine release than pancuronium. Higher doses, up to 0.4 mg/kg, have been used effectively to initiate rapid paralysis (e.g., for intubation) without untoward effects; the duration of paralysis will, however, be correspondingly prolonged.

Vitamin K_1 (Aqua-Mephyton, Mephyton, Phytonadione)	*Vitamin K deficiency:* 1–2 mg/dose IV/IM × 1 or 2–5 mg/dose po × 1.	po, IV.	IV dose must be infused slowly, maximum rate of 1 mg/min. Menadiol *(Vitamin K_4)* IM, IV, or SC–2.5–5 mg/dose in infants, 5–10 mg/dose in children—is preferred for patients with liver disease or malabsorption.

*NS = normal saline; IV = intravenous; HR = heart rate; ETT = endotracheal tube; D_5 = 5% dextrose solution; BP = blood pressure; EtOH = alcohol; PTT = partial thromboplastin time; CVP = central venous pressure; ECG = electrocardiogram; CNS = central nervous system; ICP = intracranial pressure; LR = lactated Ringer's; AAP = American Academy of Pediatrics; SVT = supraventricular tachycardia; INH = isoniazid; UTI = urinary tract infection; D_5W = 5% aqueous dextrose solution.

Antibiotic Drugs*

Name	Dose	Route	Notes
Acyclovir (Zovirax)	15–30 mg/kg/day or 750–1,500 mg/M^2/day divided into q8h doses. Administer over 1 hr.	IV.	To minimize phlebitis: dilute to ≤7 mg/mL for infants and children, to ≤1 mg/mL for neonates.
Amphotericin B (Fungizone)	*Test dose:* 0.1 mg/kg, maximum dose 0.5 mg. If no problems arise, follow test dose with therapeutic dose.	IV.	Amphotericin must be mixed with D_5W to a concentration of 0.1 mg/mL for administration; it will precipitate in the presence of electrolytes. Administer dose over 4–6 hr. Adverse reactions are common: fever, chills, malaise, nausea, and vomiting are very common reactions; hypokalemia and renal failure are common complications. Acetaminophen and diphenhydramine should be given before administering amphotericin to minimize adverse reactions; meperidine or morphine sulfate may be administered before amphotericin or halfway through the infusion if shaking chills or pain develops.
	Therapeutic doses: 0.1–0.25 mg/kg. Increase daily (commonly by 0.1 mg/kg/day) to a maximum of 1 mg/kg/day.	IV.	

Ampicillin	*Neonates ≤7 days:* Sepsis, meningitis: 200 mg/kg/day divided q12h.	IM, IV.	Meningitis dose may be raised up to 400 mg/kg/day when used as the sole β-lactam agent against a moderately sensitive organism, such as group B *Streptococcus* or *Enterococcus*.
	Neonates >7 days: Sepsis: 200 mg/kg/day divided q6–8h. *Meningitis:* 200 mg/kg/day divided q12h.		
	Infants, children: Sepsis: 100–150 mg/kg/day divided q6h. *Meningitis:* 200–300 mg/kg/day divided q6h. Maximum daily dose: 12 g.	IM, IV.	
Cefazolin (Ancef, Kefzol)	20 mg/kg q8h. Maximum daily dose: 6 g.	IV.	Administer over minimum of 5 min. Maximum concentration 100 mg/mL.
Cefotaxime (Claforan)	*Neonates ≤7 days: Sepsis, meningitis:* 150–200 mg/kg/day divided q12h. *Neonates >7 days: Sepsis, meningitis:* 150–200 mg/kg/day divided q8h. *Infants, children: Sepsis:* 100 mg/kg/day divided q6–8h.	IM, IV.	Administer over minimum of 5 min. Maximum concentration 100 mg/mL.

(Continued.)

Antibiotic Drugs* (cont'd.).

Name	Dose	Route	Notes
	Meningitis: 200 mg/kg/day divided q6h. Maximum daily dose: 12 g.		
Ceftazidime (Fortaz, Tazidime)	*Sepsis:* 90–150 mg/kg/day divided q8h.	IV.	Most active third-generation cephalosporin active against *Pseudomonas*.
	Meningitis: 200 mg/kg/day divided q6h. Maximum daily dose: 6 g.		
Ceftriaxone (Rocephin)	*Sepsis:* 50–70 mg/kg/day divided q12h.	IM, IV.	Not recommended for use in neonates. Ceftriaxone is the least painful injected IM.
	Meningitis: 100 mg/kg/day divided q12h. Maximum daily dose 4 g.		
Cefuroxime (Zinacef)	*Sepsis:* 75–150 mg/kg/day divided q8h.	IV.	Not recommended for meningitis (better antibiotics are available). Not recommended for infants <3 mo old.
	Meningitis: 200–240 mg/kg/day divided q6–8h. Maximum daily dose 6 g.		

Chloramphenicol (Chloromycetin)	*Neonates:* ≤*7 days:* 25 mg/kg/dose q24h. >*7 days:* 25 mg/kg/dose q12h.	po, IV.	The po route is the preferred route for immediately life-threatening infections.
	Infants, children: Sepsis: 50–75 mg/kg/day divided q6h. *Meningitis:* 75–100 mg/kg/day divided q6h. Maximum dose 4 g/24h.	po, IV.	
Clindamycin (Cleocin)	*Neonates:* 15–20 mg/kg/day divided q6–8h.	IM, IV.	IV administration: maximum concentration of 12 mg/mL; administer over 20–60 min.
	Infants, children: 25–40 mg/kg/day divided q6–8h. Maximum daily dose. 4 g.		
Erythromycin	20–50 mg/kg/day divided q6h. Maximum daily dose: 4 g.	po, IV.	IV infusion: dilute to ≤5 mg/mL; infuse IV over 1 hr.
Gentamicin (Garamycin)	*Neonates* ≤*7 days:* 2.5 mg/kg IV q12h.	IM, IV.	IV infusion: dilute to ≤2 mg/mL; infuse over 30 min.
	Infants >*7 days, children:* 2.5 mg/kg q8h. Maximum daily dose: 300 mg.		
Metronidazole (Flagyl)	*Anaerobic infection:* Loading dose: 15 mg/kg; Follow with daily dose: *Neonates:* 15–30 mg/kg/day divided q12h. *Infants, children:* 30 mg/kg/day divided q6h.	po, IV.	IV Metronidazole is dispensed as a ready-to-use solution, 5 mg/mL solution; the drug should be infused without further dilution over 60 min.

(Continued.)

Antibiotic Drugs* (cont'd.).

Name	Dose	Route	Notes
Nafcillin (Unipen)	*Neonates ≤7 days:* 50 mg/kg/day divided q8h.	IV.	Maximum concentration for IV infusion: 30 mg/mL; infuse over 30–60 min.
	Neonates >7 days: 75 mg/kg/day divided q6h. *Infants, children:* 150–200 mg/kg/day divided q4–6h. Maximum daily dose: 12 g.		
Oxacillin (Bactocill, Prostaphlin)	*Neonates ≤7 days: Sepsis:* 50 mg/kg/day divided q12h. *Meningitis:* 100 mg/kg/day divided q12h.	IM, IV.	
	Neonate >7 days: Sepsis: 75 mg/kg/day divided q8h. *Meningitis:* 150 mg/kg/day divided q8h. *Infants, children:* 100–200 mg/kg/day divided q6h. Maximum daily dose: 12 g.	IM, IV.	
Penicillin G potassium (aqueous penicillin)	*Neonates: Sepsis:* 25–50,000 units/kg q8–12h. *Meningitis:* 50–100,000 units/kg q6–12h.	IM, IV.	125 mg of penicillin (G or V) is approximately equivalent to 200,000 units of penicillin G potassium.

	Infants, children: Sepsis, pneumonia: 100–200,000 units/kg/day divided q4–6h. *Meningitis:* 200–400,000 units/kg/day divided q4–6h.		
Rifampin (Rifadin, Rimactane)	*Meningitis prophylaxis: Haemophilus influenzae:* 20 mg/kg/day, up to maximum dose of 600 mg/day, qday × 4 days.	po.	
	Meningitis prophylaxis: Neisseria meningitidis: ≤1 mo old: 10 mg/kg/day divided bid × 2 days. *>1 mo old:* 20 mg/kg/day, up to maximum dose of 600 mg/day, divided bid × 2 days.	po.	
Tobramycin (Nebcin)	*Neonates ≤7 days:* 2.5 mg/kg q12h. *Infants >7 days, children:* 2–2.5 mg/kg/dose q8h. Maximum daily dose: 300 mg.	IM, IV.	For IV administration: dilute to ≤2 mg/mL; administer over 30 min.

(Continued.)

Antibiotic Drugs* (cont'd.).

Name	Dose	Route	Notes
Trimethoprim-sulfamethoxazole (TMP-SMZ, a.k.a. cotrimoxazole; Bactrim, Septra)	*Neonates:* use is relatively contraindicated. *Children >2 mo: Otitis, UTI:* 8–10 mg/kg/day of TMP divided q12h. *Serious infection:* 15–20 mg/kg/day of TMP divided q6h.	po, IV.	IV administration: the IV preparation should be diluted to a ratio of 1 mL of drug in 25 mL D_5W; administer drug IV over 60–90 min. When fluid restriction is important, the drug may be diluted to a ratio of 1 mL of drug in 15 mL D_5W.
Vancomycin (Vancocin)	*Neonates:* 15–30 mg/kg/day divided q12–24h. *Infants, children: Sepsis:* 40 mg/kg/day divided q6–12h. *Meningitis:* 50 mg/kg/day divided q6h.	IV.	Dilute to ≤5 mg/mL for infusion. Administer dose over 60 min. For patients very sensitive to histamine release: may premedicate with diphenhydramine and/or extend administration time to 90–120 min.

*NS = normal saline; IV = intravenous; HR = heart rate; ETT = endotracheal tube; D_5 = 5% dextrose solution; BP = blood pressure; EtOH = alcohol; PTT = partial thromboplastin time; CVP = central venous pressure; ECG = electrocardiogram; CNS = central nervous system; ICP = intracranial pressure; LR = lactated Ringer's; AAP = American Academy of Pediatrics; SVT = supraventricular tachycardia; INH = isoniazid; UTI = urinary tract infection; D_5W = 5% aqueous dextrose solution.

II. Sedation

A. Narcotics

1. *Morphine sulfate:*
   Morphine is the gold standard of the sedative world. The dose is 0.05–0.2 mg/kg/dose (most use 0.1 mg/kg/dose) as an IV, IM, or SC injection q1–4h. The onset of action is rapid (minutes) though the respiratory suppression may not manifest itself for 20–30 minutes. It may be given as a drip using 0.01–0.2 mg/kg/hour. Patients taking MSO_4 for extended periods of time may require much higher doses of MSO_4 to achieve the same levels of sedation/analgesia. Side effects of MSO_4 include hypotension (MSO_4 is a powerful venodilator), respiratory suppression, and histamine release.
2. *Fentanyl (sublimaze)1:*
   Fentanyl is a narcotic derivative approximately 100 times more powerful than MSO_4. The dose is 1–4 μg/kg/dose IV or IM q½–2h. Fentanyl may be used as a drip at 1–2 μg/kg/hour. The peak level is reached in 10–20 minutes. Side effects include hypotension (less than with MSO_4), bradycardia, respiratory suppression, and chest wall rigidity that interferes with the ability to breathe (this most commonly occurs after a rapid IV push; it may require use of a neuromuscular blocker or naloxone for reversal).
3. *Meperidine (Demerol):*
   Meperidine is another opiate derivative used primarily for pain relief, not sedation. The dose is 1 mg/kg/dose IV, IM, SC, or po given q3–4h as needed. The peak effect is reached in 30 min–1 hour with a 2–4 hour duration. Side effects include mood changes, decreased cardiac contractility, and lowered seizure threshold.
4. *Naloxone (Narcan):*
   Narcotics are reversible. To reverse narcotic effects, use naloxone (Narcan), 0.01 mg/kg IV, IM, or SC. NOTE: The duration of naloxone's effect is only 20 minutes; dose may be repeated prn and may be increased to 0.1 mg/kg.

B. Benzodiazepines

1. *Diazepam (Valium):*
   Diazapam is the gold standard of the benzodiazepines. Advantages of benzodiazepines are that they are antianxiety drugs and they are amnestic; they are also excellent anticonvulsants. The usual dose of diazepam is 0.1–0.3 mg/

kg/dose IV, IM (painful), or po. The peak level is reached in 15–30 minutes, and the duration of effect is 1–3 hours. Side effects include respiratory suppression, which is dramatically increased in the setting of barbiturate use and narcotic use and in younger children.

2. *Lorazepam (Ativan):*
   Lorazepam is longer acting than diazepam with essentially the same advantages and side effects. The dose is 0.05–0.1 mg/kg/dose IV, IM (painful), or po q6–8h.
3. *Midazolam (Versed):*
   Midazolam is the newest and shortest acting of the benzodiazepines. The usual dose is 0.05–0.1 mg/kg/dose IV or IM. The peak level is reached in 15 minutes, and the duration of effect is 1–3 hours. Midazolam may be given as a continuous infusion at 0.05–0.1 mg/kg/hour. The side effects are the same as those of diazepam, except for some data that indicate that the respiratory suppression of midazolam may be greater than caused by diazepam.

C. Barbiturates

1. *Thiopental (Pentothal):*
   The usual IV dose of thiopental is 2–4 mg/kg/dose. Its onset of action is immediate, and its duration of effect is short. Its side effects include myocardial depression, respiratory suppression, and arrhythmias. Thiopental is also an excellent anticonvulsant. As with all barbiturates, patients rapidly develop tolerance to it. It is generally not available for transport.
2. *Methohexital (Brevital):*
   The dose of methohexital is 0.5–1.0 mg/kg/dose IV or 30 mg/kg/dose pr. In contrast to thiopental, methohexital may actually cause seizures. Its other side effects are similar. It is not generally available for transport.
3. *Pentobarbital (Nembutal):*
   Pentobarbital is an excellent sedative given IV. The usual dose is 2–5 mg/kg/dose IV, IM, or PO. Side effects are similar to thiopental.

D. Other drugs

1. *Chloral hydrate (Noctec, Somnos):*
   Chloral hydrate's mechanism of action is unknown. Chloral hydrate is a good sedative/hypnotic with no analgesic properties and minimal respiratory depression. The dose is 20–100 mg/kg/dose po or pr; the maximum one-time dose

is 1 g. The peak level occurs in 20–60 minutes, and the duration of effect is 4–10 hours. It may cause ataxia, nausea, or vomiting; respiratory depression may occasionally occur, especially in very small or ill infants. It should be avoided in hepatic disease.

2. *Diphenhydramine (Benadryl):*
   Diphenhydramine is an antihistamine that may be used for mild sedation. It is also helpful to give diphenhydramine in conjunction with a narcotic because it potentiates the narcotic action, as well as blocks some of its histamine side effects. The dose is 0.2–1.0 mg/kg/dose IV or IM q4–6h or 5 mg/kg/day po divided into 4–6 doses.

Appendix I

MANAGEMENT SUMMARIES

APPENDIX I–1.

Pediatric Endotracheal Tubes (ETTs)

A. Laryngoscope blades for intubation:
1. Straight blade for infants and children 4–6 years: Miller 0, 1, 2; Wis-Hipple 1.5.
2. Curved blade for children >4–6 years: Macintosh 2, 3.

B. Guidelines for ETT use (Table I–1):
1. Mnemonic for ETT size in children ≥2 years:

$$\text{ETT size (mm ID)} = \frac{16 + \text{Age (yr)}}{4}$$

2. Cuffed vs. uncuffed ETT: Uncuffed ETTs should be used in children <7–8 years.
3. ETT size in upper airway obstruction: Use an *uncuffed* ETT smaller than the usual size by ≥1 mm. Use *nasal length* ETT.
4. ETT insertion distance (lip-to-tip guideline): When an appropriate-sized ETT is used and with the ETT tip in good position, the distance at the lip (in centimeters) is usually about 3 × the ETT size (which is given in millimeters).

TABLE I–1.
Guidelines for Pediatric Endotracheal Tube Use

Patient Age	Internal Diameter (mm)	Distance to Lips (cm)	Suction Catheter (F)
Newborn	3.0 uncuffed	9	6
1–6 mo	3.5 uncuffed	10	8
6–18 mo	4.0 uncuffed	11	8
1.5–2 yr	4.5 uncuffed	12	8
3–4 yr	5.0 uncuffed	14	10
5–6 yr	5.5 uncuffed	16	10
7–8 yr	6.0 uncuffed	18	10
9 yr	6.0 cuffed	18	10
10–11 yr	6.5 cuffed	20	10
12+ yr	7.0 cuffed	22	10

APPENDIX I–2

Pediatric Emergency Intubation and Ventilation Guidelines

A. **Oxygen:** Use fraction of inspired oxygen (Fio_2) 100%.

B. **Provide bag-valve-mask ventilation** until the patient's airway is intubated.

C. **Intubation:** Use **oral** route! Suction equipment is essential.
   1. A stylet may increase the chance of success in small children.
   2. Consider the use of a neuromuscular relaxant (to be used only by a person skilled in intubation). See the section on facilitated intubation (p. 443).
   3. Listen to chest after successful intubation: Right mainstem bronchus intubation is very common in children.

D. **Ventilation: Ventilate manually.**
   1. **Tidal volume (TV) and pressure:**
      a. *Chest movement* is the measure of adequacy of TV. Use whatever pressure is needed to produce good chest movement.
      b. Positive end-expiratory pressure (PEEP): Physiologic PEEP is 3–4 cm H_2O pressure.
   2. **Ventilation rate:** Suggested initial rates.
      a. Suggested minimum initial rates are used for children with neuromuscular weakness in the absence of cardiorespiratory disease (e.g., infantile botulism, child who needs intubation/ventilation/sedation for head CT scan).
      b. Initial rate should be 1.5–2 times the rates provided for children with cardiorespiratory failure, CNS failure, or significant acidosis.

c. Minimum initial ventilation rates (breaths/min):

Neonate, young infant	30–40
Toddler, preschooler	20–30
School age (preadolescent)	16–20
Adolescent:	12–16

E. Obtain arterial blood gas (ABG) values. Aim for:

1. Partial pressure of oxygen (Po_2) ≥ 80 mm Hg. Do not be concerned about very high Po_2 values.
2. pH ≥ 7.35. pH values up to 7.59 are generally safe.
   (1) Partial pressure of carbon dioxide (Pco_2) as low as 20 mm Hg is safe. Use hypocarbia to compensate for metabolic acidosis.

F. Mechanical ventilation: Optional after patient is stabilized; manual ventilation is fine.

1. Pressure ventilator: Use in infants up to 5–10 kg.
   a. Select the pressure that produces adequate chest movement.
2. Volume ventilator: Use in children >5 kg.
   a. Use *delivered* TV 10–15 mL/kg. Confirm the adequacy of TV by chest movement.
3. After adequate TV is obtained, change ventilation rate to attain desired pH and Pco_2.

G. Controlled ventilation: Mechanically providing all or most of the patient's breathing is highly advisable and desirable in most cases, even when the patient begins to make respiratory efforts.

1. If the patient continues to struggle and/or fight the ventilator, provide sedation. (First be certain that the patient is not struggling because of hypoxia or acidosis.)
   a. Sedation: morphine sulfate, diazepam, or midazolam, 0.1 mg/kg IV q1–2h as needed. More than a single agent may be needed in some patients.
   b. Neuromuscular relaxants: vecuronium or pancuronium, 0.1 mg/kg prn movement; sedation must also be provided.

APPENDIX I–3.

Pharmacologic Facilitation of Endotracheal Intubation and Special Intubation Sequences

A. General guidelines:

1. Administer a single sedative/amnestic agent:
   a. Midazolam (Versed) 0.1–0.3 mg/kg.
   b. Alternatives for specific circumstances:
      (1) Thiopental (Pentothal) 3–5 mg/kg.
      NOTE: Thiopental is contraindicated in the presence of hypotension.
      (2) Ketamine (Ketalar) 0.5–3.0 mg/kg.
      NOTE: Ketamine is contraindicated in patients with increased ICP or with ocular injury. Atropine may help diminish the increased secretions that occur with Ketamine. Ketamine is useful for intubation in patients with bronchospasm.
      (3) Diazepam (Valium) 0.2–0.3 mg/kg.
2. Administer a single muscle relaxant.
   a. Depolarizing agent:
      (1) Succinylcholine (Anectine): 1–2 mg/kg.
         (a) Precede with atropine 0.02 mg/kg (minimum dose 0.1 mg, maximum dose 0.5 mg).
         NOTE: Succinylcholine is contraindicated in the presence of neuromuscular disease, significant ocular injury, burns, hyperkalemia, or >24 hours after major injury; hyperkalemia, significant cardiac dysrhythmias may occur in these patients. Succinylcholine can also produce bradycardia; premedication with atropine decreases this risk.
   b. Nondepolarizing agent:
      (1) Vecuronium (Norcuron) 0.1–0.2 mg/kg.
      (2) Pancuronium (Pavulon) 0.1–0.15 mg/kg.
3. Optional supplemental medications.
   a. Narcotics:

(1) Fentanyl (Sublimaze) 1.0–5.0 μg/kg.
(2) Morphine sulfate 0.1–0.15 mg/kg.

B. Intubation in selected special cases.

1. **Rapid-sequence intubation:** Indicated in the patient with trauma or with possible full stomach.
   a. Sequence:
      (1) Midazolam 0.1–0.2 mg/kg.
      (2) Pancuronium 0.01 mg/kg (defasciculating dose).
      (3) Atropine 0.02 mg/kg (minimum dose 0.1 mg).
      (4) Succinylcholine 1–2 mg/kg.
   b. Alternative sequence:
      (1) Midazolam 0.1–0.2 mg/kg.
      (2) Vecuronium 0.2 mg/kg, or pancuronium 0.1–0.15 mg/kg.
2. **Head trauma (potential for increased ICP):** First hyperventilate with bag-valve-mask and FiO_2 100%.
   a. Sequence when there is no evidence of hypovolemia:
      (1) Thiopental 3–5 mg/kg.
      (2) Atropine 0.02 mg/kg (minimum dose 0.1 mg).
      (3) Succinylcholine 1–2 mg/kg.
   b. Sequence when hypovolemia is present:
      (1) Midazolam 0.1–0.3 mg/kg.
      (2) Vecuronium 0.1–0.2 mg/kg, or pancuronium 0.1–0.15 mg/kg.
      (3) Fentanyl 1–5 μg/kg.
3. **Asthma.**
   a. Sequence:
      (1) Ketamine 1–2 mg/kg.
      (2) Vecuronium 0.1–0.2 mg/kg, or pancuronium 0.1–0.15 mg/kg.
   b. Alternative sequence:
      (1) Midazolam 0.1–0.3 mg/kg.
      (2) Vecuronium 0.1–0.2 mg/kg, or pancuronium 0.1–0.15 mg/kg.
   c. May choose to add fentanyl, 1–5 μg/kg, to either sequence or immediately after intubation.

APPENDIX I–4

Essential Therapy of Shock

A. **Provide oxygen.** Intubate, ventilate as needed.
B. **Patient position:** supine; may elevate legs in hypovolemic shock.
C. **Establish vascular access** (intravenous [IV] line, intraosseous line or central line).
D. **Assess type of shock:** hypovolemic vs. cardiogenic.
   1. Use history, physical examination.
   2. Use following parameters if history and physical examination are insufficient:
      a. Hypovolemic shock: absence of gallop, jugular venous distention, hepatosplenomegaly; small heart, diminished pulmonary vessels on chest radiograph.
      b. Cardiogenic shock: gallop; jugular venous distention; hepatosplenomegaly; cardiomegaly, pulmonary vascular congestion on chest radiograph.
E. **Restore circulation:** specific therapy.
   1. Hypovolemic shock: plasma volume expander:
      a. Normal saline (NS) or lactated Ringer's (LR) solution to start; may use 5% albumin, fresh frozen plasma (FFP), blood later as needed.
      b. Start with minimum 20 mL/kg IV *push;* repeat prn. May need 40–60 mL/kg in severe hypovolemia, even more with large ongoing losses.
      c. Add inotrope therapy if large volume pushes fail to restore circulation.
   2. Cardiogenic shock: inotrope infusion (see Appendix II).
      a. For tachycardic patient: dopamine or dobutamine, 5–30 μg/kg/min. Titrate dose.
      b. For patient with normal or low heart rate: isoproterenol, 0.05–1.0 μg/kg/min. Titrate dose.
      c. Add second, third inotrope as needed if first one fails to produce desired response.
      d. May need to exceed usual recommended maximum doses if patient still fails to respond appropriately.

F. Correct negative inotropic conditions.
1. Acidosis: ventilation; sodium bicarbonate.
2. Hypoglycemia: glucose (see p. 73).
3. Hypocalcemia: calcium gluconate (see p. 74).

G. Treat underlying problem (e.g., infection).

H. Postresuscitation care:
1. Monitor patient for recurring shock.
2. Monitor patient for postresuscitation problems.

APPENDIX I–5

Postresuscitation Problems

Numerous problems may arise after resuscitation. In this outline, they are presented in the order of frequency with which they generally occur in children. As a rule, the younger the child, the more severe the insult, the greater the chance that the child is likely to encounter these difficulties; for this child, these problems are more likely to appear early in this period and be greater in severity. These are problems that one must anticipate and monitor. The management of problems that do arise is found in Chapter 4.

A. Cardiovascular system: Recurrent shock.
1. Commonly occurs in the first 12–24 hours, may continue for up to 72 hours.
2. Recurring shock is secondary to:
   a. Capillary leaks: may not peak for up to 48 hours; leaks may be massive.
   b. Myocardial dysfunction: secondary to myocardial hypoxic injury; may take up to 24–48 hours to evolve.

B. Metabolic disturbances:
1. Glucose: Variable initial findings.
   a. Hyperglycemia: Usual acute response. No therapy of it is required. BEWARE: May produce large osmotic diuresis.

b. Hypoglycemia: Glucose problem of major concern. Frequently develops in the first 6–24 hours, may be profound; can be especially severe after severe shock and in very young patients.

2. Calcium: hypocalcemia.
   a. Hypocalcemia commonly develops in the first 12–24 hours after insult; may appear earlier; can severely depress myocardial contractility.
3. Metabolic acidosis: Sign of tissue hypoxia, damage.

C. Renal dysfunction:

1. Abnormal renal metabolic values: Commonly seen, even without obvious oliguria.
   a. Elevated blood urea nitrogen (BUN) and creatinine levels are the most commonly recognized abnormalities.
   b. Elevated uric acid, phosphate, and potassium levels may be seen.
   c. Maintenance of cardiac output and urine output eventually corrects this problem.
2. Oliguria and anuria develop after severe prolonged shock.
   a. Associated with profund metabolic abnormalities; attempt to restore urine output as soon as circulation is restored.

D. Liver:

1. Elevated transaminase levels are common, nonspecific findings.
2. More severe insult: Prolonged coagulation times, hypofibrinogenemia, hypoalbuminemia, hypoglycemia.

E. Gastrointestinal (GI) tract:

1. Ileus: Present in all instances.
2. GI bleeding, sloughing of intestinal mucosa, necrosis occur after severe hypoxia.
3. For reasons listed:
   a. Keep patient NPO during acute illness, and possibly for several days thereafter.
   b. Provide antacids, H_2 blockers for bleeding.

F. Hematologic system:

1. Anemia: common for several days secondary to increased red blood cell (RBC) breakdown, depressed bone marrow, possible blood loss.
2. Thrombocytopenia: commonly occurs. Platelet count may continue to fall for as long as 1 week after a severe insult.

G. Lungs:

1. Pulmonary dysfunction: ABG values.
2. Pulmonary edema, adult respiratory distress syndrome (ARDS) can develop several days after a severe injury/illness.

H. Central nervous system:

1. Depressed level of consciousness; coma in severe illness/injury.
2. Severe hypoxic injury can produce necrosis, cerebral atrophy.

I. Muscles:

1. Weakness common. Profound weakness occurs in shock! Very important medical consideration.
   a. Respiratory support (intubation and ventilation) may provide valuable help by assuring better oxygenation/ventilation, decreasing oxygen needs.
   b. Significant muscle weakness may last for days to weeks after shock, other severe illnesses.

APPENDIX I–6

Approach in Actively Seizing Child

A. Provide Fio_2 100%, assure airway patency, assist ventilation if needed.

B. Obtain rapid-test glucose determination; provide glucose if needed.

C. Anticonvulsants:

1. First-line, rapid-acting anticonvulsants:
   a. Lorazepam 0.05–0.2 mg/kg IV or IM, **or**
   b. Diazepam 0.1–0.4 mg/kg IV or deep IM.
      (1) Highly associated with respiratory suppression in pediatric patients.

2. Long-acting and other anticonvulsants for additional seizure control.
   a. Phenobarbital 20 mg/kg IV or IM 15–20 minutes after first-line drug.
      (1) Give additional 10 mg/kg ×2 if necessary.
      (2) If the patient is already receiving phenobarbital, obtain phenobarbital level, then give 5 mg/kg IV or IM.
   b. Phenytoin 20 mg/kg IV 15–20 minutes after first-line drug. Administer drug no faster than 1–2 mg/kg/minute (maximum infusion rate 50 mg/min). Do not give IM.
      (1) Phenytoin is the drug of choice for seizures associated with head trauma.
   c. Valproic acid (Depakene) 20 mg/kg rectally. Dilute PO syrup 1:1 with water and give as a retention enema.
   d. Paraldehyde 0.3 mL/kg mixed with equal volume of cottonseed or olive oil; administer rectally.
3. NOTE: Phenobarbital and diazepam in combination can cause hypotension, respiratory depression.
4. See p. 130 for further treatment and evaluation of seizure etiology.

APPENDIX I–7

Approach in Unconscious Child

A. Causes of unconsciousness.

1. Common causes:
   a. Ingestion.
   b. Infection: Meningitis; sepsis.
   c. Head trauma.
   d. Seizure or postictal state.
   e. Hypoglycemia or diabetic ketoacidosis.

2. Less common causes:
    a. Intussusception.
    b. Other metabolic aberration, including Reye's syndrome.
    c. Intracranial catastrophe: Tumor; nontraumatic vascular accident.

B. Immediate therapy:

1. Assure airway patency. Protect the cervical spines in trauma.
2. Provide respiratory assistance, if needed.
3. Assure adequate perfusion.
4. Obtain test-strip glucose assessment.
    a. Administer glucose, 0.25–0.5 g/kg, if needed.
5. Administer naloxone, 0.01 mg/kg IM.
6. Evaluate for:
    a. Increased ICP (see p. 420).
    b. Glasgow Coma Score (see p. 437).

C. Further emergent assessment and therapy:

1. Obtain history to evaluate etiology. If the etiology is clear, refer to the relevant section for evaluation and treatment.
2. If the etiology is unclear, obtain the following studies:
    a. Serum electrolyte, glucose, BUN, creatinine, alanine aminotransferase (ALT), aspartate aminotransferase (AST), and ammonia levels.
    b. Complete blood cell (CBC) count.
    c. ABG values.
    d. Serum, urine, and gastric toxicology screen (regardless of negative history for poisons in the home).
    e. Consider blood cultures, lumbar puncture (only if the patient is *stable* and is without evidence of increased ICP), computed axial tomography (CAT) scan.
3. Consider administering broad-spectrum antibiotics.
4. Monitor the patient continuously for changes in respiratory, cardiovascular, and neurologic status.

APPENDIX I–8

Signs of Increased ICP and Impending Herniation

This situation is potentially reversible but requires *immediate* recognition and treatment. If it is left unrecognized and untreated, death or permanent neurologic devastation may result.

A. **Recognition** of increased ICP, herniation:
   1. Early clinical signs:
      a. Headache.
      b. Nausea and vomiting.
      c. Progressive alteration in mental status.
   2. Late clinical signs:
      a. Blown pupil.
      b. Posturing.
      c. Cushing's triad: Bradycardia, hypertension, abnormal respiratory pattern.
         (1) NOTE: Bradycardia initially may be the only sign.

B. **Specific treatment** of elevated ICP:
   1. Treatment of early signs of elevated ICP:
      a. Assure good respiratory function (i.e., good blood gas values).
      b. Maintain adequate perfusion: Provide volume expanders/inotropes as needed. Without blood flow to the brain, all other maneuvers are futile.
      c. If perfusion and cardiovascular status are good, keep fluid infusion to low-maintenance levels to avoid fluid overload, which will increase cerebral edema.
      d. Elevate the head of the bed 30 degrees; maintain head and neck in the midline position.
      e. Consider the appropriateness of mannitol, 0.25–1.0 g/kg, or furosemide (Lasix), 1 mg/kg, for the situation.
   2. Treatment of late signs of elevated ICP.
      a. In addition to the following measures, use the measures listed above.
      b. Intubation: Use the regimen for facilitated intubation for head trauma (p. 413).

c. Hyperventilation: Maintain P_{CO_2} between 20 and 25 mm Hg. (Continue to use F_{IO_2} 100% in the emergency setting.)
d. Use neuromuscular relaxant to paralyze the patient as needed for optimizing ventilation, ICP reduction.
e. Sedate the patient with an intubated airway:
   (1) Midazolam: 0.1 mg/kg qh, and/or
   (2) Narcotic, e.g., fentanyl, 1–5 μg/kg qh.

Appendix II

REFERENCE TABLES

APPENDIX II–1.
Pediatric Age-Size Guide

Age	Weight* kg	Weight* lb	Body Surface Area (m^2)
Newborn	3.2	7	0.22
2 mo	5	11	0.27
6 mo	8	18	0.41
9 mo	9	20	0.44
1 yr	10	22	0.47
2 yr	12	27	0.55
3 yr	14	31	0.62
4 yr	16	36	0.69
5 yr	18	40	0.74
6 yr	20	44	0.80
7 yr	22	49	0.86
8 yr	25	55	0.95
9 yr	28	62	1.00
10 yr	33	73	1.15
11 yr	36	80	1.20
12 yr	40	89	1.30
13 yr	45	100	1.40
14 yr	50	111	1.50
15 yr	55	122	1.60
16 yr	60	133	1.6(F) 1.7(M)

*Approximate weight at 50th percentile.

APPENDIX II–2.

Pediatric IV Fluid Volumes

	Maintenance Volume		Restricted (two thirds) Volume	
Patient Wt (kg)	24-Hr Total	Rate/Hr	24-Hr Total	Rate/Hr
3	300	12	200	8
4	400	16	268	11
5	500	21	335	14
6	600	25	400	16
7	700	29	469	19
8	800	33	536	22
9	900	37	600	25
10	1,000	41	670	28
12	1,100	46	737	31
14	1,200	50	800	33
16	1,300	54	871	36
18	1,400	58	938	39
20	1,500	62	1,000	41
25	1,600	66	1,072	44
30	1,700	71	1,139	47
35	1,800	75	1,200	50
40	1,900	79	1,273	53
45	2,000	83	1,340	56
50	2,100	87	1,400	58
55	2,200	91	1,474	61
60	2,300	96	1,541	64
65	2,400	100	1,600	66
70	2,500	104	1,675	69

Usual IV maintenance solutions: 5% dextrose (5%) in ¼NS solution + 20–30 mEq KCl/L or 5% dextrose in ⅓NS solution + 20–30 mEq KCl/L. *Do not use D_5W as a maintenance solution!*

APPENDIX II–3

Vasoactive Infusions

A. Instructions for vasoactive drug tables:

1. Vasoactive drug infusion doses are given in "μg/kg/min" units, whereas the drugs are provided in "mg/mL" units. To reduce the confusion that arises from converting one unit of measurement to the other during preparation of these infusions, one widely used method of weight-specific constant infusions is presented.
2. The preparations are based on the "rule of 6" and its variations. The basic steps in using this rule follow.
   a. 100 mL of infusion is prepared at a time.
   b. The number of milligrams of the vasoactive drug to be placed in this solution equals patient weight (in kilograms) × 6.
   c. When it is prepared in this manner, administering the IV infusion solution at 1 mL/hr provides 1 μg/kg/min drug. Multiples of this number hold true (e.g., running the IV at 8 mL/hr provides 8 μg/kg/min drug).
3. Using this formulation, one can prepare the appropriate infusion solution for the patient and know the appropriate IV rate to select for a chosen drug infusion dose.
   a. The rule of 6 unmodified is used for dopamine and dobutamine.
   b. The rule of 6 modified is used for other drugs:
      (1) *Epinephrine, isoproterenol, and norepinephrine drips:* The factor used for drug preparation is *0.06* rather than 6, because these drugs are very potent and require low initial doses for safety. With these preparations, 1 mL/hr = 0.01 μg/kg/min and 10 mL/hr = 0.1 μg/kg/min.
      (2) *Sodium nitroprusside:* The factor used is 3, so 1 mL/hr = 0.5 μg/kg/min and 2 mL/hr = 1.0 μg/kg/min. This factor was used so that the initial recommended doses can be provided with accuracy by most pumps and maintain IV patency.

(3) *Lidocaine:* The factor used is 12, where 1 mL/hr = 2 μg/kg/min.

4. The specific preparation for each drug is presented individually in Tables II–3, A through I. Although any infusion can be prepared from scratch from the formulas, reference to these tables can be helpful, especially when these medications are not used with regularity. An overview of the summarized information on each page is presented, and other information on use of vasoactive infusions follows.

B. Infusion preparation:

1. The formula for preparation is given for the specific drug: the rule of 6 or its variant.
2. Know the patient's weight or have the best estimate available. A good estimated weight suffices well for the emergency situation; small variations in weight matter little because the drug dose is titrated to patient response. In the critical situation, it may be expedient to select the weight from the table that is closest to the patient's known or estimated weight to expedite preparation of the solution.
3. Prepare the solution in a burette for accuracy. Clamp the volutrol, add some IV solution, then add the correct amount of vasoactive solution; add more IV solution to make a *total of 100 mL* solution. Shake the contents to mix the medication and solution, then run the vasoactive solution through the end of the IV tubing. Attach the IV tubing to the patient, and infuse the medication via a pump for accurate control of infusion rate.
4. The vasoactive drugs can be prepared with most commonly used IV solutions: combinations of dextrose, sodium chloride, and/or potassium chloride. One IV additive must be avoided—sodium bicarbonate, which inactivates medications such as dopamine. Sodium nitroprusside requires added precaution: The manufacturer recommends preparation with only 5% aqueous dextrose solution (D_5W).

C. Administration and use of infusion:

1. In most instances, begin with a dose at the low end or middle range of that recommended.
2. In critical situations, observe the response for 2 to 5 minutes. If the response is not satisfactory, increase the infusion rate and repeat the process as needed. If the response is excessive or if profound side effects such as dysrhythmias appear, the dose can be stopped or reduced. The un-

desired response will usually subside or decrease within 5 minutes of reducing the infusion rate.

3. Infusion compatibilities: When more than 1 infusion is required, all of the vasoactive infusions, even sodium nitroprusside, can be infused through a common IV site using T-connectors and stopcocks (see Drug Infusion Compatibility Chart (Appendix II–5).

D. Modification of infusion preparations after stabilization: After the patient is stabilized, the infusion preparation can be modified. Most commonly this is done because of concerns about fluid volumes. The infusion concentration can be raised by a factor of X; the infusion rate must then be decreased by the same factor X to keep the drug infusion dose unchanged.

Example: A 6 kg child is given an epinephrine drip at 30 mL/hour = 0.3 μg/kg/min. To decrease the IV rate to 6 mL/hour is to decrease the IV rate by a factor of 5; the epinephrine preparation must be increased by a factor of 5 to continue to provide 0.3 μg/kg/min. Therefore, the new preparation must contain 6 kg × 0.06 × 5 = 1.8 mg of epinephrine in 100 mL of solution; 1 mL/hour = 0.05 μg/kg/min and 6 mL/hour = 0.3 μg/kg/min.

TABLE II–3, A.

Dopamine Drip: Weight-Specific Preparations

Preparation of 100 mL dopamine drip in a burette:

1. Start with nearly empty burette.
2. Add appropriate amount (mg) of dopamine; fill with IV fluid to 100 mL. (mg dopamine = weight (kg) × 6 mg/kg)
3. Shake solution; run solution through tubing, then attach to IV line.

Patient Weight (kg)	Dopamine (mg)	Dopamine* (mL)
3.0	18.00	
5.0	30.00	
7.5	45.00	
10.0	60.00	
12.5	75.00	
15.0	90.00	
17.5	105.00	
20.0	120.00	
25.0	150.00	
30.0	180.00	
35.0	210.00	
40.0	240.00	
45.0	270.00	
50.0	300.00	
55.0	330.00	
60.0	360.00	
65.0	390.00	
70.0	420.00	

*Dopamine is available in several concentrations (40, 80, 160 mg/mL). Use the form found in your institution; fill in this column based on that information.

Dopamine drip concentration and dose:

1. Concentration: 1 mL/hr = 1 μg/kg/min.
2. Usual dose: 2–30 μg/kg/min = 2–30 mL/hr.
3. Start at 5–10 μg/kg/min = 5–10 mL/hr; titrate dose.

TABLE II–3, B.

Dobutamine Drip: Weight-Specific Preparations

Preparation of 100 mL dopamine drip in a burette:

1. Start with nearly empty burette.
2. Add appropriate amount (mg) of dobutamine; fill with IV fluid to 100 mL. (mg dobutamine = weight (kg) × 6 mg/kg)
3. Shake solution; run solution through tubing, then attach to IV line.

Patient Weight (kg)	Dobutamine (mg)	Dobutamine* (mL)
3.0	18.00	1.4
5.0	30.00	2.4
7.5	45.00	3.6
10.0	60.00	4.8
12.5	75.00	6.0
15.0	90.00	7.2
17.5	105.00	8.4
20.0	120.00	9.6
25.0	150.00	12.0
30.0	180.00	14.4
35.0	210.00	16.8
40.0	240.00	19.2
45.0	270.00	21.6
50.0	300.00	24.0
55.0	330.00	26.4
60.0	360.00	28.8
65.0	390.00	31.2
70.0	420.00	33.6

*Concentration of stock dobutamine = 12.5 mg/mL

Dobutamine drip concentration and dose:

1. Concentration: 1 mL/hr = 1 μg/kg/min.
2. Usual dose: 2–20 μg/kg/min = 2–20 mL/hr.
3. Start at 5–10 μg/kg/min = 5–10 mL/hr; titrate dose.

TABLE II–3, C.
Isoproterenol Drip: Weight-Specific Preparations

Preparation of 100 mL isoproterenol (Isuprel) drip in burette:
1. Start with nearly empty burette.
2. Add appropriate amount (mg) of isoproterenol; fill with IV fluid to 100 mL. (mg isoproterenol = weight (kg) × 0.06 mg/kg)
3. Shake solution; run solution through tubing, then attach to IV line.

Patient Weight (kg)	Isoproterenol (mg)	Isoproterenol* (mL)
3.0	0.18	0.90
5.0	0.30	1.50
7.5	0.45	2.25
10.0	0.60	3.00
12.5	0.75	3.75
15.0	0.90	4.50
17.5	1.05	5.25
20.0	1.20	6.0
25.0	1.50	7.5
30.0	1.80	9.0
35.0	2.10	10.5
40.0	2.40	12.0
45.0	2.70	13.5
50.0	3.00	15.0
55.0	3.30	16.5
60.0	3.60	18.0
65.0	3.90	19.5
70.0	4.20	21.0

*Concentration of stock isoproterenol = 0.2 mg/mL.
Isoproterenol drip concentration and dose:
1. Concentration: 1 mL/hr = 0.01 μg/kg/min.
2. Usual dose: 0.05–1.0 μg/kg/min = 5–100 mL/hr.
3. Start at 0.05–0.1 μg/kg/min = 5–10 mL/hr; titrate dose. (If patient is found to require high-dose isoproterenol, switch to *concentrated Isoproterenol drip* to reduce fluid volume; see p. 51).

TABLE II–3, D.
Epinephrine Drip: Weight-Specific Preparations

Preparation of 100 mL epinephrine solution in burette:
1. Start with nearly empty burette.
2. Add appropriate amount (mg) of epinephrine; fill with IV fluid to 100 mL. (mg epinephrine = weight (kg) × 0.06 mg/kg)
3. Shake solution; run solution through tubing, then attach to IV line.

Patient Weight (kg)	Epinephrine (mg)	Epinephrine* (mL)
3.0	0.18	0.18
5.0	0.30	0.30
7.5	0.45	0.45
10.0	0.60	0.60
12.5	0.75	0.75
15.0	0.90	0.90
17.5	1.05	1.05
20.0	1.20	1.20
25.0	1.50	1.50
30.0	1.80	1.80
35.0	2.10	2.10
40.0	2.40	2.40
45.0	2.70	2.70
50.0	3.00	3.00
55.0	3.30	3.30
60.0	3.60	3.60
65.0	3.90	3.90
70.0	4.20	4.20

*Concentration of epinephrine (1:1,000 preparation) = 1 mg/mL.
Epinephrine preparation concentration and dose:
1. Concentration: 1 mL/hr rate = 0.01 μg/kg/min.
2. Usual dose: 0.05–1.0 μg/kg/min = 5–100 mL/hr rate.
3. Start at 0.05–0.1 μg/kg/min = 5–10 mL/hr; titrate dose. (If patient requires high-dose epinephrine, switch to *concentrated epinephrine preparation* to reduce fluid volume; see p. 432).

TABLE II–3, E.
Epinephrine (Concentrated) Drip

Preparation of 100 mL concentrated epinephrine drip in burette:
1. Start with nearly empty burette.
2. Add appropriate amount (mg) of epinephrine; fill with IV fluid to 100 mL.
 (mg epinephrine = weight (kg) × 0.30 mg/kg)
3. Shake solution; run solution through tubing, then attach to IV line.

Patient Weight (kg)	Epinephrine (mg)	Epinephrine* (mL)
3.0	0.90	0.90
5.0	1.50	1.50
7.5	2.25	2.25
10.0	3.00	3.00
12.5	3.75	3.75
15.0	4.50	4.50
17.5	5.25	5.25
20.0	6.0	6.00
25.0	7.50	7.50
30.0	9.00	9.00
35.0	10.50	10.50
40.0	12.00	12.00
45.0	13.50	13.50
50.0	15.00	15.00
55.0	16.50	16.50
60.0	18.00	18.00
65.0	19.50	19.50
70.0	21.00	21.00

*Concentration of stock epinephrine (1:1,000 form) = 1 mg/mL.
Epinephrine (concentrated form) drip concentration and dose:
1. Concentration: 1 mL/hr = 0.05 μg/kg/min.
2. Usual dose: 0.05–1.0 μg/kg/min = 1–20 mL/hr.
3. Start at 0.05–0.1 μg/kg/min = 1–2 mL/hr; titrate dose.

TABLE II–3, F.
Norepinephrine (Levarterenol) Drip

Preparation of 100 mL norepinephrine drip in burette:
1. Start with nearly empty burette.
2. Add appropriate amount (mg) norepinephrine; fill with IV fluid to 100 mL. (mg norepinephrine = weight (kg) × 0.06 mg/kg)
3. Shake solution; run solution through tubing, then attach to IV line.

Patient Weight (kg)	Norepinephrine (mg)	Norepinephrine* (mL)
3.0	0.18	0.18
5.0	0.30	0.30
7.5	0.45	0.45
10.0	0.60	0.60
12.5	0.75	0.75
15.0	0.90	0.90
17.5	1.05	1.05
20.0	1.20	1.20
25.0	1.50	1.50
30.0	1.80	1.80
35.0	2.10	2.10
40.0	2.40	2.40
45.0	2.70	2.70
50.0	3.00	3.00
55.0	3.30	3.30
60.0	3.60	3.60
65.0	3.90	3.90
70.0	4.20	4.20

*Concentration of stock norepinephrine = 1 mg/mL.
Norepinephrine drip concentration and dose:
1. Concentration: 1 mL/hr = 0.01 μg/kg/min.
2. Usual dose: 0.05–1.0 μg/kg/min = 5–100 mL/hr.
3. Start at 0.05–0.1 μg/kg/min = 5–10 mL/hr; titrate dose. (If high dose is needed, see *concentrated norepinephrine drip;* see p. 434).

TABLE II–3, G.
Norepinephrine (Concentrated Drip)

Preparation of 100 mL concentrated norepinephrine drip in burette:

1. Start with nearly empty burette.
2. Add appropriate amount (mg) of norepinephrine; fill with IV fluid to 100 mL. (mg norepinephrine = weight (kg) × 0.30 mg/kg)
3. Shake solution; run solution through tubing, then attach to IV line.

Patient Weight (kg)	Norepinephrine (mg)	Norepinephrine* (mL)
3.0	0.90	0.90
5.0	1.50	1.50
7.5	2.25	2.25
10.0	3.00	3.00
12.5	3.75	3.75
15.0	4.50	4.50
17.5	5.25	5.25
20.0	6.00	6.00
25.0	7.50	7.50
30.0	9.00	9.00
35.0	10.50	10.50
40.0	12.00	12.00
45.0	13.50	13.50
50.0	15.00	15.00
55.0	16.50	16.50
60.0	18.00	18.00
65.0	19.50	19.50
70.0	21.00	21.00

*Concentration of stock norepinephrine = 1 mg/mL.

Norepinephrine (concentrated) drip concentration and dose:

1. Concentration: 1 mL/hr = 0.05 μg/kg/min.
2. Usual dose: 0.05–1.0 μg/kg/min = 1–20 mL/hr.
3. Start at 0.05–0.1 μg/kg/min = 1–2 mL/hr; titrate dose.

TABLE II–3, H.
Sodium Nitroprusside (SNP) Drip

Preparation of 100 mL SNP drip in burette:
1. IV solution for SNP drip: D_5W.
2. Start with nearly empty burette.
3. Add appropriate amount (mg) of SNP; fill with IV fluid to 100 mL.
   (mg sodium nitroprusside = weight (kg) × 3 mg/kg)
4. Shake solution; run solution through tubing, then attach to IV line.
5. Protect solution from light: cover volutrol, tubing with foil, etc.

Patient Weight (kg)	Nitroprusside (mg)	Nitroprusside* (mL)
3.0	9.0	
5.0	15.0	
7.5	22.5	
10.0	30.0	
12.5	37.5	
15.0	45.0	
17.5	52.5	
20.0	60.0	
25.0	75.0	
30.0	90.0	
35.0	105.0	
40.0	120.0	
45.0	135.0	
50.0	150.0	
55.0	165.0	
60.0	180.0	
65.0	195.0	
70.0	210.0	

*Concentration of stock sodium nitroprusside varies. After determining your facility's stock SNP, column may be filled in.

Sodium nitroprusside drip concentration and dose:
1. Concentration: 1 mL/hr = 0.5 μg/kg/min.
2. Usual dose: 0.5–7.0 μg/kg/min = 1–14 mL/hr.
3. Start at 0.5–1.0 μg/kg/min = 1–2 mL/hr; titrate dose.

TABLE II–3, I.
Lidocaine Drip: Weight-Specific Preparations

Preparation of 100 mL lidocaine drip in burette:
1. Start with nearly empty burette.
2. Add appropriate amount (mg) of lidocaine; fill with IV fluid to 100 mL.
   (mg lidocaine = weight (kg) × 12 mg/kg)
3. Shake solution; run solution through tubing, then attach to IV line.

Patient Weight (kg)	Lidocaine (mg)	Lidocaine* (mL)
3.0	36	
5.0	60	
7.5	90	
10.0	120	
12.5	150	
15.0	180	
17.5	210	
20.0	240	
25.0	300	
30.0	360	
35.0	420	
40.0	480	
45.0	540	
50.0	600	
55.0	660	
60.0	720	
65.0	780	
70.0	840	

*Concentration of stock lidocaine varies: 0.5%–20% solution = 5–200 mg lidocaine/mL. Suggest 2% or 4% (20 or 40 mg/mL) solution for lidocaine drip preparation. Fill in table column accordingly.

Lidocaine drip concentration and dose:
1. Concentration: 1 mL/hr = 2 μg/kg/min.
2. Usual dose: 20–50 μg/kg/min = 10–25 mL/hr.
3. Start lidocaine drip after a bolus dose of lidocaine. Start at 10–15 mL/hr = 20–30 μg/kg/min; titrate dose.

APPENDIX II–4

A. Glasgow Coma Scale

Activity	Score
1. Eye opening:	
a. Spontaneous	4
b. To speech	3
c. To pain	2
d. None	1
2. Best verbal response:	
a. Oriented	5
b. Confused	4
c. Inappropriate words	3
d. Incomprehensible sounds	2
e. None	1
3. Best motor response:	
a. Obeys	6
b. Localizes pain	5
c. Withdraws to pain	4
d. Abnormal flexion	3
e. Abnormal extension	2
f. None	1

B. Modified Coma Scale for Infants

Activity	Score
1. Eye opening:	
a. Spontaneous	4
b. To speech	3
c. To pain	2
d. None	1
2. Best verbal response:	
a. Coos, babbles	5
b. Irritable	4
c. Cries to pain	3
d. Moans to pain	2
e. None	1
3. Best motor response	
a. Normal movements	6
b. Withdraws to touch	5
c. Withdraws to pain	4
d. Abnormal flexion	3
e. Abnormal extension	2
f. None	1

APPENDIX II–5

Drug Infusion Compatibility

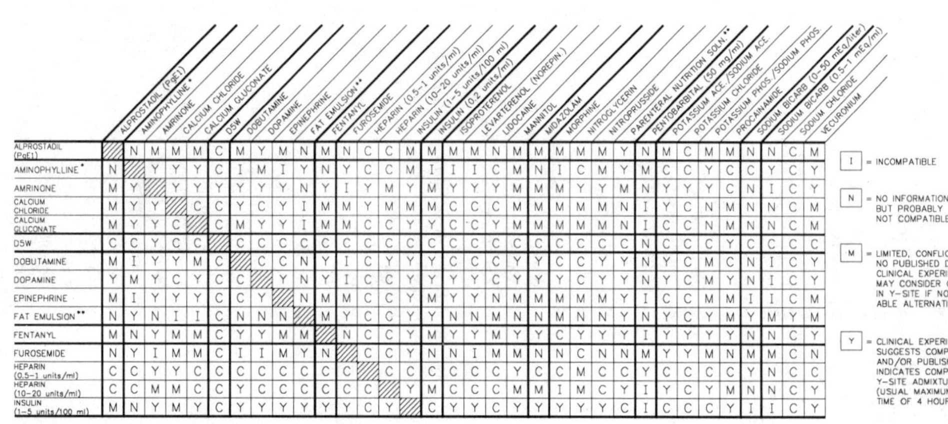

	ALPROSTADIL (PgE1)	AMINOPHYLLINE*	AMRINONE	CALCIUM CHLORIDE	CALCIUM GLUCONATE	D5W	DOBUTAMINE	DOPAMINE	EPINEPHRINE	FAT EMULSION**	FENTANYL	FUROSEMIDE	HEPARIN (0.5–1 units/ml)	HEPARIN (10–20 units/ml)	INSULIN (1–5 units/100 ml)	INSULIN (0.2 units/ml)	ISOPROTERENOL	LEVARTERENOL (NOREPIN.)	LIDOCAINE	MANNITOL	MIDAZOLAM	MORPHINE	NITROGLYCERIN	NITROPRUSSIDE	PARENTERAL NUTRITION SOLN.**	PENTOBARBITAL (50 mg/ml)	POTASSIUM ACE./SODIUM ACE.	POTASSIUM CHLORIDE	POTASSIUM PHOS./SODIUM PHOS.	PROCAINAMIDE	SODIUM BICARB (0–50 mEq/liter)	SODIUM BICARB (0.5–1 mEq/ml)	SODIUM CHLORIDE	VECURONIUM
ALPROSTADIL (PgE1)		N	M	M	M	C	M	Y	M	N	M	N	C	C	M	M	M	M	N	M	M	M	M	M	Y	N	M	C	M	M	N	N	C	M
AMINOPHYLLINE*	N		Y	Y	Y	C	I	M	I	Y	N	Y	C	C	M	I	I	I	C	M	N	I	C	M	Y	M	C	C	Y	C	C	Y	C	Y
AMRINONE	M	Y		Y	Y	Y	Y	Y	Y	N	Y	I	Y	M	Y	M	Y	Y	Y	M	M	M	Y	Y	M	N	Y	Y	Y	C	N	I	C	Y
CALCIUM CHLORIDE	M	Y	Y		C	C	Y	C	Y	I	M	M	Y	M	M	M	C	C	C	M	M	M	M	M	N	I	Y	C	N	M	N	N	C	M
CALCIUM GLUCONATE	M	Y	Y	C		C	M	Y	Y	I	M	M	C	C	Y	Y	C	C	Y	M	M	M	M	M	N	I	C	C	N	M	N	N	C	M
D5W	C	C	Y	C	C		C	C	C	C	C	C	C	C	C	C	C	C	C	C	C	C	C	C	C	N	C	C	C	Y	C	C	C	C
DOBUTAMINE	M	I	Y	Y	M	C		C	C	N	Y	I	C	Y	Y	Y	C	C	C	Y	Y	C	C	Y	Y	N	Y	C	M	C	N	I	C	Y
DOPAMINE	Y	M	Y	C	Y	C	C		Y	N	Y	I	C	C	Y	Y	Y	Y	C	Y	Y	Y	C	Y	Y	N	Y	C	M	Y	N	I	C	Y
EPINEPHRINE	M	I	Y	Y	Y	C	C	Y		N	M	M	C	C	Y	M	Y	Y	N	M	M	M	M	M	Y	I	C	C	M	M	I	I	C	M
FAT EMULSION**	N	Y	N	I	I	C	N	N	N		M	Y	C	C	Y	Y	N	N	M	N	N	M	N	N	Y	N	Y	C	Y	M	Y	M	Y	M
FENTANYL	M	N	Y	M	M	C	Y	Y	M	M		N	C	C	Y	M	Y	Y	M	Y	Y	C	Y	Y	Y	I	Y	Y	Y	Y	N	N	C	Y
FUROSEMIDE	N	Y	I	M	M	C	I	I	M	Y	N		C	C	Y	N	N	I	M	M	N	N	C	N	N	M	Y	Y	M	N	M	M	C	N
HEPARIN (0.5–1 units/ml)	C	C	Y	Y	C	C	C	C	C	C	C	C		C	C	C	C	C	C	Y	C	C	M	C	C	Y	C	C	C	C	Y	N	C	C
HEPARIN (10–20 units/ml)	C	C	M	M	C	C	Y	C	C	C	C	C	C		Y	M	C	C	C	M	M	I	M	C	Y	I	Y	C	Y	M	N	N	C	Y
INSULIN (1–5 units/100 ml)	M	N	Y	M	Y	C	Y	Y	Y	Y	Y	Y	C	Y		C	Y	Y	C	Y	Y	Y	Y	Y	C	I	C	C	C	Y	I	I	C	Y

I = INCOMPATIBLE

N = NO INFORMATION BUT PROBABLY NOT COMPATIBLE

M = LIMITED, CONFLICTING, OR NO PUBLISHED DATA OR CLINICAL EXPERIENCE; MAY CONSIDER COMPATIBLE IN Y-SITE IF NO REASONABLE ALTERNATIVE

Y = CLINICAL EXPERIENCE SUGGESTS COMPATIBLE AND/OR PUBLISHED DATA INDICATES COMPATIBLE IN Y-SITE ADMIXTURE (USUAL MAXIMUM CONTACT TIME OF 4 HOURS)

INSULIN (0.2 units/ml)	M	I	M	M	Y	C	Y	Y	M	Y	M	N	C	M	C		M	M	C	M	M	M	M	M	Y	I	Y	Y	Y	M	I	I	C	M
ISOPROTERENOL	M	I	Y	C	C	C	C	Y	Y	N	Y	N	C	C	Y	M		Y	Y	M	Y	Y	Y	Y	C	N	C	C	C	M	I	I	C	Y
LEVARTERENOL (NOREPINEPHRINE)	M	I	Y	C	C	C	C	Y	Y	N	Y	I	C	C	Y	M	Y		N	M	M	M	M	M	Y	I	Y	C	Y	M	I	I	C	Y
LIDOCAINE	N	C	Y	C	Y	C	C	C	N	M	M	M	C	C	C	C	Y	N		M	N	M	C	M	Y	M	Y	C	Y	C	Y	N	C	Y
MANNITOL	M	M	M	M	M	C	Y	Y	M	N	Y	M	Y	M	Y	M	M	M	M		Y	M	M	M	M	N	Y	Y	M	M	M	I	C	Y
MIDAZOLAM	M	N	M	M	M	C	Y	Y	M	N	Y	N	C	M	Y	M	Y	M	N	Y		C	M	Y	Y	I	Y	Y	N	M	N	N	C	Y
MORPHINE	M	I	M	M	M	C	C	Y	M	M	C	N	C	I	Y	M	Y	M	M	M	C		M	M	Y	I	Y	Y	Y	M	I	I	C	Y
NITROGLYCERIN	M	C	Y	M	M	C	C	C	M	N	Y	C	M	M	Y	M	Y	M	C	M	M	M		Y	Y	N	Y	Y	M	M	N	N	C	Y
NITROPRUSSIDE	M	M	Y	M	M	C	Y	Y	M	N	Y	N	C	C	Y	M	Y	M	M	M	Y	M	Y		Y	N	Y	Y	Y	M	N	N	C	Y
PARENTERAL NUTRITION SOLN.**	Y	Y	M	N	N	C	Y	Y	Y	Y	Y	N	C	Y	C	Y	C	Y	Y	M	Y	Y	Y	Y		N	C	C	C	M	I	I	C	Y
PENTOBARBITAL (50 mg/ml)	N	M	N	I	I	N	N	N	I	N	I	M	Y	I	I	I	N	I	M	N	I	I	N	N	N		I	I	N	N	I	I	C	N
POTASSIUM ACETATE/ SODIUM ACETATE	M	C	Y	Y	C	C	Y	Y	C	Y	Y	Y	C	Y	C	Y	C	Y	Y	Y	Y	Y	Y	Y	C	I		C	C	Y	C	Y	C	C
POTASSIUM CHLORIDE	C	C	Y	C	C	C	C	C	C	C	Y	Y	C	C	C	Y	C	C	C	Y	Y	Y	Y	Y	C	I	C		C	C	C	Y	C	C
POTASSIUM PHOSPHATE/ SODIUM PHOSPHATE	M	Y	Y	N	N	C	M	M	M	Y	Y	M	C	Y	C	Y	C	Y	Y	M	N	Y	M	Y	C	N	C	C		Y	Y	M	C	C
PROCAINAMIDE	M	C	C	M	M	Y	C	Y	M	M	Y	N	C	M	Y	M	M	M	C	M	M	M	M	M	M	N	Y	C	Y		N	N	C	M
SODIUM BICARBONATE (0–50 mEq/liter)	N	C	N	N	N	C	N	N	I	Y	N	M	Y	N	I	I	I	I	Y	M	N	I	N	N	I	I	C	C	Y	N		C	C	N
SODIUM BICARBONATE (0.5–1 mEq/ml)	N	Y	I	N	N	C	I	I	I	M	N	M	N	N	I	I	I	I	N	I	N	I	N	N	I	I	Y	Y	M	N	C		C	N
SODIUM CHLORIDE	C	C	C	C	C	C	C	C	C	Y	C	C	C	C	C	C	C	C	C	C	C	C	C	C	C	C	C	C	C	C	C	C		C
VECURONIUM	M	Y	Y	M	M	C	Y	Y	M	M	Y	N	C	Y	Y	M	Y	Y	Y	Y	Y	Y	Y	Y	N	C	C	C	M	N	N	C	Y	

C = COMPATIBLE

NOTES:

* Premixed commercial Theophylline solutions in D5W may not have the same compatibility profile as Aminophylline solutions.

** Fat Emulsion compatibility profile altered to more closely resemble that of PN solution when the two are admixed in Y-site (limited experience or data available); PN solution is assumed to contain calcium gluconate and sodium phosphate or potassium phosphate.

AUGUST 1991
FAYE LUNDERGAN, PHARM D
JUDY BROSZ, PHARM D.

APPENDIX II–6

CPR Tables

TABLE II–6, A.
Compressions and Ventilation

Age	Chest Compression Technique	Depth of Compression (inch)	Compression Rate	Compression/ Ventilation Rate*
Infant	Hand-encircling or 2-finger	0.5–1.0	100–120	5:1
Young child	Heel of 1 hand	1–1.5	80–100	5:1
Older child	1 or 2 hands	1.5–2.0	80–100	5:1

*American Heart Association recommends this compression/ventilation ratio. In actual practice, after bag-valve-mask ventilation or intubation and ventilation are instituted, compressions are commonly performed at the rate listed, whereas ventilation is provided at an independent and higher rate, as suggested on p. 27.

TABLE II–6, B.

CPR Medications*

Medication	Dose	Preparation(s)	Comments
Epinephrine	0.01 mg/kg = 0.1 mL/kg	1:10,000 = 0.1 mg/mL	Repeat q5min.
Sodium bicarbonate	1 mEq/kg = 1 mL/kg	1 mEq/mL (8.4% solution)	Use only after adequate ventilation is achieved. Dilute 1:1 with sterile water for neonates.
Atropine	0.02 mg/kg = 0.2 mL/kg (Minimum dose = 0.1 mg.)	0.1 mg/mL	Indicated for bradycardia unresponsive to oxygenation and ventilation.
Glucose	0.25 g/kg = 1 mL/kg D_{25}	D_{10} = 0.10 g/mL (10 g/100 mL) D_{25} = 0.25 g/mL (25 g/100 mL) D_{50} = 0.50 g/mL (50 g/100 mL)	May be especially necessary in the neonate and infant; higher dextrose concentrations are sclerosing to veins.

*See weight-specific CPR sheets in Table II–6, C. Each sheet provides (1) patient age and 50th percentile weight for age, (2) endotracheal tube size for age/size, and (3) weight-specific medication doses.

APPENDIX II–6C

Weight-specific Code Sheets: Suggested Use

This section contains weight-specific code sheets. Each page has an identifying patient weight at the top and the doses/sizes of medications/interventions used in resuscitation that are appropriate for a child of that weight.

Use of these sheets eliminates two major sources of difficulty in pediatric codes: the need to recall dosage formulas and the need to calculate weight-appropriate doses. When used, they permit the code leader to concentrate on assessment and interventions needed and the medication dispenser to quickly and accurately provide the appropriate medication doses by referring to the page before him or her.

A. **To use these sheets** in the manner envisioned, the following are suggested:
   1. Keep these sheets on each emergency or code cart for immediate and ready access.
   2. Know the child's weight; estimate the weight if it is not known at the time of the code. An estimated weight that is off by several kilograms rarely causes significant problems in a resuscitation.
   3. Turn to the resuscitation page with the weight closest to the patient's known or estimated weight, then use the drug doses and equipment sizes recommended. (The formulas from which these doses were derived are provided on p. 441.)

B. **Guide to using code sheets:**
   1. Top line: Identifying information.
      a. Patient weight is provided at the top.
      b. In the parentheses next to the weight is the age most children of this size will be (the 50th percentile weight for age).
      c. Endotracheal tube (ETT) recommendations: size; cuffed vs. uncuffed.
      d. Recommended delivered tidal volume (10 mL/kg).

2. Drugs.
   a. Drug doses are provided.
   b. Inotrope infusions: Preparation of infusions specific for the child's weight is given. The intravenous (IV) rate at which the drip should be run is given; the dose is to be titrated against patient response. (Specific preparation guides for each inotrope infusion can be found in Appendix II–3.)
3. Suggestions to further individualize the code sheets for your unit/institution:
   a. Many of the code medications are commercially available in differing concentrations (sodium bicarbonate, atropine, lidocaine, dopamine). Find out what preparation will be used for your codes and use these preparations consistently for codes.
   b. After identifying these preparations (concentrations), write in the corresponding *volume (milliliters)* next to the drug dose. This will further ease medication administration by eliminating the need to calculate drug volumes after the drug doses and drug preparations.

TABLE II–6, C

Emergency Medications:		2 kg (newborn)	ETT: 3.0 uncuffed Vt(del):
First-line drugs			
Epinephrine 1:10,000	0.2 mL	IV, ETT	q5min. Double dose for ETT administration.
Sodium bicarbonate	2 mEq	IV	q10min of continued arrest. Dilute 1:1 with H_2O if < 1 yr old.
Calcium chloride 10%	0.4 mL	IV	Give over 5–10 min.
Antiarrhythmics			
Atropine	0.1 mg	IV, ETT	q5min. Double dose for ETT administration.
Lidocaine	2 mg	IV, ETT	q5–10min. Double dose for ETT administration. If needed more than twice, proceed to continuous lidocaine infusion.
Lidocaine infusion	10–25 mL/hr	IV	**24 mg lidocaine** in total **100 mL fluid** Result: 1 mL/hr = 2 μg/kg/min. Dose: 20–50 μg/kg/min; titrate.
Bretylium (V. fib)	10 mg push	IV	Follow with defibrillation. If unsuccessful, give 20 mg IV, defibrillate. May repeat this step in 15 min.
Bretylium (V. tach)	10–20 mg	IV	Give over 8–10 min.
Defibrillation	4 J		Double dose if first attempt unsuccessful.
Plasma volume expanders			
LR, NS, 5% albumin, FFP, or blood	20–40 mL	IV	Give as a push, repeat prn.

Inotrope infusions			
Dopamine	5–30 mL/hr	IV	**12 mg dopamine** in total **100 mL fluid.** Result: 1 mL/hr = 1 μg/kg/min. Dose: 5–30 μg/kg/min; titrate.
Dobutamine	5–20 mL/hr	IV	**12 mg dobutamine** in total **100 mL fluid.** Result: 1 mL/hr = 1 μg/kg/min. Dose: 5–20 μg/kg/min; titrate
Isoproterenol	5–100 mL/hr	IV	**0.12 mg isoproterenol** in total **100 mL fluid.** Result: 10 mL/hr = 0.1 μg/kg/min. Dose: 0.05–1.0 μg/kg/min; titrate.
Epinephrine	5–100 mL/hr	IV	**0.12 mg epinephrine** in total **100 mL fluid.** Result: 10 mL/hr = 0.1 μg/kg/min. Dose: 0.05–1.0 μg/kg/min; titrate.
Miscellaneous			
Glucose 50%	2 mL	IV	Mix 1:1 with sterile H_2O if < 1 yr old.
Diazepam	0.2–0.6 mg	IV	q15min for status epilepticus.
Phenytoin	20–40 mg	IV	Give over 10–20 min. Precipitates in glucose.
Phenobarbital	20–40 mg	IV, IM	
Pancuronium bromide	0.2–0.4 mg	IV	prn movement.
Vecuronium	0.2–0.4 mg	IV	prn movement.
Morphine sulfate	0.2 mg	IV, IM	q1–2h prn.
Mannitol	1–2	IV	Insert bladder catheter.

(Continued.)

TABLE II–6, C (cont.)

Emergency Medications:		3 kg (newborn)	ETT: 3.5 uncuffed Vt(del):
First-line drugs			
Epinephrine 1:10,000	0.3 mL	IV, ETT	q5min. Double dose for ETT administration.
Sodium bicarbonate	3 mEq	IV	q10min of continued arrest. Dllute 1:1 with H_2O if < 1 yr old.
Calcium chloride 10%	0.6 mL	IV	Give over 5–10 min.
Antiarrhythmics			
Atropine	0.1 mg	IV, ETT	q5min. Double dose for ETT administration.
Lidocaine	3 mg	IV, ETT	q5–10 min. Double dose for ETT administration. If needed more than twice, proceed to continuous lidocaine infusion.
Lidocaine infusion	10–25 mL/hr	IV	**36 mg lidocaine** in total **100 mL fluid.** Result: 1 mL/hr = 2 μg/kg/min. Dose: 20–50 μg/kg/min; titrate.
Bretylium (V. fib)	15 mg push	IV	Follow with defibrillation. If unsuccessful, 30 mg IV, defibrillate. May repeat this step in 15 min.
Bretylium (V. tach)	15–30 mg	IV	Give over 8–10 min.
Defribrillation	6 J		Double dose if first attempt unsuccessful.
Plasma volume expanders			
LR, NS, 5% albumin, FFP, or blood	30–60 mL	IV	Give as a push, repeat prn.

Inotrope infusions			
Dopamine	5–30 mL/hr	IV	**18 mg dopamine** in total **100 mL fluid.** Result: 1 mL/hr = 1 μg/kg/min. Dose: 5–30 μg/kg/min; titrate.
Dobutamine	5–20 mL/hr	IV	**18 mg dobutamine** in total **100 mL fluid.** Result: 1 mL/hr = 1 μg/kg/min. Dose: 5–20 μg/kg/min; titrate.
Isoproterenol	5–100 mL/hr	IV	**0.18 mg isoproterenol** in total **100 mL fluid.** Result: 10 mL/hr = 0.1 μg/kg/min. Dose: 0.05–1.0 μg/kg/min; titrate.
Epinephrine	5–100 mL/hr	IV	**0.18 mg epinephrine** in total **100 mL fluid.** Result: 10 mL/hr = 0.1 μg/kg/min. Dose: 0.05–1.0 μg/kg/min; titrate.
Miscellaneous			
Glucose 50%	3 mL	IV	Mix 1:1 with sterile H_2O if < 1 yr old.
Diazepam	0.3–0.9 mg	IV	q15min for status epilepticus.
Phenytoin	30–60 mg	IV	Give over 10–20 min. Precipitates in glucose.
Phenobarbital	30–60 mg	IV, IM	
Pancuronium bromide	0.3–0.6 mg	IV	prn movement.
Vecuronium	0.3–0.6 mg	IV	prn movement.
Morphine sulfate	0.3 mg	IV, IM	q1–2h prn.
Mannitol	1.5–3 g	IV	Insert bladder catheter.

(Continued.)

TABLE II–6, C (cont.).

Emergency Medications:		4 kg (newborn–1 mo)	ETT: 3.5 uncuffed Vt(del):
First-line drugs			
Epinephrine 1:10,000	0.4 mL	IV, ETT	q5min. Double dose for ETT administration.
Sodium bicarbonate	4 mEq	IV	q10min of continued arrest. Dilute 1:1 with H_2O if < 1 yr old.
Calcium chloride 10%	0.8 mL	IV	Give over 5–10 min.
Antiarrhythmics			
Atropine	0.1 mg	IV, ETT	q5min. Double dose for ETT administration.
Lidocaine	4 mg	IV, ETT	q5–10min. Double dose for ETT administration. If needed more than twice, proceed to continuous lidocaine infusion.
Lidocaine infusion	10–25 mL/hr	IV	**48 mg lidocaine** in total **100 mL fluid.** Result: 1 mL/hr = 2 μg/kg/min. Dose: 20–50 μg/kg/min; titrate.
Bretylium (V. fib)	20 mg push	IV	Follow with defibrillation. If unsuccessful, give 40 mg IV, defibrillate. May repeat this step in 15 min.
Bretylium (V. tach)	20–40 mg	IV	Give over 8–10 min.
Defibrillation	8 J		Double dose if first attempt unsuccessful.
Plasma volume expanders			
LR, NS, 5% albumin, FFP, or blood	40–80 mL	IV	Give as a push, repeat prn.

Inotrope infusions			
Dopamine	5–30 mL/hr	IV	**24 mg dopamine** in total **100 mL fluid.** Result: 1 mL/hr = 1 μg/kg/min. Dose: 5–30 μg/kg/min; titrate.
Dobutamine	5–20 mL/hr	IV	**24 mg dobutamine** in total **100 mL fluid.** Result: 1 mL/hr = 1 μg/kg/min. Dose: 5–20 μg/kg/min; titrate.
Isoproterenol	5–100 mL/hr	IV	**0.24 mg isoproterenol** in total **100 mL fluid.** Result: 10 mL/hr = 0.1 μg/kg/min. Dose: 0.05–1.0 μg/kg/min; titrate.
Epinephrine	5–100 mL/hr	IV	**0.24 mg epinephrine** in total **100 mL fluid.** Result: 10 mL/hr = 0.1 μg/kg/min. Dose: 0.05–1.0 μg/kg/min; titrate.
Miscellaneous			
Glucose 50%	4 mL	IV	Mix 1:1 with sterile H_2O if < 1 yr old.
Diazepam	0.4–1.2 mg	IV	q15min for status epilepticus.
Phenytoin	40–80 mg	IV	Give over 10–20 min. Precipitates in glucose.
Phenobarbital	40–80 mg	IV, IM	
Pancuronium bromide	0.4–0.8 mg	IV	prn movement.
Vecuronium	0.4–0.8 mg	IV	prn movement.
Morphine sulfate	0.4 mg	IV, IM	q1–2h prn.
Mannitol	2–4 g	IV	Insert bladder catheter.

(Continued.)

TABLE II–6, C (cont.)

Emergency Medications:		5 kg (2 mo)	ET: 3.5 uncuffed Vt(del): 50 cc
First-line drugs			
Epinephrine 1:10,000	0.5 mL	IV, ETT	q5min. Double dose for ETT administration.
Sodium bicarbonate	5 mEq	IV	q10min of continued arrest. Dilute 1:1 with H_2O if < 1 yr old.
Calcium chloride, 10%	1.0 mL	IV	Give over 5–10 min.
Antiarrhythmics			
Atropine	0.1 mg	IV, ETT	q5min. Double dose for ETT administration.
Lidocaine	5 mg	IV, ETT	q5–10 min. Double dose for ETT administration. If needed more than twice, proceed to continuous lidocaine infusion.
Lidocaine infusion	10–25 mL/hr	IV	**60 mg lidocaine** in total **100 mL fluid.** Result: 1 mL/hr = 2 μg/kg/min. Dose: 20–50 μg/kg/min; titrate.
Bretylium (V. fib)	25 mg push	IV	Follow with defibrillation. If unsuccessful, give 50 mg IV, defibrillate. May repeat this step in 15 min.
Bretylium (V. tach)	25–50 mg	IV	Give over 8–10 min.
Defibrillation	10 J		Double dose if first attempt unsuccessful.
Plasma volume expanders			
LR, NS, 5% albumin, FFP, or blood	50–100 mL	IV	Give as a push, repeat prn.

Inotrope infusions			
Dopamine	5–30 mL/hr	IV	**30 mg dopamine** in total **100 mL fluid.** Result: 1 mL/hr = 1 μg/kg/min. Dose: 5–30 μg/kg/min; titrate.
Dobutamine	5–20 mL/hr	IV	**30 mg dobutamine** in total **100 mL fluid.** Result: 1 mL/hr = 1 μg/kg/min. Dose: 5–20 μg/kg/min; titrate.
Isoproterenol	5–100 mL/hr	IV	**0.30 mg Isoproterenol** in total **100 mL fluid.** Result: 10 mL/hr = 0.1 μg/kg/min. Dose: 0.05–1.0 μg/kg/min; titrate.
Epinephrine	5–100 mL/hr	IV	**0.30 mg epinephrine** in total **100 mL fluid.** Result: 10 mL/hr = 0.1 μg/kg/min. Dose: 0.05–1.0 μg/kg/min; titrate.
Miscellaneous			
Glucose 50%	5 mL	IV	Mix 1:1 with sterile H_2O if < 1 yr old.
Diazepam	0.5–1.5 mg	IV	q15min for status epilepticus.
Phenytoin	50–100 mg	IV	Give over 10–20 min. Precipitates in glucose.
Phenobarbital	50–100 mg	IV, IM	
Pancuronium bromide	0.5–1.0 mg	IV	prn movement.
Vercuronium	0.5–1.0 mg	IV	prn movement.
Morphine sulfate	0.5 mg	IV, IM	q1–2h prn.
Mannitol	2.5–5 g	IV	Insert bladder catheter.

(Continued.)

TABLE II–6, C (cont.)

Emergency Medications:		6 kg (3 mo)	ETT: 3.5 uncuffed Vt(del): 60 cc
First-line drugs			
Epinephrine 1:10,000	0.6 mL	IV, ETT	q5min. Double dose for ETT administration.
Sodium bicarbonate	6 mEq	IV	q10min of continued arrest. Dilute 1:1 with H_2O if < 1 yr old.
Calcium chloride 10%	1.2 mL	IV	Give over 5–10 min.
Antiarrhythmics			
Atropine	0.1–0.12 mg	IV, ETT	q5min. Double dose for ETT administration.
Lidocaine	6 mg	IV, ETT	q5–10min. Double dose for ETT administration. If needed more than twice, proceed to continuous lidocaine infusion.
Lidocaine infusion	10–25 mL/hr	IV	**72 mg lidocaine** in total **100 mL fluid.** Result: 1 mL/hr = 2 μg/kg/min. Dose: 20–50 μg/kg/min; titrate.
Bretylium (V. fib)	30 mg push	IV	Follow with defibrillation. If unsuccessful, give 60 mg IV, defibrillate. May repeat this step in 15 min.
Bretylium (V. tach)	30–60 mg	IV	Give over 8–10 min.
Defibrillation	12 J		Double dose if first attempt unsuccessful.
Plasma volume expanders			
LR, NS, 5% albumin, FFP, or blood	60–120 mL	IV	Give as a push, repeat prn.

Inotrope infusions			
Dopamine	5–30 mL/hr	IV	**36 mg dopamine** in total **100 mL fluid.** Result: 1 mL/hr = 1 μg/kg/min. Dose: 5–30 μg/kg/min; titrate.
Dobutamine	5–20 mL/hr	IV	**36 mg dobutamine** in total **100 mL fluid.** Result: 1 mL/hr = 1 μg/kg/min. Dose: 5–20 μg/kg/min; titrate.
Isoproterenol	5–100 mL/hr	IV	**0.36 mg isoproterenol** in total **100 mL fluid.** Result: 10 mL/hr = 0.1 μg/kg/min. Dose: 0.05–1.0 μg/kg/min; titrate.
Epinephrine	5–100 mL/hr	IV	**0.36 mg epinephrine** in total **100 mL fluid.** Result: 10 mL/hr = 0.1 μg/kg/min. Dose: 0.05–1.0 μg/kg/min; titrate.
Miscellaneous			
Glucose 50%	6 mL	IV	Mix 1:1 with sterile H_2O if < 1 yr old.
Diazepam	0.6–1.8 mg	IV	q15min for status epilepticus.
Phenytoin	60–120 mg	IV	Give over 10–20 min. Precipitates in glucose.
Phenobarbital	60–120 mg	IV, IM	
Pancuronium bromide	0.6–1.2 mg	IV	prn movement.
Vecuronium	0.6–1.2 mg	IV	prn movement.
Morphine sulfate	0.6 mg	IV, IM	q1–2h prn.
Mannitol	3–6 g	IV	Insert bladder catheter.

(Continued.)

TABLE II–6, C (cont.)

Emergency Medications:		7 kg (4–5 mo)	ETT: 3.5 uncuffed Vt(del): 70 cc
First-line drugs			
Epinephrine 1:10,000	0.7 mL	IV, ETT	q5min. Double dose for ETT administration.
Sodium bicarbonate	7 mEq	IV	q10min of continued arrest.
Calcium chloride 10%	1.4 mL	IV	Dilute 1:1 with H_2O if < 1 yr old. Give over 5–10 min.
Antiarrhythmics			
Atropine	0.1–0.14 mg	IV, ETT	q5min. Double dose for ETT administration.
Lidocaine	7 mg	IV, ETT	q5–10min. Double dose for ETT administration. If needed more than twice, proceed to continuous lidocaine infusion.
Lidocaine infusion	10–25 mL/hr	IV	**84 mg lidocaine** in total **100 mL fluid.** Result: 1 mL/hr = 2 μg/kg/min. Dose: 25–50 μg/kg/min; titrate.
Bretylium (V. fib)	35 mg push	IV	Follow with defibrillation. If unsuccessful, give 70 mg IV, defibrillate. May repeat this step in 15 min.
Bretylium (V. tach)	35–70 mg	IV	Give over 8–10 min.
Defibrillation	14 J		Double dose if first attempt unsuccessful.
Plasma volume expanders			
LR, NS, 5% albumin, FFP, or blood	70–140 mL	IV	Give as a push, repeat prn.

Inotrope infusions			
Dopamine	5–30 mL/hr	IV	**42 mg dopamine** in total **100 mL fluid.** Result: 1 mL/hr = 1 μg/kg/min. Dose: 5–30 μg/kg/min; titrate.
Dobutamine	5–20 mL/hr	IV	**42 mg dobutamine** in total **100 mL fluid.** Result: 1 mL/hr = 1 μg/kg/min. Dose: 5–20 μg/kg/min; titrate.
Isoproterenol	5–100 mL/hr	IV	**0.42 mg isoproterenol** in total **100 mL fluid.** Result: 10 mL/hr = 0.1 μg/kg/min. Dose: 0.05–1.0 μg/kg/min; titrate.
Epinephrine	5–100 mL/hr	IV	**0.42 mg epinephrine** in total **100 mL fluid.** Result: 10 mL/hr = 0.1 μg/kg/min. Dose: 0.05–1.0 μg/kg/min; titrate.
Miscellaneous			
Glucose 50%	7 mL	IV	Mix 1:1 with sterile H_2O if $<$ 1 yr old.
Diazepam	0.7–2.1 mg	IV	q15min for status epilepticus.
Phenytoin	70–140 mg	IV	Give over 10–20 min. Precipitates in glucose.
Phenobarbital	70–140 mg	IV, IM	
Pancuronium bromide	0.7–1.4 mg	IV	prn movement.
Vecuronium	0.7–1.4 mg	IV	prn movement.
Morphine sulfate	0.7 mg	IV, IM	q1–2h prn.
Mannitol	3.5–7 g	IV	Insert bladder catheter.

(Continued.)

TABLE II–6, C (cont.)

Emergency Medications:		8 kg (6–7 months)	ETT: 3.5 uncuffed Vt(del): 80 cc
First-line drugs			
Epinephrine 1:10,000	0.8 mL	IV, ETT	q5min. Double dose for ETT administration.
Sodium bicarbonate	8 mEq	IV	q10min of continued arrest. Dilute 1:1 with H_2O if < 1 yr old.
Calcium chloride 10%	1.6 mL	IV	Give over 5–10 min.
Antiarrhythmics			
Atropine	0.1–0.16 mg	IV, ETT	q5min. Double dose for ETT administration.
Lidocaine	8 mg	IV, ETT	q5–10min. Double dose for ETT administration. If needed more than twice, proceed to continuous lidocaine infusion.
Lidocaine infusion	10–25 mL/hr	IV	**96 mg lidocaine** in total **100 mL fluid.** Result: 1 mL/hr = 2 μg/kg/min. Dose: 20–50 μg/kg/min; titrate.
Bretylium (V. fib)	40 mg push	IV	Follow with defibrillation. If unsuccessful, 80 mg IV, defibrillate. May repeat this step in 15 min.
Bretylium (V. tach)	40–80 mg	IV	Give over 8–10 min.
Defibrillation	16 J		Double dose if first attempt unsuccessful.
Plasma volume expanders			
LR, NS, 5% albumin, FFP, or blood	80–160 mL	IV	Give as a push, repeat prn.

Inotrope infusions			
Dopamine	5–30 mL/hr	IV	**48 mg dopamine** in total **100 mL fluid.** Result: 1 mL/hr = 1 μg/kg/min. Dose: 5–30 μg/kg/min; titrate.
Dobutamine	5–20 mL/hr	IV	**48 mg dobutamine** in total **100 mL fluid.** Result: 1 mL/hr = 1 μg/kg/min. Dose: 5–20 μg/kg/min; titrate.
Isoproterenol	5–100 mL/hr	IV	**0.48 mg isoproterenol** in total **100 mL fluid.** Result: 10 mL/hr = 0.1 μg/kg/min. Dose: 0.05–1.0 μg/kg/min; titrate.
Epinephrine	5–100 mL/hr	IV	**0.48 mg epinephrine** in total **100 mL fluid.** Result: 10 mL/hr = 0.1 μg/kg/min. Dose: 0.05–1.0 μg/kg/min; titrate.
Miscellaneous			
Glucose 50%	8 mL	IV	Mix 1:1 with sterile H_2O if < 1 yr old.
Diazepam	0.8–2.4 mg	IV	q15min for status epilepticus.
Phenytoin	80–160 mg	IV	Give over 10–20 min. Precipitates in glucose.
Phenobarbital	80–160 mg	IV, IM	
Pancuronium bromide	0.8–1.6 mg	IV	prn movement.
Vecuronium	0.8–1.6 mg	IV	prn movement.
Morphine sulfate	0.8 mg	IV, IM	q1–2h prn.
Mannitol	4–8 g	IV	Insert bladder catheter.

(Continued.)

TABLE II–6, C (cont.)

Emergency Medications:		9 kg (8–9 mo)	ET: 4.0 uncuffed Vt(del): 90 cc
First-line drugs			
Epinephrine 1:10,000	0.9 mL	IV, ETT	q5min. Double dose for ETT administration.
Sodium bicarbonate	9 mEq	IV	q10min of continued arrest.
Calcium chloride 10%	1.8 mL	IV	Dilute 1:1 with H_2O if < 1 yr old. Give over 5–10 min.
Antiarrhythmics			
Atropine	0.1–0.18 mg	IV, ETT	q5min. Double dose for ETT administration.
Lidocaine	9 mg	IV, ETT	q5–10min. Double dose for ETT administration. If needed more than twice, proceed to continuous lidocaine infusion.
Lidocaine infusion	10–25 mL/hr	IV	**108 mg lidocaine** in total **100 mL fluid.** Result: 1 mL/hr = 2 μg/kg/min. Dose: 20–50 μg/kg/min; titrate.
Bretylium (V. fib)	45 mg push	IV	Follow with defibrillation. If unsuccessful, give 90 mg IV, defibrillate. May repeat this step in 15 min.
Bretylium (V. tach)	45–90 mg	IV	Give over 8–10 min.
Defibrillation	18 J		Double dose if first attempt unsuccessful.
Plasma volume expanders			
LR, NS, 5% albumin, FFP, or blood	90–180 mL	IV	Give as a push, repeat prn.

Inotrope infusions			
Dopamine	5–30 mL/hr	IV	**54 mg dopamine** in total **100 mL fluid.** Result: 1 mL/hr = 1 μg/kg/min. Dose: 5–30 μg/kg/min; titrate.
Dobutamine	5–20 mL/hr	IV	**54 mg dobutamine** in total **100 mL fluid.** Result: 1 mL/hr = 1 μg/kg/min. Dose: 5–20 μg/kg/min; titrate.
Isoproterenol	5–100 mL/hr	IV	**0.54 mg isoproterenol** in total **100 mL fluid.** Result: 10 mL/hr = 0.1 μg/kg/min. Dose: 0.05–1.0 μg/kg/min; titrate.
Epinephrine	5–100 mL/hr	IV	**0.54 mg epinephrine** in total **100 mL fluid.** Result: 10 mL/hr = 0.1 μg/kg/min. Dose: 0.05–1.0 μg/kg/min; titrate.
Miscellaneous			
Glucose 50%	9 mL	IV	Mix 1:1 with sterile H_2O if < 1 yr old.
Diazepam	0.9–2.7 mg	IV	q15min for status epilepticus.
Phenytoin	90–180 mg	IV	Give over 10–20 min. Precipitates in glucose.
Phenobarbital	90–180 mg	IV, IM	
Pancuronium bromide	0.9–1.8 mg	IV	prn movement.
Vecuronium	0.9–1.8 mg	IV	prn movement.
Morphine sulfate	0.9 mg	IV, IM	q1–2h prn.
Mannitol	4.5–9 g	IV	Insert bladder catheter.

(Continued.)

TABLE II–6, C (cont.)

Emergency Medications:		**10 kg (12 mo)**	ETT: 4.0 uncuffed Vt(del): 100 cc
First-line drugs			
Epinephrine 1:10,000	1.0 mL	IV, ETT	q5min. Double dose for ETT administration.
Sodium bicarbonate	10 mEq	IV	q10min of continued arrest. Dilute 1:1 with H_2O if < 1 yr old.
Calcium chloride 10%	2.0 mL	IV	Give over 5–10 min.
Antiarrhythmics			
Atropine	0.1–0.2 mg	IV, ETT	q5min. Double dose for ETT administration.
Lidocaine	10 mg	IV, ETT	q5–10min. Double dose for ETT administration. If needed more than twice, proceed to continuous lidocaine infusion.
Lidocaine infusion	10–25 mL/hr	IV	**120 mg lidocaine** in total **100 mL fluid.** Result: 1 mL/hr = 2 μg/kg/min. Dose: 20–50 μg/kg/min; titrate.
Bretylium (V. fib)	50 mg push	IV	Follow with defibrillation. If unsuccessful, give 100 mg IV, defibrillate. May repeat this step in 15 min.
Bretylium (V. tach)	50–100 mg	IV	Give over 8–10 min.
Defibrillation	20 J		Double dose if first attempt unsuccessful.
Plasma volume expanders			
LR, NS, 5% albumin, FFP, or blood	100–200 mL	IV	Give as a push, repeat prn.

Inotrope infusions			
Dopamine	5–30 mL/hr	IV	**60 mg dopamine** in total **100 mL fluid.** Result: 1 mL/hr = 1 μg/kg/min. Dose: 5–30 μg/kg/min; titrate.
Dobutamine	5–20 mL/hr	IV	**60 mg dobutamine** in total **100 mL fluid.** Result: 1mL/hr = 1 μg/kg/min. Dose: 5–20 μg/kg/min; titrate.
Isoproterenol	5–100 mL/hr	IV	**0.60 mg isoproterenol** in total **100 mL fluid.** Result: 10 mL/hr = 0.1 μg/kg/min. Dose: 0.05–1.0 μg/kg/min; titrate.
Epinephrine	5–100 mL/hr	IV	**0.60 mg epinephrine** in total **100 mL fluid.** Result: 10 mL/hr = 0.1 μg/kg/min. Dose: 0.05–1.0 μg/kg/min; titrate.
Miscellaneous			
Glucose 50%	10 mL	IV	Mix 1:1 with sterile H_2O if < 1 yr old.
Diazepam	1.0–3.0 mg	IV	q15min for status epilepticus.
Phenytoin	100–200 mg	IV	Give over 10–20 min. Precipitates in glucose.
Phenobarbital	100–200 mg	IV, IM	
Pancuronium bromide	1.0–2.0 mg	IV	prn movement.
Vecuronium	1.0–2.0 mg	IV	prn movement.
Morphine sulfate	1.0 mg	IV, IM	q1–2h prn.
Mannitol	5–10 g	IV	Insert bladder catheter.

(Continued.)

TABLE II–6, C (cont.)

Emergency Medications:		**12 kg (18 mo)**	ETT: 4.5 uncuffed Vt(del): 120 cc
First-line drugs			
Epinephrine 1:10,000	1.2 mL	IV, ETT	q5min. Double dose for ETT administration.
Sodium bicarbonate	12 mEq	IV	q10min of continued arrest. Dilute: 1:1 with H_2O if < 1 yr old.
Calcium chloride 10%	2.4 mL	IV	Give over 5–10 min.
Antiarrhythmics			
Atropine	0.12–0.24 mg	IV, ETT	q5min. Double dose for ETT administration.
Lidocaine	12 mg	IV, ETT	q5–10min. Double dose for ETT administration. If needed more than twice, proceed to continuous lidocaine infusion.
Lidocaine infusion	10–25 mL/hr	IV	**144 mg lidocaine** in total **100 mL fluid.** Result: 1 mL/hr = 2 μg/kg/min. Dose: 20–50 μg/kg/min; titrate.
Bretylium (V. fib)	60 mg push	IV	Follow with defibrillation. If unsuccessful, give 120 mg IV, defibrillate. May repeat this step in 15 min.
Bretylium (V. tach)	60–120 mg	IV	Give over 8–10 min.
Defibrillation	24 J		Double dose if first attempt unsuccessful.
Plasma volume expanders			
LR, NS, 5% albumin, FFP, or blood	120–240 mL	IV	Give as a push, repeat prn.

Inotrope infusions			
Dopamine	5–30 mL/hr	IV	**72 mg dopamine** in total **100 mL fluid.** Result: 1 mL/hr = 1 μg/kg/min. Dose: 5–30 μg/kg/min; titrate.
Obutamine	5–20 mL/hr	IV	**72 mg dobutamine** in total **100 mL fluid.** Result: 1 mL/hr = 1 μg/kg/min. Dose: 5–20 μg/kg/min; titrate.
Isoproterenol	5–100 mL/hr	IV	**0.72 mg isoproterenol** in total **100 mL fluid.** Result: 10 mL/hr = 0.1 μg/kg/min. Dose: 0.05–1.0 μg/kg/min; titrate.
Epinephrine	5–100 mL/hr	IV	**0.72 mg epinephrine** in total **100 mL fluid.** Result: 10 mL/hr = 0.1 μg/kg/min. Dose: 0.05–1.0 μg/kg/min; titrate.
Miscellaneous			
Glucose 50%	12 mL	IV	Mix 1:1 with sterile H_2O if < 1 yr old.
Diazepam	1.2–3.6 mg	IV	q15min for status epilepticus.
Phenytoin	120–240 mg	IV	Give over 10–20 min. Precipitates in glucose.
Phenobarbital	120–240 mg	IV, IM	
Pancuronium bromide	1.2–2.4 mg	IV	prn movement.
Vecuronium	1.2–2.4 mg	IV	prn movement.
Morphine sulfate	1.2 mg	IV, IM	q1–2h prn.
Mannitol	6–12 g	IV	Insert bladder catheter.

(Continued.)

TABLE II–6, C (cont.)

Emergency Medications:		**13 kg (2 yr)**	ETT: 4.5 uncuffed Vt(del): 130 cc
First-line drugs			
Epinephrine 1:10,000	1.3 mL	IV, ETT	q5min. Double dose for ETT administration.
Sodium bicarbonate	13 mEq	IV	q10min of continued arrest. Dilute 1:1 with H_2O if < 1 yr old.
Calcium chloride 10%	2.6 mL	IV	Give over 5–10 min.
Antiarrhythmics			
Atropine	0.13–0.26 mg	IV, ETT	q5min. Double dose for ETT administration.
Lidocaine	13 mg	IV, ETT	q5–10min. Double dose for ETT administration. If needed more than twice, proceed to continuous lidocaine infusion.
Lidocaine infusion	10–25 mL/hr	IV	**156 mg lidocaine** in total **100 mL fluid.** Result: 1 mL/hr = 2 μg/kg/min. Dose: 20–50 μg/kg/min; titrate.
Bretylium (V. fib)	65 mg push	IV	Follow with defibrillation. If unsuccessful, give 130 mg IV, defibrillate. May repeat this step in 15 min.
Bretylium (V. tach)	65–130 mg	IV	Give over 8–10 min.
Defibrillation	26 J		Double dose if first attempt unsuccessful.
Plasma volume expanders			
LR, NS, 5% albumin, FFP, or blood	130–260 mL	IV	Give as a push, repeat prn.

Inotrope infusions			
Dopamine	5–30 mL/hr	IV	**78 mg dopamine** in total **100 mL fluid.** Result: 1 mL/hr = 1 μg/kg/min. Dose: 5–30 μg/kg/min; titrate.
Dobutamine	5–20 mL/hr	IV	**78 mg dobutamine** in total **100 mL fluid.** Result: 1 mL/hr = 1 μg/kg/min. Dose: 5–20 μg/kg/min; titrate.
Isoproterenol	5–100 mL/hr	IV	**0.78 mg isoproterenol** in total **100 mL fluid.** Result: 10 mL/hr = 0.1 μg/kg/min. Dose: 0.05–1.0 μg/kg/min; titrate.
Epinephrine	5–100 mL/hr	IV	**0.78 mg epinephrine** in total **100 mL fluid.** Result: 10 mL/hr = 0.1 μg/kg/min. Dose: 0.05–1.0 μg/kg/min; titrate.
Miscellaneous			
Glucose 50%	13 mL	IV	Mix 1:1 with sterile H_2O if < 1 yr old.
Diazepam	1.3–3.9 mg	IV	q15min for status epilepticus.
Phenytoin	130–260 mg	IV	Give over 10–20 min. Precipitates in glucose.
Phenobarbital	130–260 mg	IV, IM	
Pancuronium bromide	1.3–2.5 mg	IV	prn movement.
Vecuronium	1.3–2.5 mg	IV	prn movement.
Morphine sulfate	1.3 mg	IV, IM	q1–2h prn.
Mannitol	6.5–13 g	IV	Insert bladder catheter.

(Continued.)

TABLE II–6, C (cont.)

Emergency Medications:		15 kg (3 yr)	ETT: 4.5 uncuffed Vt(del): 150 cc
First-line drugs			
Epinephrine 1:10,000	1.5 mL	IV, ETT	q5min. Double dose for ETT administration.
Sodium bicarbonate	15 mEq	IV	q10min of continued arrest. Dilute 1:1 with H_2O if < 1 yr old.
Calcium chloride 10%	3.0 mL	IV	Give over 5–10 min.
Antiarrhythmics			
Atropine	0.15–0.3 mg	IV, ETT	q5min. Double dose for ETT administration.
Lidocaine	15 mg	IV, ETT	q5–10min. Double dose for ETT administration. If needed more than twice, proceed to continuous lidocaine infusion.
Lidocaine infusion			**180 mg lidocaine** in total **100 mL fluid.** Result: 1 mL/hr = 2 μg/kg/min. Dose: 20–50 μg/kg/min; titrate.
Bretylium (V. fib)	75 mg push	IV	Follow with defibrillation. If unsuccessful, give 150 mg IV, defibrillate. May repeat this step in 15 min.
Bretylium (V. tach)	75–150 mg	IV	Give over 8–10 min.
Defibrillation	30 J		Double dose if first attempt unsuccessful.
Plasma volume expanders			
LR, NS, 5% albumin, FFP, or blood	150–300 mL	IV	Give as a push, repeat prn.

Inotrope infusions			
Dopamine	5–30 mL/hr	IV	**90 mg dopamine** in total **100 mL fluid.** Result: 1 mL/hr = 1 μg/kg/min. Dose: 5–30 μg/kg/min; titrate.
Dobutamine	5–20 mL/hr	IV	**90 mg dobutamine** in total **100 mL fluid.** Result: 1 mL/hr = 1 μg/kg/min. Dose: 5–20 μg/kg/min; titrate.
Isoproterenol	5–100 mL/hr	IV	**0.9 mg isoproterenol** in total **100 mL fluid.** Result: 10 mL/hr = 0.1 μg/kg/min. Dose: 0.05–1.0 μg/kg/min; titrate.
Epinephrine	5–100 mL/hr	IV	**0.9 mg epinephrine** in total **100 mL fluid.** Result: 10 mL/hr = 0.1 μg/kg/min. Dose: 0.05–1.0 μg/kg/min; titrate.
Miscellaneous			
Glucose 50%	15 mL	IV	Mix 1:1 with sterile H_2O if < 1 yr old.
Diazepam	1.5–4.5 mg	IV	q15min for status epilepticus.
Phenytoin	150–300 mg	IV	Give over 10–20 min. Precipitates in glucose.
Phenobarbital	150–300 mg	IV, IM	
Pancuronium bromide	1.5–2.5 mg	IV	prn movement.
Vecuronium	1.5–2.5 mg	IV	prn movement.
Morphine sulfate	1.5 mg	IV, IM	q1–2h prn.
Mannitol	7.5–15 g	IV	Insert bladder catheter.

(Continued.)

TABLE II–6, C (cont.)

Emergency Medications:		17 kg (4 yr)	ETT: 5.0 uncuffed Vt(del): 170 cc
First-line drugs			
Epinephrine 1:10,000	1.7 mL	IV, ETT	q5min. Double dose for ETT administration.
Sodium bicarbonate	17 mEq	IV	q10min of continued arrest. Dilute 1:1 with H_2O if < 1 yr old.
Calcium chloride 10%	3.4 mL	IV	Give over 5–10 min.
Antiarrhythmics			
Atropine	0.17–0.34 mg	IV, ETT	q5min. Double dose for ETT administration.
Lidocaine	17 mg	IV, ETT	q5–10min. Double dose for ETT administration. If needed more than twice, proceed to continuous lidocaine infusion.
Lidocaine infusion	10–25 mL/hr	IV	**204 mg lidocaine** in total **100 mL fluid.** Result: 1 mL/hr = 2 μg/kg/min. Dose: 20–50 μg/kg/min; titrate.
Bretylium (V. fib)	85 mg push	IV	Follow with defibrillation. If unsuccessful, give 170 mg IV, defibrillate. May repeat this step in 15 min.
Bretylium (V. tach)	85–170 mg	IV	Give over 8–10 min.
Defibrillation	34 J		Double dose if first attempt unsuccessful.
Plasma volume expanders			
LR, NS, 5% albumin, FFP, or blood	170–340 mL	IV	Give as a push, repeat prn.

Inotrope infusions			
Dopamine	5–30 mL/hr	IV	**102 mg dopamine** in total **100 mL fluid.** Result: 1 mL/hr = 1 μg/kg/min. Dose: 5–30 μg/kg/min; titrate.
Dobutamine	5–20 mL/hr	IV	**102 mg dobutamine** in total **100 mL fluid.** Result: 1 mL/hr = 1 μg/kg/min. Dose: 5–20 μg/kg/min; titrate.
Isoproterenol	5–100 mL/hr	IV	**1.02 mg isoproterenol** in total **100 mL fluid.** Result: 10 mL/hr = 0.1 μg/kg/min. Dose: 0.05–1.0 μg/kg/min; titrate.
Epinephrine	5–100 mL/hr	IV	**1.02 mg epinephrine** in total **100 mL fluid.** Result: 10 mL/hr = 0.1 μg/kg/min. Dose: 0.05–1.0 μg/kg/min; titrate.
Miscellaneous			
Glucose 50%	17 mL	IV	Mix 1:1 with sterile H_2O if < 1 year old.
Diazepam	1.7–5.1 mg	IV	q15min for status epilepticus.
Phenytoin	170–340 mg	IV	Give over 10–20 min. Precipitates in glucose.
Phenobarbital	170–340 mg	IV, IM	
Pancuronium bromide	1.7–2.5 mg	IV	prn movement.
Vecuronium	1.7–2.5 mg	IV	prn movement.
Morphine sulfate	1.7 mg	IV, IM	q1–2h prn.
Mannitol	8.5–17 g	IV	Insert bladder catheter.

(Continued.)

TABLE II–6, C (cont.)

Emergency Medications:		**20 kg (5 yr)**	ETT: 5.5 uncuffed Vt(del): 200 cc
First-line drugs			
Epinephrine 1:10,000	2.0 mL	IV, ETT	q5min. Double dose for ETT administration.
Sodium bicarbonate	20 mEq	IV	q10min of continued arrest. Dilute 1:1 with H_2O if < 1 yr old.
Calcium chloride 10%	4.0 mL	IV	Give over 5–10 min.
Antiarrhythmics			
Atropine	0.2–0.4 mg	IV, ETT	q5min. Double dose for ETT administration.
Lidocaine	20 mg	IV, ETT	q5–10min. Double dose for ETT administration. If needed more than twice, proceed to continuous lidocaine infusion.
Lidocaine infusion	10–25 mL/hr	IV	**240 mg lidocaine** in total **100 mL fluid.** Result: 1 mL/hr = 2 μg/kg/min. Dose: 20–50 μg/kg/min; titrate.
Bretylium (V. fib)	100 mg push	IV	Follow with defibrillation. If unsuccessful, give 200 mg IV, defibrillate. May repeat this step in 15 min.
Bretylium (V. tach)	100–200 mg	IV	Give over 8–10 min.
Defibrillation	40 J		Double dose if first attempt unsuccessful.
Plasma volume expanders			
LR, NS, 5% albumin, FFP, or blood	200–400 mL	IV	Give as a push, repeat prn.

Inotrope infusions			
Dopamine	5–30 mL/hr	IV	**120 mg dopamine** in total **100 mL fluid.** Result: 1 mL/hr = 1 μg/kg/min. Dose: 5–30 μg/kg/min; titrate.
Dobutamine	5–20 mL/hr	IV	**120 mg dobutamine** in total **100 mL fluid.** Result: 1 mL/hr = 1 μg/kg/min. Dose: 5–20 μg/kg/min; titrate.
Isoproterenol	5–100 mL/hr	IV	**1.2 mg isoproterenol** in total **100 mL fluid.** Result: 10 mL/hr = 0.1 μg/kg/min. Dose: 0.05–1.0 μg/kg/min; titrate.
Epinephrine	5–100 mL/hr	IV	**1.2 mg epinephrine** in total **100 mL fluid.** Result: 10 mL/hr = 0.1 μg/kg/min. Dose: 0.05–1.0 μg/kg/min; titrate.
Miscellaneous			
Glucose 50%	20 mL	IV	Mix 1:1 with sterile H_2O if < 1 yr old.
Diazepam	2.0–6.0 mg	IV	q15min for status epilepticus.
Phenytoin	200–400 mg	IV	Give over 10–20 min. Precipitates in glucose.
Phenobarbital	200–400 mg	IV, IM	
Pancuronium bromide	2.0–2.5 mg	IV	prn movement.
Vecuronium	2.0–2.5 mg	IV	prn movement.
Morphine sulfate	2.0 mg	IV, IM	q1–2h prn.
Mannitol	10–20 g	IV	Insert bladder catheter.

(Continued.)

TABLE II–6, C (cont.)

Emergency Medications:		**22 kg (6 yr)**	ETT: 5.5 uncuffed Vt(del): 220 cc
First-line drugs			
Epinephrine 1:10,000	2.2 mL	IV, ETT	q5min. Double dose for ETT administration.
Sodium bicarbonate	22 mEq	IV	q10min of continued arrest. Dilute 1:1 with H_2O if < 1 yr old.
Calcium chloride 10%	4.4 mL	IV	Give over 5–10 min.
Antiarrhythmics			
Atropine	0.22–0.44 mg	IV, ETT	q5min. Double dose for ETT administration.
Lidocaine	22 mg	IV, ETT	q5–10min. Double dose for ETT administration. If needed more than twice, proceed to continuous lidocaine infusion.
Lidocaine infusion	10–25 mL/hr	IV	**264 mg lidocaine** in total **100 mL fluid.** Result: 1 mL/hr = 2 μg/kg/min. Dose: 20–50 μg/kg/min; titrate.
Bretylium (V. fib)	110 mg push	IV	Follow with defibrillation. If unsuccessful, give 220 mg IV, defibrillate. May repeat this step in 15 min.
Bretylium (V. tach)	110–220 mg	IV	Give over 8–10 min.
Defibrillation	44 J		Double dose if first attempt unsuccessful.
Plasma volume expanders			
LR, NS, 5% albumin, FFP, or blood	220–440 mL	IV	Give as a push, repeat prn.

Inotrope infusions			
Dopamine	5–30 mL/hr	IV	**132 mg dopamine** in total **100 mL fluid.** Result: 1 mL/hr = 1 μg/kg/min. Dose: 5–30 μg/kg/min; titrate.
Dobutamine	5–20 mL/hr	IV	**132 mg dobutamine** in total **100 mL fluid.** Result: 1 mL/hr = 1 μg/kg/min. Dose: 5–20 μg/kg/min; titrate.
Isoproterenol	5–100 mL/hr	IV	**1.32 mg isoproterenol** in total **100 mL fluid.** Result: 10 mL/hr = 0.1 μg/kg/min. Dose: 0.05–1.0 μg/kg/min; titrate.
Epinephrine	5–100 mL/hr	IV	**1.32 mg epinephrine** in total **100 mL fluid.** Result: 10 mL/hr = 0.1 μg/kg/min. Dose: 0.05–1.0 μg/kg/min; titrate.
Miscellaneous			
Glucose 50%	22 mL	IV	Mix 1:1 with sterile H_2O if < 1 yr old.
Diazepam	2.2–6.6 mg	IV	q15min for status epilepticus.
Phenytoin	220–400 mg	IV	Give over 10–20 min. Precipitates in glucose.
Phenobarbital	220–440 mg	IV, IM	
Pancuronium bromide	2.2–2.5 mg	IV	prn movement.
Vecuronium	2.2–2.5 mg	IV	prn movement.
Morphine sulfate	2.2 mg	IV, IM	q1–2h prn.
Mannitol	11–22 g	IV	Insert bladder catheter.

(Continued.)

TABLE II–6, C (cont.)

Emergency Medications:		25 kg (7 yr)	ETT: 6.0 uncuffed Vt(del): 250 cc
First-line drugs			
Epinephrine 1:10,000	2.5 mL	IV, ETT	q5min. Double dose for ETT administration.
Sodium bicarbonate	25 mEq	IV	q10min of continued arrest. Dilute 1:1 with H_2O if < 1 yr old.
Calcium chloride 10%	5.0 mL	IV	Give over 5–10 min.
Antiarrhythmics			
Atropine	0.25–0.50 mg	IV, ETT	q5min. Double dose for ETT administration.
Lidocaine	25 mg	IV, ETT	q5–10min. Double dose for ETT administration. If needed more than twice, proceed to continuous lidocaine infusion.
Lidocaine infusion	10–25 mL/hr	IV	**300 mg lidocaine** in total **100 mL fluid.** Result: 1 mL/hr = 2 μg/kg/min. Dose: 20–50 μg/kg/min; titrate.
Bretylium (V. fib)	125 mg push	IV	Follow with defibrillation. If unsuccessful, give 250 mg IV, defibrillate. May repeat this step in 15 min.
Bretylium (V. tach)	125–250 mg	IV	Give over 8–10 min.
Defibrillation	50 J		Double dose if first attempt unsuccessful.
Plasma volume expanders			
LR, NS, 5% albumin, FFP, or blood	250–500 mL	IV	Give as a push, repeat prn.

Inotrope infusions			
Dopamine	5–30 mL/hr	IV	**150 mg dopamine** in total **100 mL fluid.** Result: 1 mL/hr = 1 μg/kg/min. Dose: 5–30 μg/kg/min; titrate.
Dobutamine	5–20 mL/hr	IV	**150 mg dobutamine** in total **100 mL fluid.** Result: 1 mL/hr = 1 μg/kg/min. Dose: 5–20 μg/kg/min; titrate.
Isoproterenol	5–100 mL/hr	IV	**1.5 mg isoproterenol** in total **100 mL fluid.** Result: 10 mL/hr = 0.1 μg/kg/min. Dose: 0.05–1.0 μg/kg/min; titrate.
Epinephrine	5–100 mL/hr	IV	**1.5 mg epinephrine** in total **100 mL fluid.** Result: 10 mL/hr = 0.1 μg/kg/min. Dose: 0.05–1.0 μg/kg/min; titrate.
Miscellaneous			
Glucose 50%	25 mL	IV	Mix 1:1 with sterile H_2O if < 1 yr old.
Diazepam	2.5–7.5 mg	IV	q15min for status epilepticus.
Phenytoin	250–450 mg	IV	Give over 10–20 min. Precipitates in glucose.
Phenobarbital	250–500 mg	IV, IM	
Pancuronium bromide	2.5 mg	IV	prn movement.
Vecuronium	2.5 mg	IV	prn movement.
Morphine sulfate	2.5 mg	IV, IM	q1–2h prn.
Mannitol	12.5–25 g	IV	Insert bladder catheter.

(Continued.)

TABLE II–6, C (cont.)

Emergency Medications:		**28 kg (8 yr)**	ETT: 6.0 cuffed Vt(del): 280 cc
First-line drugs			
Epinephrine 1:10,000	2.8 mL	IV, ETT	q5min. Double dose for ETT administration.
Sodium bicarbonate	28 mEq	IV	q10min of continued arrest. Dilute 1:1 with H_2O if < 1 yr old.
Calcium chloride 10%	5.6 mL	IV	Give over 5–10 min.
Antiarrhythmics			
Atropine	0.28–0.56 mg	IV, ETT	q5min. Double dose for ETT administration.
Lidocaine	28 mg	IV, ETT	q5–10min. Double dose for ETT administration. If needed more than twice, proceed to continuous lidocaine infusion.
Lidocaine infusion	10–25 mL/hr	IV	**336 mg lidocaine** in total **100 mL fluid.** Result: 1 mL/hr = 2 μg/kg/min. Dose: 20–50 μg/kg/min; titrate.
Bretylium (V. fib)	140 mg push	IV	Follow with defibrillation. If unsuccessful, give 280 mg IV, defibrillate. May repeat this step in 15 min.
Bretylium (V. tach)	140–280 mg	IV	Give over 8–10 min.
Defibrillation	56 J		Double dose if first attempt unsuccessful.
Plasma volume expanders			
LR, NS, 5% albumin, FFP, or blood	280–560 mL	IV	Give as a push, repeat prn.

Inotrope infusions			
Dopamine	5–30 mL/hr	IV	**168 mg dopamine** in total **100 mL fluid.** Result: 1 mL/hr = 1 μg/kg/min. Dose: 5–30 μg/kg/min; titrate.
Dobutamine	5–20 mL/hr	IV	**168 mg dobutamine** in total **100 mL fluid.** Result: 1 mL/hr = 1 μg/kg/min. Dose: 5–20 μg/kg/min; titrate.
Isoproterenol	5–100 mL/hr	IV	**1.68 mg isoproterenol** in total **100 mL fluid.** Result: 10 mL/hr = 0.1 μg/kg/min. Dose: 0.05–1.0 μg/kg/min; titrate.
Epinephrine	5–100 mL/hr	IV	**1.68 mg epinephrine** in total **100 mL fluid.** Result: 10 mL/hr = 0.1 μg/kg/min. Dose: 0.05–1.0 μg/kg/min; titrate.
Miscellaneous			
Glucose 50%	28 mL	IV	Mix 1:1 with sterile H_2O if < 1 yr old.
Diazepam	2.8–8.4 mg	IV	q15min for status epilepticus.
Phenytoin	280–500 mg	IV	Give over 10–20 min. Precipitates in glucose.
Phenobarbital	280–560 mg	IV, IM	
Pancuronium	2.8 mg	IV	prn movement.
Vecuronium	2.8 mg	IV	prn movement.
Morphine sulfate	2.8 mg	IV, IM	q1–2h prn.
Mannitol	14–28 g	IV	Insert bladder catheter.

(Continued.)

TABLE II–6, C (cont.)

Emergency Medications:		30 kg (9 yr)	ETT: 3.0 cuffed Vt(del): 300 cc
First-line drugs			
Epinephrine 1:10,000	3.0 mL	IV, ETT	q5min. Double dose for ETT administration.
Sodium bicarbonate	30 mEq	IV	q10min of continued arrest. Dilute 1:1 with sterile H_2O if $<$ 1 yr old.
Calcium chloride 10%	6.0 mL	IV	Give over 5–10 min.
Antiarrhythmics			
Atropine	0.3–0.6 mg	IV, ETT	q5min. Double dose for ETT administration.
Lidocaine	30 mg	IV, ETT	q5–10min. Double dose for ETT administration. If needed more than twice, proceed to continuous lidocaine infusion.
Lidocaine infusion	10–25 mL/hr	IV	**360 mg lidocaine** in total **100 mL fluid.** Result: 1 mL/hr = 2 μg/kg/min. Dose: 20–50 μg/kg/min; titrate.
Bretylium (V. fib)	150 mg push	IV	Follow with defibrillation. If unsuccessful, give 300 mg IV, defibrillate. May repeat this step in 15 min.
Bretylium (V. tach)	150–300 mg	IV	Give over 8–10 min.
Defibrillation	60 J		Double dose if first attempt unsuccessful.
Plasma volume expanders			
LR, NS, 5% albumin, FFP, or blood	300–600 mL	IV	Give as a push, repeat prn.

Inotrope infusions			
Dopamine	5–30 mL/hr	IV	**180 mg dopamine** in total **100 mL fluid.** Result: 1 mL/hr = 1 μg/kg/min. Dose: 5–30 μg/kg/min; titrate.
Dobutamine	5–20 mL/hr	IV	**180 mg dobutamine** in total **100 mL fluid.** Result: 1 mL/hr = 1 μg/kg/min. Dose: 5–20 μg/kg/min; titrate.
Isoproterenol	5–100 mL/hr	IV	**1.8 mg isoproterenol** in total **100 mL fluid.** Result: 10 mL/hr = 0.1 μg/kg/min. Dose: 0.05–1.0 μg/kg/min; titrate.
Epinephrine	5–100 mL/hr	IV	**1.8 mg epinephrine** in total **100 mL fluid.** Result: 10 mL/hr = 0.1 μg/kg/min. Dose: 0.05–1.0 μg/kg/min; titrate.
Miscellaneous			
Glucose 50%	30 mL	IV	Mix 1:1 with sterile H_2O if < 1 yr old.
Diazepam	3.0–9.0 mg	IV	q15min for status epilepticus.
Phenytoin	300–550 mg	IV	Give over 10–20 min. Precipitates in glucose.
Phenobarbital	300–600 mg	IV, IM	
Pancuronium	3.0 mg	IV	prn movement.
Vecuronium	3.0 mg	IV	prn movement.
Morphine sulfate	3.0 mg	IV, IM	q1–2h prn.
Mannitol	15–30 g	IV	Insert bladder catheter.

(Continued.)

TABLE II–6, C (cont.)

Emergency Medications:		**35 kg (10 yr)**	ETT: 6.5 cuffed Vt(del): 350 cc
First-line drugs			
Epinephrine 1:10,000	3.5 mL	IV, ETT	q5min. Double dose for ETT administration.
Sodium bicarbonate	35 mEq	IV	q10min of continued arrest. Dilute 1:1 with H_2O if < 1 yr old.
Calcium chloride 10%	7.0 mL	IV	Give over 5–10 min.
Antiarrhythmics			
Atropine	0.35–0.7 mg	IV, ETT	q5min. Double dose for ETT administration.
Lidocaine	35 mg	IV, ETT	q5–10min. Double dose for ETT administration. If needed more than twice, proceed to continuous lidocaine infusion.
Lidocaine infusion	10–25 mL/hr	IV	**420 mg lidocaine** in total **100 mL fluid.** Result: 1 mL/hr = 2 μg/kg/min. Dose: 20–50 μg/kg/min; titrate.
Bretylium (V. fib)	175 mg push	IV	Follow with defibrillation. If unsuccessful, give 350 mg IV, defibrillate. May repeat this step in 15 min.
Bretylium (V. tach)	175–350 mg	IV	Give over 8–10 min.
Defibrillation	70 J		Double dose if first attempt unsuccessful.
Plasma volume expanders			
LR, NS, 5% albumin, FFP, or blood	350–700 mL	IV	Give as a push, repeat prn.

Inotrope infusions			
Dopamine	5–30 mL/hr	IV	**210 mg dopamine** in total **100 mL fluid.** Result: 1 mL/hr = 1 μg/kg/min. Dose: 5–30 μg/kg/min; titrate.
Dobutamine	5–20 mL/hr	IV	**210 mg dobutamine** in total **100 mL fluid.** Result: 1 mL/hr = 1 μg/kg/min. Dose: 5–20 μg/kg/min; titrate.
Isoproterenol	5–100 mL/hr	IV	**2.1 mg isoproterenol** in total **100 mL fluid.** Result: 10 mL/hr = 0.1 μg/kg/min. Dose: 0.05–1.0 μg/kg/min; titrate.
Epinephrine	5–100 mL/hr	IV	**2.1 mg epinephrine** in total **100 mL fluid.** Result: 10 mL/hr = 0.1 μg/kg/min. Dose: 0.05–1.0 μg/kg/min; titrate.
Miscellaneous			
Glucose 50%	35 mL	IV	Mix 1:1 with sterile H_2O if < 1 yr old.
Diazepam	3.5–10 mg	IV	q15min for status epilepticus.
Phenytoin	350–600 mg	IV	Give over 10–20 min. Precipitates in glucose.
Phenobarbital	350–700 mg	IV, IM	
Pancuronium	3.5 mg	IV	prn movement.
Vecuronium	3.5 mg	IV	prn movement.
Morphine sulfate	3.5 mg	IV, IM	q1–2h prn.
Mannitol	17–35 g	IV	Insert bladder catheter.

(Continued.)

TABLE II–6, C (cont.)

Emergency Medications:		40 kg (11 yr)	ETT: 6.5 cuffed Vt(del): 400 cc
First-line drugs			
Epinephrine 1:10,000	4.0 mL	IV, ETT	q5min. Double dose for ETT administration.
Sodium bicarbonate	40 mEq	IV	q10min of continued arrest. Dilute 1:1 with H_2O if < 1 yr old.
Calcium chloride 10%	8.0 mL	IV	Give over 5–10 min.
Antiarrhythmics			
Atropine	0.4–0.8 mg	IV, ETT	q5min. Double dose for ETT administration.
Lidocaine	40 mg	IV, ETT	q5–10min. Double dose for ETT administration. If needed more than twice, proceed to continuous lidocaine infusion.
Lidocaine infusion	10–25 mL/hr	IV	**480 mg lidocaine** in total **100 mL fluid.** Result: 1 mL/hr = 2 μg/kg/min. Dose: 20–50 μg/kg/min; titrate.
Bretylium (V. fib)	200 mg push	IV	Follow with defibrillation. If unsuccessful, give 400 mg IV, defibrillate. May repeat this step in 15 min.
Bretylium (V. tach)	200–400 mg	IV	Give over 8–10 min.
Defibrillation	80 J		Double dose if first attempt unsuccessful.
Plasma volume expanders			
LR, NS, 5% albumin, FFP, or blood	400–800 mL	IV	Give as a push, repeat prn.

Inotrope infusions			
Dopamine	5–30 mL/hr	IV	**240 mg dopamine** in total **100 mL fluid.** Result: 1 mL/hr = 1 μg/kg/min. Dose: 5–30 μg/kg/min; titrate.
Dobutamine	5–20 mL/hr	IV	**240 mg dobutamine** in total **100 mL fluid.** Result: 1 mL/hr = 1 μg/kg/min. Dose: 5–20 μg/kg/min; titrate.
Isoproterenol	5–100 mL/hr	IV	**2.4 mg isoproterenol** in total **100 mL fluid.** Result: 10 mL/hr = 0.1 μg/kg/min. Dose: 0.05–1.0 μg/kg/min; titrate.
Epinephrine	5–100 mL/hr	IV	**2.4 mg epinephrine** in total **100 mL fluid.** Result: 10 mL/hr = 0.1 μg/kg/min. Dose: 0.05–1.0 μg/kg/min; titrate.
Miscellaneous			
Glucose 50%	40 mL	IV	Mix 1:1 with sterile H_2O if < 1 yr old.
Diazepam	4.0–10 mg	IV	q15min for status epilepticus.
Phenytoin	400–650 mg	IV	Give over 10–20 min. Precipitates in glucose.
Phenobarbital	400–800 mg	IV, IM	
Pancuronium	4.0 mg	IV	prn movement.
Vecuronium	4.0 mg	IV	prn movement.
Morphine sulfate	4.0 mg	IV, IM	q1–2h prn.
Mannitol	20–40 g	IV	Insert bladder catheter.

(Continued.)

TABLE II–6, C (cont.)

Emergency Medications:		45 kg (12 yr)	ETT: 7.0 cuffed Vt(del): 450 cc
First-line drugs			
Epinephrine 1:10,000	4.5 mL	IV, ETT	q5min. Double dose for ETT administration.
Sodium bicarbonate	45 mEq	IV	q10min of continued arrest. Dilute 1:1 with H_2O if $<$ 1 yr old.
Calcium chloride 10%	9.0 mL	IV	Give over 5–10 min.
Antiarrhythmics			
Atropine	0.45–0.9 mg	IV, ETT	q5min. Double dose for ETT administration.
Lidocaine	45 mg	IV, ETT	q5–10min. Double dose for ETT administration. If needed more than twice, proceed to continuous lidocaine infusion.
Lidocaine infusion	10–25 mL/hr	IV	**540 mg lidocaine** in total **100 mL fluid.** Result: 1 mL/hr = 2 μg/kg/min. Dose: 20–50 μg/kg/min; titrate.
Bretylium (V. fib)	225 mg push	IV	Follow with defibrillation. If unsuccessful, give 450 mg IV, defibrillate. May repeat this step in 15 min.
Bretylium (V. tach)	225–450 mg	IV	Give over 8–10 min.
Defibrillation	90 J		Double dose if first attempt unsuccessful.
Plasma volume expanders			
LR, NS, 5% albumin, FFP, or blood	450–900 mL	IV	Give as a push, repeat prn.

Inotrope infusions			
Dopamine	5–30 mL/hr	IV	**270 mg dopamine** in total **100 mL fluid.** Result: 1 mL/hr = 1 μg/kg/min. Dose: 5–30 μg/kg/min; titrate.
Dobutamine	5–20 mL/hr	IV	**270 mg dobutamine** in total **100 mL fluid.** Result: 1 mL/hr = 1 μg/kg/min. Dose: 5–20 μg/kg/min; titrate.
Isoproterenol	5–100 mL/hr	IV	**2.7 mg isoproterenol** in total **100 mL fluid.** Result: 10 mL/hr = 0.1 μg/kg/min. Dose: 0.05–1.0 μg/kg/min; titrate.
Epinephrine	5–100 mL/hr	IV	**2.7 mg epinephrine** in total **100 mL fluid.** Result: 10 mL/hr = 0.1 μg/kg/min. Dose: 0.05–1.0 μg/kg/min; titrate.
Miscellaneous			
Glucose 50%	45 mL	IV	Mix 1:1 with sterile H_2O if < 1 yr old.
Diazepam	4.5–10 mg	IV	q15min for status epilepticus.
Phenytoin	450–700 mg	IV	Give over 10–20 min. Precipitates in glucose.
Phenobarbital	450–900 mg	IV, IM	
Pancuronium	4.5 mg	IV	prn movement.
Vecuronium	4.5 mg	IV	prn movement.
Morphine sulfate	4.5 mg	IV, IM	q1–2h prn.
Mannitol	22–45 g	IV	Insert bladder catheter.

(Continued.)

TABLE II–6, C (cont.)

Emergency Medications:		50 kg (Adolescent–Adult)	ETT: 7.0 cuffed Vt(del): 500 cc
First-line drugs			
Epinephrine 1:10,000	5.0 mL	IV, ETT	q5min. Double dose for ETT administration.
Sodium bicarbonate	50 mEq	IV	q10min of continued arrest. Dilute 1:1 with H_2O if < 1 yr old.
Calcium chloride 10%	10.0 mL	IV	Give over 5–10 min.
Antiarrhythmics			
Atropine	05–1.0 mg	IV, ETT	q5min. Double dose for ETT administration.
Lidocaine	50 mg	IV, ETT	q5–10min. Double dose for ETT administration. If needed more than twice, proceed to continuous lidocaine infusion.
Lidocaine infusion	10–25 mL/hr	IV	**600 mg lidocaine** in total **100 mL fluid.** Result: 1 mL/hr = 2 μg/kg/min. Dose: 20–50 μg/kg/min; titrate.
Bretylium (V. fib)	250 mg push	IV	Follow with defibrillation. If unsuccessful, give 500 mg IV, defibrillate. May repeat this step in 15 min.
Bretylium (V. tach)	250–500 mg	IV	Give over 8–10 min.
Defibrillation	100 J		Double dose if first attempt unsuccessful.
Plasma volume expanders			
LR, NS, 5% albumin, FFP, or blood	500–1,000 mL	IV	Give as a push, repeat prn.

Inotrope infusions			
Dopamine	5–30 mL/hr	IV	**300 mg dopamine** in total **100 mL fluid.** Result: 1 mL/hr = 1 μg/kg/min. Dose: 5–30 μg/kg/min; titrate.
Dobutamine	5–20 mL/hr	IV	**300 mg dobutamine** in total **100 mL fluid.** Result: 1 mL/hr = 1 μg/kg/min. Dose: 5–20 μg/kg/min; titrate.
Isoproterenol	5–100 mL/hr	IV	**3.0 mg isoproterenol** in total **100 mL fluid.** Result: 10 mL/hr = 0.1 μg/kg/min. Dose: 0.05–1.0 μg/kg/min; titrate.
Epinephrine	5–100 mL/hr	IV	**3.0 mg epinephrine** in total **100 mL fluid.** Result: 10 mL/hr = 0.1 μg/kg/min. Dose: 0.05–1.0 μg/kg/min; titrate.
Miscellaneous			
Glucose 50%	50 mL	IV	Mix 1:1 with sterile H_2O if < 1 yr old.
Diazepam	5.0–10 mg	IV	q15min for status epilepticus.
Phenytoin	500–750 mg	IV	Give over 10–20 min. Precipitates in glucose.
Phenobarbital	500–1,000 mg	IV, IM	
Pancuronium	5.0 mg	IV	prn movement.
Vecuronium	5.0 mg	IV	prn movement.
Morphine sulfate	5.0 mg	IV, IM	q1–2h prn.
Mannitol	25–50 g	IV	Insert bladder catheter.

(Continued.)

TABLE II–6, C (cont.)

Emergency Medications:		55 kg (Adolescent–Adult)	ETT: 7.0 cuffed Vt(del): 550 cc
First-line drugs			
Epinephrine 1:10,000	5.5 mL	IV, ETT	q5min. Double dose for ETT administration.
Sodium bicarbonate	50 mEq	IV	q10min of continued arrest. Dilute 1:1 with H_2O if < 1 yr old.
Calcium chloride 10%	10.0 mL	IV	Give over 5–10 min.
Antiarrhythmics			
Atropine	0.55–1.0 mg	IV, ETT	q5min. Double dose for ETT administration.
Lidocaine	55 mg	IV, ETT	q5–10min. Double dose for ETT administration. If needed more than twice, proceed to continuous lidocaine infusion.
Lidocaine infusion	10–25 mL/hr	IV	**660 mg lidocaine** in total **100 mL fluid.** Result: 1 mL/hr = 2 μg/kg/min. Dose: 20–50 μg/kg/min; titrate.
Bretylium (V. fib)	250 mg push	IV	Follow with defibrillation. If unsuccessful, give 500 mg IV, defibrillate. May repeat this step in 15 min.
Bretylium (V. tach)	250–500 mg	IV	Give over 8–10 min.
Defibrillation	110 J		Double dose if first attempt unsuccessful.
Plasma volume expanders			
LR, NS, 5% albumin, FFP, or blood	550–1,100 mL	IV	Give as a push, repeat prn.

Inotrope infusions			
Dopamine	5–30 mL/hr	IV	**330 mg dopamine** in total **100 mL fluid.** Result: 1 mL/hr = 1 μg/kg/min. Dose: 5–30 μg/kg/min; titrate.
Dobutamine	5–20 mL/hr	IV	**330 mg dobutamine** in total **100 mL fluid.** Result: 1 mL/hr = 1 μg/kg/min. Dose: 5–20 μg/kg/min; titrate.
Isoproterenol	5–100 mL/hr	IV	**3.3 mg isoproterenol** in total **100 mL fluid.** Result: 10 mL/hr = 0.1 μg/kg/min. Dose: 0.05–1.0 μg/kg/min; titrate.
Epinephrine	5–100 mL/hr	IV	**3.3 mg epinephrine** in total **100 mL fluid.** Result: 10 mL/hr = 0.1 μg/kg/min. Dose: 0.05–1.0 μg/kg/min; titrate.
Miscellaneous			
Glucose 50%	50 mL	IV	Mix 1:1 with sterile H_2O if < 1 yr old.
Diazepam	5.5–10 mg	IV	q15min for status epilepticus.
Phenytoin	550–825 mg	IV	Give over 10–20 min. Precipitates in glucose.
Phenobarbital	550–1,000 mg	IV, IM	
Pancuronium	5.5 mg	IV	prn movement.
Vecuronium	5.5 mg	IV	prn movement.
Morphine sulfate	5.5 mg	IV, IM	q1–2h prn.
Mannitol	27–55 g	IV	Insert bladder catheter.

(Continued.)

TABLE II–6, C (cont.)

Emergency Medications:		**60 kg (Adolescent–Adult)**	ETT: 7.0 cuffed Vt(del): 600 cc
First-line drugs			
Epinephrine 1:10,000	6.0 mL	IV, ETT	q5min. Double dose for ETT administration.
Sodium bicarbonate	50 mEq	IV	q10min of continued arrest. Dilute 1:1 with H_2O if < 1 yr old.
Calcium chloride 10%	10.0 mL	IV	Give over 5–10 min.
Antiarrhythmics			
Atropine	06–1.0 mg	IV, ETT	q5min. Double dose for ETT administration.
Lidocaine	60 mg	IV, ETT	q5–10min. Double dose for ETT administration. If needed more than twice, proceed to continuous lidocaine infusion.
Lidocaine infusion	10–25 mL/hr	IV	**720 mg lidocaine** in total **100 mL fluid.** Result: 1 mL/hr = 2 μg/kg/min. Dose: 20–50 μg/kg/min; titrate.
Bretylium (V. fib)	300 mg push	IV	Follow with defibrillation. If unsuccessful, give 600 mg IV, defibrillate. May repeat this step in 15 min.
Bretylium (V. tach)	300–600 mg	IV	Give over 8–10 min.
Defibrillation	120 J		Double dose if first attempt unsuccessful.
Plasma volume expanders			
LR, NS, 5% albumin, FFP, or blood	600–1,200 mL	IV	Give as a push, repeat prn.

Inotrope infusions			
Dopamine	5–30 mL/hr	IV	**360 mg dopamine** in total **100 mL fluid.** Result: 1 mL/hr = 1 μg/kg/min. Dose: 5–30 μg/kg/min; titrate.
Dobutamine	5–20 mL/hr	IV	**360 mg dobutamine** in total **100 mL fluid.** Result: 1 mL/hr = 1 μg/kg/min. Dose: 5–20 μg/kg/min; titrate.
Isoproterenol	5–100 mL/hr	IV	**3.6 mg isoproterenol** in total **100 mL fluid.** Result: 10 mL/hr = 0.1 μg/kg/min. Dose: 0.05–1.0 μg/kg/min; titrate.
Epinephrine	5–100 mL/hr	IV	**3.6 mg epinephrine** in total **100 mL fluid.** Result: 10 mL/hr = 0.1 μg/kg/min. Dose: 0.05–1.0 μg/kg/min; titrate.
Miscellaneous			
Glucose 50%	50 mL	IV	Mix 1:1 with sterile H_2O if $<$ 1 yr old.
Diazepam	6.0–10 mg	IV	q15min for status epilepticus.
Phenytoin	600–900 mg	IV	Give over 10–20 min. Precipitates in glucose.
Phenobarbital	600–1,000 mg	IV, IM	
Pancuronium	6.0 mg	IV	prn movement.
Vecuronium	6.0 mg	IV	prn movement.
Morphine sulfate	6.0 mg	IV, IM	q1–2h prn.
Mannitol	30–60 g	IV	Insert bladder catheter.

(Continued.)

TABLE II–6, C (cont.)

Emergency Medications:		**65 kg (Adolescent–Adult)**	ETT: 7.0 cuffed Vt(del): 650 cc
First-line drugs			
Epinephrine 1:10,000	6.5 mL	IV, ETT	q5min. Double dose for ETT administration.
Sodium bicarbonate	50 mEq	IV	q10min of continued arrest. Dilute 1:1 with H_2O if < 1 yr old.
Calcium chloride 10%	10.0 mL	IV	Give over 5–10 min.
Antiarrhythmics			
Atropine	0.65–1.0 mg	IV, ETT	q5min. Double dose for ETT administration.
Lidocaine	65 mg	IV, ETT	q5–10min. Double dose for ETT administration. If needed more than twice, proceed to continuous lidocaine infusion.
Lidocaine infusion	10–25 mL/hr	IV	**780 mg lidocaine** in total **100 mL fluid.** Result: 1 mL/hr = 2 μg/kg/min. Dose: 20–50 μg/kg/min; titrate.
Bretylium (V. fib)	325 mg push	IV	Follow with defibrillation. If unsuccessful, give 650 mg IV, defibrillate. May repeat this step in 15 min.
Bretylium (V. tach)	325–650 mg	IV	Give over 8–10 min.
Defibrillation	130 J		Double dose if first attempt unsuccessful.
Plasma volume expanders			
LR, NS, 5% albumin, FFP, or blood	650–1,300 mL	IV	Give as a push, repeat prn.

Inotrope infusions			
Dopamine	5–30 mL/hr	IV	**390 mg dopamine** in total **100 mL fluid.** Result: 1 mL/hr = 1 μg/kg/min. Dose: 5–30 μg/kg/min; titrate.
Dobutamine	5–20 mL/hr	IV	**390 mg dobutamine** in total **100 mL fluid.** Result: 1 mL/hr = 1 μg/kg/min. Dose: 5–20 μg/kg/min; titrate.
Isoproterenol	5–100 mL/hr	IV	**3.9 mg isoproterenol** in total **100 mL fluid.** Result: 10 mL/hr = 0.1 μg/kg/min. Dose: 0.05–1.0 μg/kg/min; titrate.
Epinephrine	5–100 mL/hr	IV	**3.9 mg epinephrine** in total **100 mL fluid.** Result: 10 mL/hr = 0.1 μg/kg/min. Dose: 0.05–1.0 μg/kg/min; titrate.
Miscellaneous			
Glucose 50%	50 mL	IV	Mix 1:1 with sterile H_2O if < 1 yr old.
Diazepam	6.5–10 mg	IV	q15min for status epilepticus.
Phenytoin	650–950 mg	IV	Give over 10–20 min. Precipitates in glucose.
Phenobarbital	650–1,000 mg	IV, IM	
Pancuronium	6.5 mg	IV	prn movement.
Vecuronium	6.5 mg	IV	prn movement.
Morphine sulfate	6.5 mg	IV, IM	q1–2h prn.
Mannitol	32–65 g	IV	Insert bladder catheter.

(Continued.)

TABLE II–6, C (cont.)

Emergency Medications:		≥70 kg (Adolescent–Adult)	ETT: 7.0 cuffed Vt(del): 700 cc
First-line drugs			
Epinephrine 1:10,000	7.0–10.0 mL	IV, ETT	q5min. Double dose for ETT administration.
Sodium bicarbonate	50 mEq	IV	q10min of continued arrest. Dilute 1:1 with H_2O if < 1 yr old.
Calcium chloride 10%	10.0 mL	IV	Give over 5–10 min.
Antiarrhythmics			
Atropine	0.7–1.0 mg	IV, ETT	q5min. Double dose for ETT administration.
Lidocaine	70 mg	IV, ETT	q5–10min. Double dose for ETT administration. If needed more than twice, proceed to continuous lidocaine infusion.
Lidocaine infusion	10–25 mL/hr	IV	**840 mg lidocaine** in total **100 mL fluid.** Result: 1 mL/hr = 2 μg/kg/min. Dose: 20–50 μg/kg/min; titrate.
Bretylium (V. fib)	350 mg push	IV	Follow with defibrillation. If unsuccessful, give 700 mg IV, defibrillate. May repeat this step in 15 min.
Bretylium (V. tach)	350–700 mg	IV	Give over 8–10 min.
Defibrillation	140 J		Double dose if first attempt unsuccessful.
Plasma volume expanders			
LR, NS, 5% albumin, FFP, or blood	700–1,400 mL	IV	Give as a push, repeat prn.

Inotrope infusions			
Dopamine	5–30 mL/hr	IV	**420 mg dopamine** in total **100 mL fluid.** Result: 1 mL/hr = 1 μg/kg/min. Dose: 5–30 μg/kg/min; titrate.
Dobutamine	5–20 mL/hr	IV	**420 mg dobutamine** in total **100 mL fluid.** Result: 1 mL/hr = 1 μg/kg/min. Dose: 5–20 μg/kg/min; titrate.
Isoproterenol	5–100 mL/hr	IV	**4.2 mg isoproterenol** in total **100 mL fluid.** Result: 10 mL/hr = 0.1 μg/kg/min. Dose: 0.05–1.0 μg/kg/min; titrate.
Epinephrine	5–100 mL/hr	IV	**4.2 mg epinephrine** in total **100 mL fluid.** Result: 10 mL/hr = 0.1 μg/kg/min. Dose: 0.05–1.0 μg/kg/min; titrate.
Miscellaneous			
Glucose 50%	50 mL	IV	Mix 1:1 with sterile H_2O if < 1 yr old.
Diazepam	7.0–10 mg	IV	q15min for status epilepticus.
Phenytoin	700–1,000 mg	IV	Give over 10–20 min. Precipitates in glucose.
Phenobarbital	700–1,000 mg	IV, IM	
Pancuronium	7.0 mg	IV	prn movement.
Vecuronium	7.0 mg	IV	prn movement.
Morphine sulfate	7.0 mg	IV, IM	q1–2h prn.
Mannitol	35–70 g	IV	Insert bladder catheter.

INDEX

B

E

F

J

K

N

S

U